Register Now for Online Access to Your Book!

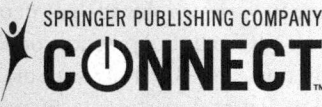
SPRINGER PUBLISHING COMPANY
CONNECT™

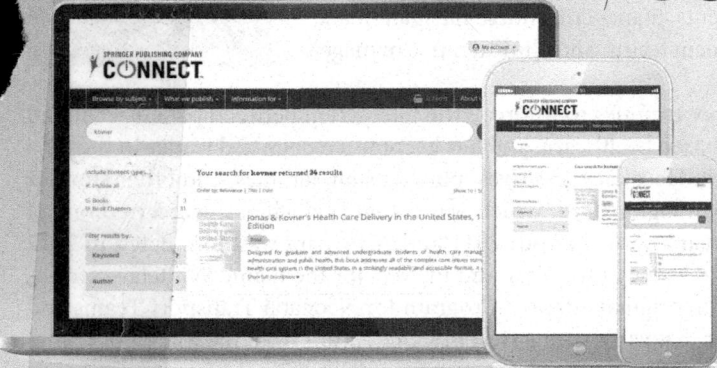

Your print purchase of *Care Coordination in the NICU* includes online access to the contents of your book—increasing accessibility, portability, and searchability!

Access today at:
http://connect.springerpub.com/
content/book/978-0-8261-4012-8
or scan the QR code at the right
with your smartphone
and enter the access code below.

1199DPVT0

*Scan here for
quick access.*

D0911338

SPRINGER PUBLISHING COMPANY
View all our products at springerpub.com

Sara L. Mosher, MHA, BSN, RN, has been in nursing practice for more than 15 years. She received a bachelor's degree from Linfield College and a master's degree in healthcare administration from the University of Phoenix. Her career has been spent as a nurse in various roles such as neonatal bedside nurse, charge nurse, NICU clinical practice coordinator, critical care neonatal flight nurse, NICU family-support specialist, manager of NICU and pediatric departments, manager of nurse navigation and inpatient case management teams, and clinical nurse manager of population health.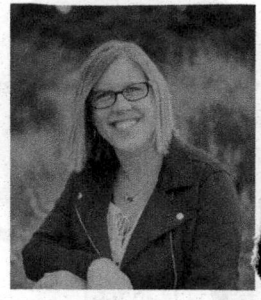

Sara is driven by opportunities to improve the interaction between patient-centered practice and evidence-based healthcare, and has become a recognized leader in the field of NICU family support. Hospital executives, nursing staff, families, and other support organizations hold her in high regard, which was recognized when she received one of Oregon's nurse of the year awards in both 2011 and 2014. Sara was nominated in 2012 for the Oregon Pediatric Nurse of the Year and in 2013 for the Elaine Whitelaw Service Award. She developed an original Support Program for Neonatal Transport Teams and received recognition for that work with a Best Practice Award from the March of Dimes in 2012. She was named a 2014 National Association of Professional Woman of the Year and received the 2015 Lloydena Grimes Award for Excellence in Nursing.

CARE COORDINATION IN THE NICU

Implementing Family-Centered Nursing Care
for Optimal Outcomes

Sara L. Mosher, MHA, BSN, RN

SPRINGER PUBLISHING COMPANY

Springer Publishing Company, LLC
11 West 42nd Street
New York, NY 10036
www.springerpub.com

Acquisitions Editor: Elizabeth Nieginski
Compositor: S4Carlisle Publishing Services

ISBN: 9780826140043
ebook ISBN: 9780826140128

The author and the publisher of this Work have made every effort to use sources believed to be reliable to provide information that is accurate and compatible with the standards generally accepted at the time of publication. Because medical science is continually advancing, our knowledge base continues to expand. Therefore, as new information becomes available, changes in procedures become necessary. We recommend that the reader always consult current research and specific institutional policies before performing any clinical procedure. The author and publisher shall not be liable for any special, consequential, or exemplary damages resulting, in whole or in part, from the readers' use of, or reliance on, the information contained in this book. The publisher has no responsibility for the persistence or accuracy of URLs for external or third-party Internet websites referred to in this publication and does not guarantee that any content on such websites is, or will remain, accurate or appropriate.

Library of Congress Cataloging-in-Publication Data

Names: Mosher, Sara L., author.
Title: Care coordination in the NICU : implementing family-centered nursing
  care for optimal outcomes / Sara L. Mosher.
Description: New York : Springer Publishing Company, [2018] | Includes
  bibliographical references.
Identifiers: LCCN 2018015139| ISBN 9780826140043 | ISBN 9780826140128 (ebook)
Subjects: | MESH: Neonatal Nursing | Family Nursing | Patient Care Management
  | Intensive Care Units, Neonatal
Classification: LCC RJ253 | NLM WY 157.3 | DDC 618.92/01--dc23
LC record available at https://lccn.loc.gov/2018015139

Contact us to receive discount rates on bulk purchases.
We can also customize our books to meet your needs.
For more information please contact: sales@springerpub.com

Printed in the United States of America.

CONTENTS

CONTRIBUTORS

Cheryl A. Milford, EdS   Educational/Neonatal Psychologist, Cheryl Milford Consulting, National Perinatal Association, Huntington Beach, California

Pat Scheans, DNP, NNP-BC   Neonatal Nurse Practitioner, Clinical Support for Neonatal Care for Legacy Health, Emanuel Medical Center, Portland, Oregon

FOREWORD

The question of nature versus nurture has been around for as long as the field of neonatology has been around, and maybe even longer. Steady gains have been made in the understanding of how the NICU environment interacts with genes to influence neurodevelopmental outcomes. Of critical import is what a big part that the family contributes to the NICU environment. This book illuminates some of the murky corners of collaborative neonatal and neuroprotective care and provides pearls of wisdom for support of the family experiencing a major life trauma—NICU admission.

The NICU of the 1970s and 1980s was a very different place than it is today. So much has changed—NICUs don't look the same, sound the same, or even smell the same now that the impact of light, noise, and noxious stimuli on the neurodevelopment of the ill and/or preterm infant has been recognized. The list of therapeutic discoveries goes on ad infinitum. There have been subtle innovations such as removal of exposure to toxins (e.g., benzyl alcohol in intravenous [IV] flush solution) and preservatives (e.g., carcinogenic estrogen interrupters in plasticizers in IV tubing). In addition, there have been crucial advances in nutrition, allowing far smaller and sicker babies to survive and thrive. Moreover, there have been major breakthroughs in therapies for respiratory illness: artificial surfactant replacement, high-frequency ventilation, nitrous oxide, and extracorporeal membrane oxygenation. Gone are the dark NICU days of inadequate parenteral nutrition, lumbar puncture to confirm intraventricular hemorrhage, and denial ("newborns don't feel pain") of postoperative and procedural pain control during the multitude of invasive procedures. Noninvasive monitoring, fat emulsions, cranial imaging, and nonpharmacological analgesia were all lacking in the primordial NICU. Imagine life in the NICU without today's technologies such as size-appropriate percutaneous catheters, telemedicine, immune therapies, and microsurgical interventions. Novel care modalities allow for the lower limits for perinatal viability to drop to a level beyond which anyone envisioned in the 1980s.

With improved survival comes the need for enhanced *intact* survival. As the late preterm infant demonstrates, every day in the uterus improves IQ and executive function. There are neonatal interventions galore to support the developing lungs; the current search is for the illusive answers to protecting the developing brain.

The benefits of the NICU providing care to the family while the family cares for their baby are clear. Improved clinical outcomes are gained by parental bonding and attachment, as well as full family participation as primary caregivers. Parents are central to the care of their baby, and steps are taken to avoid the historical negative effects the NICU can have on confidence and anxiety. The NICU is not a scary, forbidding place any longer—it is a home away from home. New NICU configuration and compassionate facility design allow for

24/7 family-integrated care that supports the caregivers (and others such as grandparents) during caregiving, allows for continuous kangaroo care, and improves communication.

Over the decades, neonatal care has come a very long way. As with all aspects of medical and nursing science, knowledge and technology have virtually (in all senses of the word) exploded in the last 30 years. From mapping of the human genome to babies with DNA contributed by three parents, it is impossible to know where we will be tomorrow. Will stem cell therapy allow regrowth of brain tissue damaged by hypoxic-ischemic encephalopathy or intraventricular hemorrhage? Will bionics or brain–computer interfaces improve the mobility of children with anomalous limbs? Will there even be anomalies? Until the future becomes the present, we still have work to do to improve the quantity and quality of life for preterm or ill newborns and their families. Read on to learn how to be part of this evolution.

Pat Scheans, DNP, NNP-BC
Neonatal Nurse Practitioner, Clinical Support
Neonatal Care for Legacy Health
Emanuel Medical Center
Portland, Oregon

BIBLIOGRAPHY

Altimier, L., & Phillips, R. (2016). The neonatal integrative developmental care model: Advanced clinical applications of the seven core measures for neuroprotective family-centered developmental care. *Newborn and Infant Nursing Reviews, 16*(4), 230–244. doi:10.1053/j.nainr.2016.09.030

Ash, J., & Williams, M. E. (2016). Policies and systems support for infant mental health in the care of fragile infants and their families. *Newborn and Infant Nursing Reviews, 16*(4), 316–321. doi:10.1053/j.nainr.2016.09.015

Barton, S. A., & White, R. D. (2016). Advancing NICU care with a new multi-purpose room concept. *Newborn and Infant Nursing Reviews, 16*(4), 222–224. doi:10.1053/j.nainr.2016.09.010

Best, K., Bogossian, F., & New, K. (2017). The impact of family integrated care on infant health outcomes in the neonatal unit. *Cochrane Database of Systematic Reviews*.

Brødsgaard, A., Helth, T., Andersen, B. L., & Petersen, M. (2017). Rallying the troops: How sharing knowledge with grandparents supports the family of the preterm infant in neonatal intensive care unit. *Advances in Neonatal Care, 17*(3), E1–E10. doi:10.1097/ANC.0000000000000360

Browne, J. V., Martinez, D., & Talmi, A. (2016). Infant mental health (IMH) in the intensive care unit: Considerations for the infant, the family and the staff. *Newborn and Infant Nursing Reviews, 16*(4), 274–280. doi:10.1053/j.nainr.2016.09.018

D'Agata, A. L., & McGrath, J. M. (2016). A framework of complex adaptive systems: Parents as partners in the neonatal intensive care unit. *Advances in Nursing Science, 39*(3), 244–256. doi:10.1097/ANS.0000000000000127

Davidson, J. E., Aslakson, R. A., Long, A. C., Puntillo, K. A., Kross, E. K., Hart, J., ... Netzer, G. (2017). Guidelines for family-centered care in the neonatal, pediatric, and adult ICU. *Critical Care Medicine, 45*(1), 103–128. doi:10.1097/CCM.0000000000002169

Duggan, M. P. (2017). Keeping compromised neonates and mothers together in integrated neonatal intensive care. *Journal of Obstetric, Gynecologic and Neonatal Nursing, 46*(3), S4–S5. doi:10.1016/j.jogn.2017.04.120

Dunn, M. S., MacMillan-York, E., & Robson, K. (2016). Single family rooms for the NICU: Pros, cons and the way forward. *Newborn and Infant Nursing Reviews, 16*(4), 218–221. doi:10.1053/j.nainr.2016.09.011

Enke, C., Oliva y Hausmann, A., Miedaner, F., Roth, B., & Woopen, C. (2017). Communicating with parents in neonatal intensive care units: The impact on parental stress. *Patient Education and Counseling, 100*(4), 710–719. doi:10.1016/j.pec.2016.11.017

Hynan, M. T. (2016). The transformation of the neonatal intensive care unit: A father's perspective over 36 years. *Newborn and Infant Nursing Reviews, 16*(4), 285–288. doi:10.1053/j.nainr.2016.09.021

Mann, D. (2016). Design, implementation, and early outcome indicators of a new family-integrated neonatal unit. *Nursing for Women's Health, 20*(2), 158–166. doi:10.1016/j.nwh.2016.01.007

Maree, C., & Downes, F. (2016). Trends in family-centered care in neonatal intensive care. *Journal of Perinatal and Neonatal Nursing, 30*(3), 265–269. doi:10.1097/JPN.0000000000000202

Milette, I., Martel, M. J., da Silva, M. R., & Coughlin McNeil, M. (2017). Guidelines for the institutional implementation of developmental neuroprotective care in the NICU. Part B: Recommendations and justification. A joint position statement from the CANN, CAPWHN, NANN, and COINN. *Canadian Journal of Nursing Research, 49*(2), 63–74. doi:10.1177/0844562117708126.

Purdy, I. B., Melwak, M. A., Smith, J. R., Kenner, C., Chuffo-Siewert, R., Ryan, D. J., ... Hall, S. (2017). Neonatal nurses NICU quality improvement: Embracing EBP recommendations to provide parent psychosocial support. *Advances in Neonatal Care, 17*(1), 33–44. doi:10.1097/ANC.0000000000000352.

Robson, K., MacMillan-York, E., & Dunn, M. S. (2016). Celebration in the face of trauma: Supporting NICU families through compassionate facility design. *Newborn and Infant Nursing Reviews, 16*(4), 225–229. doi:10.1053/j.nainr.2016.09.007

Roué, J. M., Kuhn, P., Maestro, M. L., Maastrup, R. A., Mitanchez, D., Westrup, B., & Sizun, J. (2017). Eight principles for patient-centred and family-centred care for newborns in the neonatal intensive care unit. *Archives of Disease in Childhood–Fetal and Neonatal Edition, 102*(4), F364–F368. doi:10.1136/archdischild-2016-312180

Skene, C., Gerrish, K., Price, F., Pilling, E., & Bayliss, P. (2016). Developing family-centred care in a neonatal intensive care unit: An action research study protocol. *Journal of Advanced Nursing, 72*(3), 658–668. doi:10.1111/jan.12863

White, R. D. (2016). The next big ideas in NICU design. *Journal of Perinatology, 36*(4), 259–263. doi:10.1038/jp.2016.6

PREFACE

I still remember what it was like walking into the NICU for the very first time, and that day was over 15 years ago. I remember the sounds, the sights, the smells, and the feeling my heart felt when I saw the smallest and most fragile little babies lying there in their beds with countless wires and tubes connecting them to machines and pumps. I vividly remember standing beside a patient who was 26 weeks at birth, and I was awestruck at the translucency of her skin and couldn't fathom how a life so small and so delicate was able to survive in such a loud and invasive environment. What was more unbelievable to me, above all of the medical and technological advances that amazed me, was that there were families coming in and out of this place and calling these infants their babies. How did these parents have the strength to enter this foreign world and function? How did they push past the fear and the uncertainty they most certainly had to have and pour out enough love that these babies needed to grow and thrive?

As I began and continued on my career in nursing, these questions were answered. Parents, whose infants were in a high-risk situation, walked into that unit day after day. They came in blindly at the mercy of the staff and entrusted their precious children's lives in the hands of complete strangers. Families relied on the doctors and nurses not only to care for their baby, but also to care for them as parents and to teach them how to parent in this new reality they were facing. They brought with them strength and courage in amounts I had never witnessed before in my life or in my nursing training. Later, when I became a parent myself, I realized that the way parents could come into this foreign world and pour out enough love to help their babies grow and thrive was because they were parents. They came into that frightening and overwhelming unit to protect and shield their child from everything they possibly could. Despite feeling scared, isolated, depressed, overwhelmed, exhausted, and hopeless, these parents showed up for their babies. I have always had the utmost respect for these parents and admire them in ways they will never fully understand.

My entire career, since 2001, has been dedicated to helping those brave families have a less stressful experience when they have to journey through the NICU with their child. The reality is that as nurses, we chose the profession we go into. I chose to walk into that NICU so many years ago; parents don't make that choice willingly. After seeing that very first family sit with their child, I knew I wanted nothing more than to help families in that situation feel more supported, more educated, less isolated, and more empowered to be included in their child's life so that the NICU wouldn't seem so scary and overwhelming.

Over the years, I have been honored to receive some very humbling recognition; these recognitions have all stemmed from the work I have done supporting families and traveling the country speaking at conferences on family-centered care topics. My career has been incredibly rewarding, and although these recognitions have been gratifying, the most satisfying aspect of all of my work has been being trusted by the hundreds of families to care for their precious children and the countless incredible professionals I have worked with and met along the way.

The main goal of this text is to provide education, tools, and support for caregivers who care for high-risk maternal and neonatal patients so that they, too, can learn how to effectively and successfully provide high-quality care coordination and family-centered care to patients and families in their daily care practice. Each chapter is formatted in the following manner:

GENERAL INTRODUCTION

Each chapter starts with a general overview of the topic, including supporting data and information.

CHAPTER SECTIONS

The chapter has several sections that dive deeper into more information and more detailed descriptions about the topic at hand.

AUTHOR'S PERSONAL STORY

Throughout my entire 15+ year career as a nurse, no matter what role I was in, my goal and passion were always to find ways to improve the patient and family experience and to teach my colleagues how to better care for families through care coordination and family support. I share stories, some partially fictionalized, from the many families I have had the honor to walk alongside in their journey. The goal is to share these important topics from the care provider perspective.

FAMILY STORY

I feel that the real learning can happen from reading the stories from families that have lived the high-risk labor and delivery and/or NICU experience. Families are by far the real experts in this journey and are the one voice that tends to be left out when we should be asking to hear them first. Eighteen families have shared their very personal stories and experiences to increase the depth of this book, and their words have not been altered. You will read their very words directly from their hearts.

RECOMMENDATIONS/SUGGESTIONS FOR BEST PRACTICE

Within this section of each chapter, a summary of tips, strategies, and best practice recommendations are listed on how staff can support families when they encounter each particular situation. The list provides a glimpse into the main points covered in the introduction of each topic in a numbered-list format and is meant to act as a quick reference guide.

RECOMMENDED RESOURCES

A list of recommended resources is given within each chapter to provide further education and support, including, but not limited to:

- Books
- Journal articles
- Websites
- Apps
- Educational opportunities

CASE STUDIES

To further enhance the benefit of this text, the last section of each chapter contains a case scenario formulated by Pat Scheans, DNP, NNP-BC. Dr. Scheans has been practicing neonatal medicine for over 34 years. As a sought-after speaker by the Association of Women's Health, Obstetric and Neonatal Nurses, a worldwide neonatal resuscitation trainer, and a frequent author for *Neonatal Network*, Scheans is regarded as a leading expert in the field of neonatal practice. The Case-Based Learning section provides detailed case studies describing a typical real-world scenario and encourages readers to build their knowledge on how they would approach the situation. Several recommendations for this section of the text include:

- Use the case studies to foster group discussions in a classroom setting where students can begin to discuss the importance of family support concepts in the real-world setting.
- Use the case studies to promote discussion and policy change at the unit level in staff meetings, unit practice committee meetings, and/or quality meetings.
- Use the case studies to enhance personal growth by reflecting on how individuals would react; journaling thoughts, feelings, and even personal experiences for each situation; and examining how the reflection impacts future feelings and behaviors related to family-centered care.

This text looks at the high-risk antepartum patient stay, the high-risk delivery, the NICU admission, the NICU journey, the discharge home, special situations in the NICU, palliative and bereavement in the perinatal and neonatal period, and caring for the caregiver. Each chapter focuses on one of these areas, and you will be provided real-world examples of care situations, positive care-coordination efforts, and exceptional psychosocial support provided to patients and families. You may even come across a few examples of where care coordination and psychosocial support did not go as well as it could have. The goal and main objective of this text are to present best practice recommendations in a way that is easy to read, is placed in the context of actual scenarios, brings a little humor in from time to time, and advocates for the interdisciplinary collaborative approach among teams.

This text is intended primarily for the nursing and nurse practitioner audience, yet that is not to say that it would not be a beneficial read for anyone who works with NICU families. The reality is that each and every discipline that partners with the NICU department has a very important role in impacting a patient's experience. Everyone who interacts with a NICU family or visitor in one way or another impacts the family's perspective of the NICU journey. Everyone in the hospital that a family interacts with has the ability to positively impact a family's experience and could benefit from reading these practice recommendations to reflect on how their own interactions with patients and visitors may influence a patient's experience.

If each provider and individual who interacted with a NICU family adopted care-coordination and family-centered care practices into their daily routine, care would be revolutionized!

The hope is that this text, along with the additional resources included, will genuinely help the reader fully implement new practices into daily care of patients and families. There is no reason that patients and families should have a less than optimal experience in your care after you take the time to read, understand, implement, and support some key practice changes.

I hope you enjoy this text, and I also hope you will help me thank the many families who were courageous enough to share their personal experiences to help you have a firsthand glimpse into how our care directly impacts their lives forever.

Sara L. Mosher

ACKNOWLEDGMENTS

I would like to thank my husband, Christopher, who has been with me from the moment my career started, has supported me at home so that I could support families, and has never let me give up on my dreams of finding ways to stay connected to what I love.

Thank you to my boys, Andrew and Wyatt, who have been ever so patient with their mother who has spent hours on the computer writing this manuscript (and has maybe not always been the most patient during the process). They have taught me how much strength parental love can give a person and have brought me more joy in this life than I ever knew was possible.

Thank you to my parents, Wayne and Patricia, for supporting me financially, emotionally, and physically, through nursing school and in all of life, and to my in-laws, David and Christine, who have been a constant source of support and encouragement.

I would like to thank my entire extended family as well, for always being there to provide reassurance and encouragement and for being good role models as to what true love and acceptance are.

Thank you, Dr. Weaver, my advisor in nursing school, and Amber Nelson, who both continuously encouraged me to stick it out when the going got tough and kept me on the path to nursing graduation. Thank you to the Portland Providence St. Vincent staff who welcomed me as a new graduate, and to all my inspirational mentors I've had along the way.

Thank you also to Maggs, for dedicating countless hours proofreading these chapters, and for being the best thing that has happened to me every year since 2014. To Car-Los, who has provided genuine friendship, invaluable advice, and the best humor! To the HFVBC, who bring me laughter, joy, and an outlet anytime I need one!

I want to thank the hundreds of families I have cared for, who have allowed me to walk beside them on their difficult journeys and have trusted me with the pieces of their broken hearts. To the angels who have left this earth far too soon, but whom I was blessed enough to know and care for during their short time here. You will never be forgotten.

I also extend thanks to my grandmother and best friend, who has led by example to show what it means to care and deliver compassion to others. She has always been there to share more love than she has received, has been ever gracious with her time, and has never put her own desires above anyone else's. She is the one who has instilled the best qualities within me that have made me the nurse that I am.

CARE COORDINATION AND
FAMILY-CENTERED CARE

1

NURSING HISTORY, CARE COORDINATION, AND FAMILY-CENTERED CARE: AN OVERVIEW

When many think back to the beginning of the nursing profession, they picture Florence Nightingale, a brave and beautiful woman who pulled together a team of other young women and went into a British hospital to improve the unsanitary conditions, treat wounded soldiers, and decrease the death toll of the men fighting for their country. Her writing "sparked worldwide healthcare reform. In 1860 she established St. Thomas' Hospital and the Nightingale Training School for Nurses" (History.com, 2009, para. 1). However, nursing had started well before Florence became the iconic symbol.

Nursing was born from the marriage of practices from both religious and military personnel. It was the nuns and other religious figures who would tend to their ill and sickly patrons because it was considered the honorable thing to do, and in times of war and conflict, the need became very apparent to tend to the wounded and those stricken by outbreaks of disease. Gradually, it was realized that there was a real need for experts who could come in and fulfill the role of caretaker to address both the physical and spiritual needs of those in distress, so nursing became a proper line of work.

Nightingale was the one who was instrumental in formalizing nursing into a profession and was the one responsible for opening the first nurse training school in London, in the year 1860, complete with a full curriculum on nursing practices. For the first time in history, nursing education was defined. In 1885, Japan opened the first nursing institute, and the United States followed in its footsteps the following year (History.com, 2009).

When you look up the definition of *nurse*, you will see that it is "one that looks after, fosters, or advises" and "a person who cares for the sick or infirm; specifically: a licensed health-care professional who practices independently or is supervised by a physician, surgeon, or dentist and who is skilled in promoting and maintaining health" (Nurse, n.d.). This definition, however, is just the beginning of what a nurse is or does. A nurse provides care, communicates care, and coordinates care for a host of patients all at once with compassion, empathy, and understanding. A nurse removes barriers to care and assists patients in finding ways to become empowered to care for themselves and meet self-care goals. Nurses are a comfort to patients who find themselves in need in their most vulnerable moments.

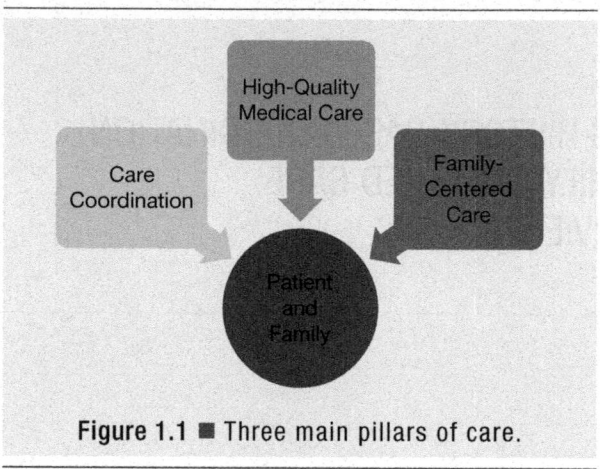

Figure 1.1 ■ Three main pillars of care.

Beyond what they are to patients and their families, nurses serve a great purpose to organizations and healthcare systems as well. Nurses are highly responsible for three main pillars of care that lead to optimal health: high-quality medical care, care coordination, and family-centered care, as seen in Figure 1.1. To ensure improved long-term health outcomes and higher patient satisfaction rates, all providers who interact with and care for patients and their families need to focus on these three main pillars.

I will mention here that I could write an entire book on the importance of care coordination in the outpatient setting. There is critical significance to the role that care management plays in outpatient obstetrical care, outpatient postpartum care, and outpatient pediatric world post-NICU discharge. Some clinics are really well versed in their care-coordination practices, whereas others are still naive about what the concept means. For the purposes of this text, however, we are not going to dive into the outpatient setting but will rather focus on inpatient units and ways to care for high-risk patients once they arrive in the labor and delivery departments and the NICU. Please do not let this lead you to believe that outpatient care coordination is not important. In fact, it is so important that I encourage you to further your knowledge and seek to understand what type of care coordination occurs in the clinics that feed into your units or in the clinics your hospital feeds out into. What works well? What are the areas for improvement? If areas have been identified as necessitating improvement, work with leaders in your organization and in the clinics to find ways to improve care-coordination efforts to improve transitions of care.

When time and effort are put into identifying ways to improve communication and standardize shared care plans for high-risk patients between clinics and hospital settings, you will see that you can produce numerous benefits for your organization, including, but certainly not limited to, the following:

- Thought-out care plans that are communicated prior to emergencies
- More accurate and shared data and medical records

- Reduction in care fragmentation
- Safe and timely care delivered to patients
- Methodical allocation of resources to departments
- Ordering and availability of equipment and supplies for high-risk and/or rare upcoming cases
- Reduction in duplication of testing (e.g., radiologic, laboratory)
- Early and proper consultation with specialists
- Support of patients: "Decreases in threats to quality and safety by providing patients and caregivers with tools and support to encourage them to more actively participate in their care transition" (Coleman, Parry, Chalmers, & Min, 2006, "Essential Features of the Care" section)
- Cost savings from the reduction of waste, reduction of duplicative services, more appropriate allocation of resources, and improved collaboration of care
- Improved patient satisfaction

When I think back to Florence Nightingale and her team of nurses, the differences are so poignantly dramatic. Florence and her peers practiced in nursing wards with poor sanitary conditions, were general practitioners, likely had minimal charting requirements (if any), and focused solely on treating the injured and ill. Nursing now has advanced to where nurses are practicing in very specialized fields and in extremely high-tech environments, have precise documentation requirements, are in positions where they have to worry about patient-satisfaction scores and the ramifications of low scores on their organization, collaborate with a multitude of other disciplines to care for each patient, and are now being asked to put time and energy into care-coordinated efforts for high-risk patients.

As previously mentioned, some clinics and organizations are very skilled at care-coordination efforts, whereas others are not quite yet operating with functional care-coordination teams. Regardless of the care-coordination efforts at surrounding clinics, the inpatient setting must be prepared to care for women and their infants who have been, or who have not been, properly managed with care-coordination efforts during pregnancy when they arrive to deliver. Why? Because when taking the high-risk pregnant population into account, many of these women have multiple needs that, if left unaddressed, can lead to multiple negative consequences such as the following:

1. The maternal patient may suffer from poor health outcomes.
2. The fetus/newborn may suffer from poor health outcomes.
3. Maternal and newborn poor health outcomes will lead to increased healthcare costs individually.
4. Maternal and newborn poor health outcomes will lead to increased healthcare costs to society and to the healthcare system as a whole.
5. Patient satisfaction will likely be low if the maternal patient and/or her child experience poor health outcomes.

One of the primary focuses of care coordination is to deliver "health benefits to those with multiple needs, while improving their experience of the care system and driving down overall health care (and societal) costs" (Craig, Eby, & Whittington, 2011, p. 2). This concept is known to organizations as the *triple aim*: better health, better care, lower cost. Many believe that the triple aim is the only way that healthcare organizations are going to survive the changes in healthcare reform and the complexities of reimbursement models that will impact hospital systems. One of the many ways that organizations are attempting to meet the triple aim is by hiring individuals to serve as care coordinators, separately from case managers and social workers, to assist with the growing complexities of high-risk patients and with the growing emphasis on the benefits of care coordination for both patients and the organization. Leaders have made business plans for care-coordination positions that have been well received by executives and financial departments because focused care coordination has been proved to achieve the following (Camicia et al., 2013):

- Reductions in emergency department visits
- Noticeable decreases in medication costs
- Reduced inpatient charges
- Reduced overall charges
- Increased average savings per patient
- Significant increases in survival with fewer readmissions
- Increased patient confidence in self-managing care
- Improved quality of care
- Improved clinical outcomes
- Improved overall patient satisfaction

The truth of the matter is, organizations do not need to hire care coordinators to have successful care coordination for patients. Would it be nice? Sure! Just like it would be nice to have one-to-one nursing for every patient. But we all know that we do not always get what we want, and because of the growing scrutiny of productivity standards and the tightening of budgetary constraints, we have to find creative ways to supply these services. *I would argue that due to the current environment and the unknown future of how legislative change will impact healthcare practices, each and every discipline that works with patients needs to focus on improving and enhancing their role to incorporate care-coordination efforts into their daily practice.*

A white paper published by the Institute for Healthcare Improvement (IHI) in 2011 describes a care coordinator as a "provider responsible for identifying an individual's health goals and coordinating services and providers to meet those goals. Given the needs of the individual, the care coordinator may be a nurse care manager, social worker, community health worker, or lay person. Regardless of the credential, the care coordinator will have expertise in self-management and patient advocacy" (Craig et al., 2011, p. 7).

Given the IHI's definition of *care coordinator*, organizations and individual care providers should rest assured that most employees are already well trained in this role. It is probable that many managers, leaders, and even staff are hesitant at the thought of what it would take to get approval for additional staff who would offset productivity and not generate revenue. But among the caregiving professions, such as nurses and nurse practitioners, these hired professionals are already trained during their extensive schooling to focus on helping patients meet their physical, emotional, cognitive, social, and spiritual needs. They have a unique role because they are responsible for the ongoing assessment of a patient's health status and response to their plan of care, as well as the assessment of any barriers a patient may have that would hinder him or her from being able to follow through with the plan of care.

The American Nurses Association (ANA) "recognizes and promotes the integral role of registered nurses in the care coordination process to improve healthcare consumers' care quality and outcomes across patient populations and health care settings, while stewarding the efficient and effective use of health care resources" (ANA, 2012, p. 1). The ANA takes its statement even further and declares that care coordination is a "core professional standard and competency for all registered nursing practice" (ANA, 2012, p. 1). The ANA feels that nurses are "integral to patient care equality, satisfaction and the effective and efficient use of health care resources. Registered nurses are qualified and educated for the role of care coordination, especially with high risk and vulnerable populations" (ANA, 2012, p. 1).

I feel it could be argued, with this robust and clearly articulated position statement from the ANA, that any nurse in practice is already trained and ready to integrate care coordination into everyday practice with patients. According to the ANA, the "care coordination process is one aspect of processional practice through which registered nurses at every level regularly influence patient care" (ANA, 2012, p. 6).

This is quite good news because although many organizations have been successful in receiving approval for care-coordination positions, many have not. Care-management positions do not generate revenue, and showing return on investment can be quite challenging. Yet when the stakes are high for organizations to implement effective care coordination in our time of healthcare reform and when the work is so foundational to the quality health service we provide, organizations must find ways to develop care coordination with or without dedicated roles.

"Various care delivery models, including nursing-led models, have been evaluated in relation to improved clinical and financial outcomes. In general, care coordination results in better care at lower cost, particularly for populations with multiple health and social needs" (ANA, 2012, p. 5). This really backs the recommendation that each and every discipline that works with patients (especially nurses and nurse practitioners) needs to focus on improving and enhancing its role to incorporate care-coordination efforts into its daily practice. Nurses are central to coordinating the patient experience and have an opportunity to directly impact cost efficiencies and improved care outcomes for their patient population. Within maternal and neonatal nursing, this is especially true, and we are going to dive deep into how nurses and practitioners can directly impact improved outcomes through their detailed care-coordination practices. However, care coordination is not the only important aspect of care that maternal and neonatal nurses need to incorporate into their care to help improve patient outcomes.

As previously mentioned, family-centered care must also be incorporated into care practices "to lead to better outcomes and enhance efficiency and cost-effectiveness" (Institute for Patient- and Family-Centered Care, 2017, "Believe Patient and Family" section). Family-centered care within maternal and neonatal nursing is founded on the mutual understanding that the family truly plays a vital role in creating a partnership in developing care plans, making decisions, sharing information, and honoring the perspectives and choices of one another.

The Institute of Medicine (2001) published a book titled *Crossing the Quality Chasm: A New Health System for the 21st Century* that highlights the many issues that exist in our healthcare system. This book was pivotal because it reported the developed strategy that came out of the Committee on Quality of Health Care in America that was formed in June 1998 and had been "charged with developing a strategy that would result in a substantial improvement in the quality of health care over the next 10 years" (p. 1). Although family-centered care was far from the focus of this book, the topic was presented and highlighted as one of the many aims and rules that could redesign and improve care through family-centered care practices.

The year 2001 was also an impactful year for family-centered care because the March of Dimes (MOD) launched a program in which it provided information and comfort to families that found themselves on a journey through the NICU with a child. The MOD felt that if their program was able to provide focused support to families, then the overall NICU experience for families would be enhanced and prove to hospital administrators that family-centered care is associated with "numerous benefits including decreased length of stay, enhanced parent-infant attachment and bonding, improved well-being of pre-term infants, better mental health outcomes, better allocation of resources, decreased likelihood of lawsuits and greater patients and family satisfaction" (Cooper et al., 2007, "Introduction" section).

In 2007, an article titled "Impact of a family-centered care initiative on NICU care, staff and families" was published in the *Journal of Perinatology*, highlighting the impact the MOD program had in its mere 6 years in practice (Cooper et al., 2007). The authors of this publication were able to show that after several years of researching their program, "NICU family support enhances the overall quality of NICU care resulting in less stressed, more informed and confident parents" (Cooper et al., 2007, "Results" section), according to the many NICU staff members who were interviewed. Having a focused and methodical NICU family support "reduced stress and made them feel more confident as their baby's parent" (Cooper et al., 2007, "Information and Comfort" section). The MOD concluded that its NICU Family Support Program, which is available for purchase and can be licensed through its national office, has a "positive impact on the stress level, comfort level and parent confidence of NICU families. In addition, it has enhanced the receptivity of staff to the presence and benefits of family-centered care" (Cooper et al., 2007, "Conclusion" section).

In 2008, as a clinical practice coordinator in a small community NICU, I was able to find grant funding to bring the MOD NICU Family Support Program to our NICU. What I appreciated about the program is that it not only provided support to families through education, information, and programmatic validation, but also provided education and information for the neonatal staff. Since family-centered care first became a topic among healthcare providers, nurses were quite apprehensive about incorporating the practices into their daily routines. Initially, it was thought that family-centered care would take more time, cost more money, and lead to families getting in the way when nurses or other providers would be trying to care for the patient. Over the years, countless research articles have been published showing that the complete opposite is true; however, it has been difficult to get care providers to incorporate family-centered care fully into practice. Therefore, as an educator for a neonatal department, I was extremely pleased to have access to professional education for staff that was provided both online and in person and, in my opinion, made the MOD NICU Family Support Program even more valuable and successful. Staff were able to learn the benefits of family-centered care from experts in the field and become its true supporters, leading to the successful implementation of the program within our department. Since the 2007 publication, countless other scholarly articles and books have been written about the importance of family-centered care, and they have highlighted key examples of how its practices have truly impacted long-term health outcomes in a positive way.

In December 2015, there was a supplemental publication from the *Journal of Perinatology* that was written by numerous members of the National Perinatal Association (NPA), and the six key articles included in this publication highlight the incredible importance of psychosocial support for parents during their NICU journey. We will look into each of these articles in greater depth later on in this book as we focus on NICU-specific topics. These articles, which were written by a group of experts in the field of neonatology and psychology, are the best resources that I have found when it comes to best practice recommendations on how to support families during their neonatal intensive care journey and how staff can provide genuine family-centered care in their daily practice. What is even more notable about this publication is that it provides the reader with recommended actions to take to improve practice. During their initial schooling, nurses, and therefore nursing leaders, are not provided formal education and instruction on how to provide psychosocial support to NICU families. Training and guidance on how to perform and perfect this artful task have to occur independently through professional education after graduation. Thankfully, such education is beginning to emerge and become available for staff.

An organization that is leading the way in bringing educational support to staff is the NPA (www.nationalperinatal.org). The NPA brought together a team of professionals to develop the Interdisciplinary Recommendations for Psychosocial Support of NICU Parents (National Perinatal Association, 2018) and that contributed to the authorship of the articles published in the *Journal of Perinatology*. Although many organizations offer professional education for NICU staff, the NPA brings a unique offering and perspective through its multidisciplinary approach to all of the work it does. The organization is built on the foundation of the inclusion of all voices across the spectrum of perinatal care: academic professionals, parent advocates, clinicians, and students alike. Active members of the organization are representatives from the fields of nursing, neonatology, obstetrics, psychology, law, family advocacy, academia, physical therapy, and a variety of others.

In 2017, the NPA entered into a unique collaborative partnership with Patient+Family Care (www.patientfamilycare.com), an organization that provides online education and support to NICU parents and is expanding into providing education for NICU staff and the Preemie Parent Alliance (https://preemieparentalliance.org), an organization that has established itself as the leading voice for NICU parents in the country. The team of multidisciplinary professionals (neonatology, nursing, psychology, occupational therapy) and parents came together to develop an educational course based on the Interdisciplinary Recommendations for Psychosocial Support of NICU Parents (National Perinatal Association, 2018). The unified goal in creating the educational course, which is offered online and is available worldwide, is to provide caregivers with the tools they need to provide optimal support to distressed NICU parents who are dealing with the trauma of having a premature or sick newborn. The course, available at www.mynicunetwork.com, promotes potentially better practices and is clinically relevant, story driven, resource rich, family and patient centered, and parent approved.

How well do you feel you practice care coordination and family-centered care in your daily routine with patients? I would give anything to have magic powers that would allow me to collect all of your answers right now and immediately be able to share the responses. In looking at Figure 1.2, I imagine that the responses would be all over the board.

Despite the ample amount of data and research indicating the importance of these care practices, there is still a demonstrated gap between what should be and what is in many nurses' and other providers' practice. Why is that?

There are plenty of reasons why care providers are not fully integrating family-centered care into their daily practice. For example, when I have asked staff directly why they are not fully integrating family-centered care into their unit or into their routine, a few of the responses I received were as follows:

- "We are short-staffed all of the time; I just don't have the bandwidth."
- "Our leadership does not support it, and therefore I don't have the support I need at the bedside."
- "We don't have the tools on hand to provide good family support."
- "No one else I work with does it, so it's too hard to be the only one doing it."
- "We don't have any training on how to do care coordination or family-centered care, so it doesn't seem to be a priority."

All of these responses are legitimate, and I can respect these care providers for not being in a place where they feel they can fully incorporate these practices into their routine care.

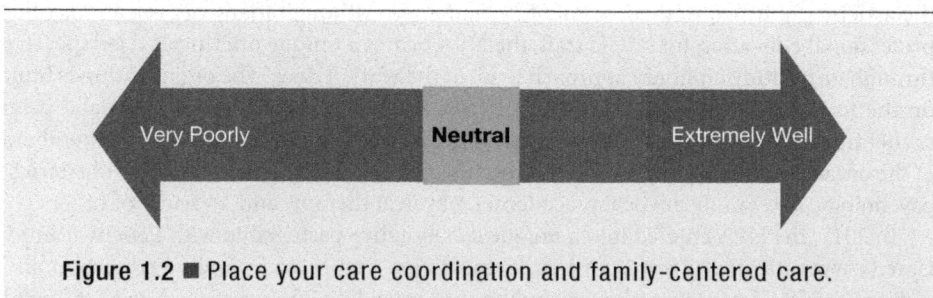

Figure 1.2 ■ Place your care coordination and family-centered care.

Yet, we know that care coordination and family-centered care, especially in the maternal and neonatal specialty care areas, are critical to ensuring the best outcomes for babies and families. So the question we need to ask is, how do we provide the right support and infrastructure to staff so that care coordination and family support in fact do become standard practice in every care provider's daily routine care plan for patients? It is the responsibility of every hospital executive, hospital leader, care provider, and patient to ask this question and then do their part to ensure that everyone has the tools, education, and ongoing support they need to perform these practices to the best of their ability every day to ensure that patients and families receive the highest quality care possible.

REFERENCES

American Nurses Association. (2012, June). *The value of nursing care coordination*. A White Paper of the American Nurses Association. Retrieved from https://www.nursingworld.org/~4afc0d/globalassets/practiceandpolicy/health-policy/care-coordination-white-paper-3.pdf

Camicia, M., Chamberlain, B., Finnie, R. R., Nalle, M., Lindeke, L. L., Lorenz, L., ... Mcmenamin, P. (2013). The value of nursing care coordination: A white paper of the American Nurses Association. *Nursing Outlook, 61*(6), 490–501. doi:10.1016/j.outlook.2013.10.006

Coleman, E. A., Parry, C., Chalmers, S., & Min, S. (2006). The care transitions intervention: Results of a randomized controlled trial. *Archives of Internal Medicine, 166*(17), 1822–1828. doi:10.1001/archinte.166.17.1822

Cooper, L. G., Gooding, J. S., Gallagher, J., Sternesky, L., Ledsky, R., & Berns, S. D. (2007). Impact of a family-centered care initiative on NICU care, staff and families. *Journal of Perinatology, 27*, S32–S37. doi:10.1038/sj.jp.7211840

Craig, C., Eby, D., & Whittington, J. (2011). *Care coordination model: Better care at lower cost for people with multiple health and social needs* (IHI Innovation Series white paper). Cambridge, MA: Institute for Healthcare Improvement.

History.com. (2009). Florence Nightingale. Retrieved from https://www.history.com/topics/womens-history/florence-nightingale

Institute for Patient- and Family-Centered Care. (2017). Advancing the practice of patient- and family-centered care in hospitals: How to get started.... Retrieved from http://www.ipfcc.org/resources/getting_started.pdf

Institute of Medicine. (2001). *Crossing the quality chasm: A new health system for the 21st century*. Washington, DC: National Academies Press. Retrieved from https://www.nap.edu/read/10027/chapter/2

National Perinatal Association. (2018). *Recommendations for support of NICU parents*. Support 4 NICU Parents. Retrieved from http://support4nicuparents.org/interdisciplinary-recommendations-for-psychosocial-support-of-nicu-parents

Nurse. (n.d.). Merriam-Webster online dictionary. Retrieved from https://www.merriam-webster.com/dictionary/nurse?utm_campaign=sd&utm_medium=serp&utm_source=jsonld

SUPPORTING PATIENTS IN HIGH-RISK PREGNANCY AND DELIVERY

SUPPORTING HIGH-RISK PREGNANCY BED-REST PATIENTS AND PREPARING THEM FOR A POTENTIAL NICU BABY

SUPPORTING HIGH-RISK PREGNANCY BED-REST PATIENTS

Patients experiencing a high-risk pregnancy sometimes find themselves admitted to an inpatient labor and delivery unit for days, weeks, or even months. The rationale for this extreme measure is that they can be intermittently or continuously monitored and be within an environment where a medical team can intervene quickly if an emergency with the pregnancy arises. The degree to which restrictive bed rest is prescribed varies in both activity restrictions and lengths of time based on provider discretion and preference, but universally providers tend to agree on the recommendation that bed rest is prescribed to "prevent preterm delivery, premature rupture of membranes, threatened abortion, multiple gestation, hypertensive diseases of pregnancy including preeclampsia, fetal growth restriction and edema" (Durrance & Guldi, 2015, p. 348). What a safe and comforting experience for these women! They have the safeguard of knowing their health, and the health of their unborn child is being constantly monitored; they are able to access room service; they get to lie in bed and be waited on hand and foot; they can catch up on daytime TV shows; they can watch their favorite movies; they can finally sit and read those books they have always wanted to read; they can knit that baby blanket they wanted to make for their little bundle of joy; and they get to have some much-needed downtime before the demands of motherhood are placed on them. Sounds amazing, doesn't it?

Well, for some mothers to be this might be the case. Yet for the majority, hospital bed rest is one of the most stressful and overwhelming experiences of their lives. These women are removed from their homes, jobs, families, maybe other children, support systems, daily routines, and daily responsibilities, and they are told to lie down and stay down until they deliver their infants.

When women are admitted to the hospital for bed rest and pregnancy monitoring, their stay can last anywhere from hours to months until the time of their delivery, and there is "growing evidence of physiologic and psychological side effects of hospitalized bed rest and inactivity" (Rubarth, Schoening, Cosimano, & Sandhurst, 2012, p. 398, para. 2). Care providers must pay close attention to the wide array of side effects that women may experience and do their best to reduce the incidence of these negative effects. More important, staff should educate long-term bed-resting patients on how they can lessen their chances of experiencing unpleasant side effects by "promote[ing] a reasonable and safe amount of patient control that may empower women in a situation where many things are beyond their control" (Rubarth et al., 2012, p. 406). Women on bed rest commonly express the feeling of being out of control, so anytime that staff can give control to the patient and family, the better they will fare. And let's be perfectly honest; the more patients can be empowered to care for themselves, the less staff are burdened with having to perform tasks that patients are capable of doing for themselves, freeing up valuable time to focus on higher-acuity patient needs.

Staff working in high-risk antepartum units must be equipped to both support and attempt to remedy medical and psychosocial side effects to ensure a healthy mom, a healthy remaining pregnancy, and a healthy baby. Although every woman has her own unique experience during bed rest and has her own emotional journey, staff should be particularly aware of some very common side effects. These include the following (Maloni, Chance, Zhang, Betts, & Gange, 1993):

- Skeletal muscle atrophy
- Weight loss
- Bone demineralization
- Increased heart rate
- Blood coagulation
- Heartburn and reflux
- Constipation
- Decreased cardiac output and stroke volume
- Glucose intolerance
- Insulin resistance in skeletal muscle
- Changes in affect, cognition, and behavior
- Sensory disturbances
- Depression
- Inability to concentrate
- Fatigue

Helping women on bed rest to cope with side effects is a crucial responsibility of the nursing team and is viewed by many as an important family-centered care task. There are many ways to address comfort, and it should be realized that comfort would mean different things to different patients. Staff should keep in mind that purposely asking patients what would help them feel more comfortable throughout their stay is what will be most impactful to mothers' satisfaction, contentment, and outcome. It is also is a way to "reduce premature births, improve infant health, and reduce the time infants spend in the costly neonatal intensive care unit (NICU)" (Durrance & Guldi, 2015, p. 346).

Let's first discuss the issues of physical discomforts that staff can address when caring for the high-risk antepartum patient, which most often include muscle soreness, joint pain, weight loss, heartburn, reflux, and constipation.

One principal way to help with physical discomfort is to motivate patients to keep moving. Depending on how strict their bed-rest orders are, they may not be able to get up and out of bed regularly, so finding ways for patients to move around in bed can help decrease joint and muscle discomfort. Movement will also help decrease a patient's risk of developing blood clots, which is noteworthy because the "relative risk of antenatal venous thromboembolism is approximately 5-fold higher in pregnant women than in non-pregnant women of the same age due to the changes in the coagulation and venous systems associated with pregnancy, but the absolute risk remains low at around 1 in 1000 pregnancies" (Greer, 2012, "Introduction" section).

It is great when individual units can create bed-rest exercise regimens that can be provided to patients and that are supported by the physician groups that have privileges at the organization. Many organizations find online bed-rest videos that they recommend their patients watch or go the extra distance to produce their own exercise video that is vetted through their medical staff as safe and appropriate for patients. One of the better practices that is becoming more widespread within the inpatient setting is integrating physical therapy into the care team of antepartum patients. These professionals visit women while they are in the hospital and use a "sophisticated clinical reasoning process that requires the ability to integrate medical information with specialized knowledge about mobility and to engage in rapid and continual assessment of patients and their responses to movement" (Masley, Havrilko, Mahnensmith, Aubert, & Jette, 2011, "Conclusion" section).

I would love to see a hospital go even further and make the effort to wheel women in their beds to a classroom located near the antepartum unit and host a bed-resting exercise class in a group setting! Can you imagine how powerful that would be? A group setting that would allow women to get exercise, see they are not alone, connect with others, build community, and have social interaction that they get cut off from once we stick them in a hospital room on bed rest. I strongly believe this would be such an influential activity. Although there are many safety risks and liability concerns with this idea, I believe it can be done and would love to hear from organizations that can make this happen!

For women who are restricted to very rigid bed-rest orders, properly supporting their body and full body weight while lying down is critical in helping them decrease discomfort. Helping patients change positions from time to time is imperative to not only aid in providing comfort, but also in decreasing the risk of developing pressure ulcers, skin injuries and skin "breakdown leading to pain, infection and other complications" (HCPro, 2012, "Integumentary" section), all of which can lead to further complicating factors and pain.

Many hospitals now provide antepartum body pillows and pregnancy positioning aids for that deliver great positioning relief to women who find it difficult to get comfortable lying down for hours. If your hospital does not offer these to patients or is not willing to make the investment to do so, encourage patients to purchase their own. Unfortunately, many patients struggle with financial stressors and are not able to purchase pregnancy positioning aids, so staff should start searching empty rooms and bring in as many single pillows as they can find to help frequently reposition their patients' limbs and abdomens. Another wonderful way to help with body aches is to provide massage for patients. In a dream world, nurses or nursing aides would have the time to do this independently for their patients, but in today's busy world, the likelihood of that being a reality is pretty slim. The best practice is to find a massage therapist who is trained in pregnancy massage and would be willing to volunteer on the antepartum unit. Routine massage therapy is a huge patient satisfier and is a therapeutic way of addressing many of the discomforts of bed rest. Of course, the massage therapist must be aware of pressure points to avoid and a patient's provider would need to approve of the therapy, but having someone come to the patient and massage joints and sore muscles does wonders for both physical and mental health alike. In fact, research has shown that massage during pregnancy has "lessened norepinephrine and anxiety during pregnancy as well as [has] produced fewer postnatal and obstetric problems afterwards" (Pacific College of Oriental Medicine, n.d., para. 3). That statistic leads me to say we should be recommending prenatal massage to every woman during pregnancy.

Another fundamental subject to prioritize with patients on bed rest is their nutritional health. Maintaining comfort can equate to providing education on the importance of maintaining a healthy diet during pregnancy. It was mentioned previously to integrate physical therapy to address the limited mobility of these patients and to decrease the risk of skin integrity issues, blood clots, muscle atrophy, and discomfort. When it comes to nutritional health, it is best to integrate hospital dieticians who can assess and treat women with the "understanding that the relation between maternal nutrition and birth outcomes may provide a basis for developing nutritional interventions that will improve birth outcomes and long-term quality of life and reduce mortality, morbidity, and health-care costs" (Abu-Saad & Fraser, 2010, "Adverse Birth Outcomes" section, para. 1). Dieticians can use their detailed knowledge and expertise to develop meal plans that the patient adheres to based on preferences and likes that also meet the nutritional demands of her and her developing fetus.

If hospital dieticians are unavailable, nursing staff can support patients by encouraging them to increase their intake of fruits and vegetables, whole grains, protein, and fiber while reducing their intake of carbohydrates, empty calories, and sugary and salty snacks. It can be difficult to maintain a healthy diet when you are limited to a hospital menu and are battling bizarre cravings, so encourage families to bring in healthy food from home that the patient enjoys. Many hospitals go above and beyond and provide miniature refrigerators in the rooms of antepartum patients so that they have access to food that is brought in from home and do not have to bother asking staff to get it from a communal patient fridge at the nurse's station. In addition to the refrigerator, those same hospitals are providing individual microwaves in the patient rooms so that patients can also heat up their own foods, providing a way for them to be more independent and, once again, have a way to be in control of their meals and meal times.

Along with healthy eating, it is so important to encourage patients to stay hydrated. Drinking enough water helps patients avoid some negative conditions that lead to further discomfort and undesirable side effects, such as headaches, constipation, bladder infections, nausea, hemorrhoids, and Braxton-Hicks contractions. A physician or overseeing provider should write orders regarding how much fluid a patient should consume per day, and nursing staff must monitor intake and output to ensure that patients adhere to what these recommendations to optimize their health.

The physical side effects of bed rest that we have just discussed are usually pretty easy to visualize, and most patients are typically comfortable enough speaking about them. The emotional and psychosocial side effects of bed rest are very real issues that are not as easily visualized and/or brought up to staff by patients. Let's now dive into how nursing staff can play a role in the support of the emotional and mental health of the antepartum high-risk patient.

Signs and symptoms that are key to monitor patients for include, but are not limited to, the following:

- Persistent sadness
- Feelings of hopelessness
- Feelings of isolation
- Increase or decrease in normal appetite
- Difficulty sleeping
- Increased irritability
- Overwhelming fears
- Constant worries

One symptom, or all of them, may be evident to the nursing staff. However, not all of them will be, so it is important to know that some patients are very good at hiding their anxiety and depression due to their desire to appear okay and having it all together. Talking about these frequent emotional side effects and normalizing them for patients may help them realize that these feelings are okay for them to feel, that they are not alone in feeling this way, and that they are not crazy for feeling this way in their situation.

When a patient is identified as facing these emotional side effects, one of the easiest things to start with is basic room comfort. Nurses can help empower patients and their families to take control of the room environment, as long as they maintain safety precautions and do not make the room unsafe for themselves or staff. Patients should be encouraged to make their room feel as comfortable as possible, and that can mean bringing in personal items to make it feel more like home. Suggest they bring in their own pillows; bed blanket; pajamas; pictures for the night stand; fabric to drape in the room; essential oils; battery-operated, nonflame candles; spiritual symbols; and other comfort items that may bring them peace. Patient should also be allowed to adjust room temperature to make themselves comfortable, so show them how to use the thermostat and allow them to make adjustments as they need to, again as long as it does not impact their care or condition. When patients have been inpatients for a long time, seek charge nurse or supervisor approval to physically change rooms to give the patient and family a change of scenery. In many units, rooms are set up the same, so such a move may not bring much change in the environment, but in other units, a room change might be a big difference. Small gestures such as these can make a big difference for patients, and the staff ought to continuously be thinking of ways to improve their environment.

A second way nurses can help is by assisting patients in getting structure to the day. Nurses can make a schedule for meals, reading, activities, sleeping, showering, and visitors, for example. Having a routine can help bring a sense of normalcy and comfort that patients might be missing. Nurses should also encourage patients and their families to prepare for baby. Although they might not be able to leave the hospital to go home and set up the nursery, they may be able to shop online. Encourage them to shop for items they still need or to set up a baby registry for their baby shower. Did they miss out on a birthing class? If so, help them find education online that they can participate in and get all of the birthing information they would have received in a local birthing class or assist in finding a book that they can check out and read. These things help them not only pass time, but also become more informed about the journey they are embarking on.

One very beneficial practice that nurses and other staff can encourage patients to participate in when experiencing emotional distress is journaling. Journaling is an ancient practice with countless benefits, including reducing stress, bringing stability, releasing pent-up emotions and thoughts, bringing empowerment, bridging inner thinking with outer effects, enhancing self-expression, healing relationships, balancing and harmonizing, offering new perspectives, and awakening inner voices. It also captures their story! What better way to help moms make sense of what is going on and have a way to go back and reflect later in their journey? Many bed-resting moms express feeling overwhelmed with confusion when trying to understand why things are happening to them the way they are. Experts say that journaling in times of stress, "translating these experiences into language, gives us a physical piece to contemplate, perhaps allowing us to better 'grasp' what's going on. In a different but related theory, the ability to construct a story from our experiences may give us the opportunity to detach ourselves and approach our situation more objectively" (Lewis, 2012, para. 7).

Many patients have told me that at the time, journaling felt like homework. All the nurses told them that the practice would be helpful to them if they stuck with it; once they got started, they soon found it to be therapeutic. Looking back, these patients view their journal as a gift because it captures everything they went through; it captures all of their milestones and celebrations, it recounts their accomplishments, and it is a part of their story that made them who they are. For long-term bed-resting patients, the nurse should provide them with a quality journal and encourage them to write! They should write down their fears, their frustrations, their goals, their dreams, their visions, and even a long list of questions.

For patients with a more severe level of emotional or mental distress, in whom journaling does not meet therapy needs, it would be beneficial to integrate another professional team member. Social work, licensed counselors, or psychology providers should be brought in any time that a patient exhibits signs of a true mental health issue or severe depression because "antepartum mental disorders are a major cause of disability among women during the perinatal period, and may have consequences for children's (intra-uterine) growth and development" (van Ravesteyn, Lambregtse-van den Berg, Hoogendijk, & Kamperman, 2017, "Introduction" section). Therefore, mental health disorders in this population put both mom's and baby's health at risk and warrant professional assessment and treatment. It becomes bedside staff's responsibility to bring support and professional help in early to get mothers the help they need.

For further encouragement, I love when hospitals provide calendars for patients that allow them to track their progress and physically see the accomplishments they make every day. We all know that every single day a baby is able to stay within the womb is an added day to their viability, which equates to an increased chance of survival and a more favorable outcome. Each of those days should be celebrated, and the mom who was able to successfully maintain that pregnancy, as difficult as it might have been and as horrible as she might have felt, should be congratulated and celebrated. Having a calendar to see that accomplishment is a visual reminder for patients that they are doing something that only they can do for their babies. Calendars can also track important tests, gestational milestones, visitors, checkups, and other events of their pregnancy, which is another great way to capture their story.

Extra supportive measures that hospitals can take for patients on long-term hospital bed rest is to produce and provide a services guide that offers a list of available amenities. The list should include all conveniences provided by the hospital and services that will deliver to the hospital from within the community. For example, many items on service lists include, but are not limited to, DVDs that can be checked out from the department, books in the hospital library, gift shop items for sale, massage therapists who see patients in the hospital, acupuncturists who provide treatments in the acute care setting, nail technicians who provide no-cost manicures and pedicures, hair stylists who provide inexpensive haircuts, food-delivery options, and nearby dry cleaners. These lists provide patients with options to have services that they may wish to have but didn't know they could have access to while they are in the hospital awaiting delivery.

On a celebratory level, nurses can support patients who are in the hospital on bed rest long term by helping them experience the pregnancy things other moms get to do. What would those things be? A baby shower and pregnancy photography are two examples that come up most often when I talk to bed-resting moms. Just because they are in the hospital doesn't mean that they should miss out on those fun pregnancy events. Baby showers, if kept small, can be hosted in a mom's antepartum room. Guests should be allowed to bring decorations, a cake, and gifts. While they are there, they may even play a few fun games! If you are lucky, you might be able to sneak in and join in for some of the fun. If the patient is stable and able to be off a monitor for a short period, a conference room at the hospital near the labor unit may be available for her group to reserve. In fact, just the nurses' break room might do if nothing else is available. Regardless, staff should encourage celebration with family and friends, and if mom and baby are stable on bed rest, every effort should be made to allow for a baby shower if the family wishes to have one prior to the delivery. As far as photography is concerned, the scenery might not be at the beautiful riverside park they imagined or in the nursery next to the baby's crib, but beautiful pregnancy photos can be taken in a hospital room. Remember that list of services referenced previously? Having a list of photographers who will come to the hospital is also helpful to have on that list! Once again, this is a way to capture their story.

Finding ways to celebrate other special days or events is an additional way to help support a patient's emotional health but doubles as a method of improving patient satisfaction. Let's look at a few specific examples of special days that tend to be popular among patients that have been particularly successful in improving satisfaction rates:

- Birthdays: A patient's birthday is really important to celebrate in the hospital. Family and friends can be encouraged to make the day special by bringing in balloons, decorations, and a cake. Families should be allowed to plan a small party in the room and invite some of the patient's best friends and family to help her celebrate her special day. If no family or friends are around or if they do not have the means to throw a celebration, staff should do what they can to make the day special by putting up a few decorations, getting some balloons from the gift shop, and seeing if the cafeteria has a piece of cake they can give the patient. Nurses should do anything to make the day special and different than the other days the patient is in the hospital. If the patient's significant other or other children have a birthday while she is in the hospital, help her make that day special by planning a celebration in the room. Patients who are on bed rest miss out on so many social events that are important to them and their families, so bringing the events to them helps them be included and, it is hoped, decreases some of the sadness they feel from being left out.

- Anniversaries: Anniversaries are special days for many couples and traditionally are days they honor by celebrating together to reflect on their relationship and love for one another. While on bed rest, they are not going to have a romantic holiday getaway, but they can certainly have an intimate evening together celebrating their relationship. If a patient has an anniversary while in the hospital, staff can help her and her partner celebrate this important day by creating a special date night in their hospital room. Many couples enjoy their special day by getting their favorite takeout, renting a movie, turning the lights off and eating by battery-operated candlelight.

- Holidays: Some holidays are more difficult and emotional to endure in the hospital than others, but all holidays should be recognized and celebrated in ways that are meaningful and significant to patients. Here are a few examples of ways to make holidays special for antepartum patients who are spending the holidays in the hospital:

  - New Year's Eve: Serve sparkling cider in plastic champagne flutes, provide fun New Year's hats, encourage patients to write their New Year resolutions, and help them count down until the New Year.

  - Valentine's Day: Decorate the room with hearts, deliver a special chocolate, and provide supplies for the patient to create handmade Valentines for special people in her life, especially her other children.

  - St. Patrick's Day: Give out paper four-leaf clovers for patients to hang up to give them "good luck" surviving more days on bed rest. Also, throughout the day, serve green foods and drinks (this is a great way to get in those green vegetables!).

  - Easter: Not all patients celebrate this religious holiday, so be sure to find out if this is a holiday they typically observe before doing anything that might be culturally insensitive. Of course, decorations are always fun, but providing ways for patients to decorate Easter eggs is a very popular activity, especially if they have other children. Invite other children to come in and have an egg-decorating event with mom. On Easter, plan an egg hunt for siblings on the unit and provide moms with an Easter basket for their unborn child with little first Easter gifts. (Ideas may include an Easter-themed book, a small stuffed bunny, and a pastel outfit.)

- Memorial and Labor Day: If patients can be taken outdoors, plan a unit BBQ or ice cream social and get all the bed-resting patients and their families together for a social event. BBQs are popular events for families on these weekends, so bringing that tradition into the hospital setting can be a fun way to bring some normalcy to the mundane routine of being in their room day after day. In addition, if family members have been in the armed services, finding ways to thank them for their service is very important.

- 4th of July: Some hospitals are located in areas where local firework displays can be seen, so having friends and family join patients to watch the light show together should be planned and encouraged. The BBQ idea previously mentioned is also a popular event on the 4th of July, and patients love having a summer themed meal with their family and friends to commemorate the holiday. If patients are not able to view a firework show or are unstable to leave their rooms, provide glow sticks that they can use to create their own version of a light show. Patients who have children especially love this adaptation and find tossing the light sticks up into the air can be just as fun as actual fireworks.

- Halloween: There are many ways to help patients have fun over the Halloween holiday. Some might get messy, but it is hoped that the housekeeping staff will forgive you and be willing to work a little extra this one time. Local grocery stores or farms may want to donate pumpkins, and patients can get creative and carve them. What can be really fun is to then put all the carved pumpkins on a cart and have them wheeled from room to room to let patients vote on their favorite. Offer prizes for the most creative, the most detailed, the silliest, and so on. If the mess is too much, provide paint and craft supplies so that patients can decorate the outside of the pumpkin. Stock up on bowls of candy and encourage patients to have their children come to the hospital to trick-or-treat. If patients give permission to have visitors, supply them with candy, and allow trick-or-treaters to enter their rooms during trick-or-treat hours. This offers children the opportunity to see that other moms are also on bed rest just like their mom and can do a lot to alleviate some of their own fears and questions. It can also be really fun to encourage patients to get into the holiday spirit by dressing up and having a costume contest.

- Thanksgiving: Thanksgiving is a holiday that can be very difficult for families because it is typically spent with extended family and is filled with long-standing traditions. Nurses should spend time talking with patients about those traditions and get creative in finding ways to making many of them possible. At minimum, departments should provide a proper Thanksgiving meal for patients and their families. A tablecloth, nice table settings, and a meal should be brought in for the immediate family so that they can enjoy the meal together. If a family is going to be gone over the dinner hour, this meal could be served at lunch. Being accommodating for families is the key and finding ways to make this day special is important. I particularly love the idea of also providing patients with a Thanksgiving Tree or Thanksgiving Turkey. These are simple paper items and can be hung up in the room or placed on their bedside table. With either of these options, patients can write down on the paper leaves or paper feathers all of the things they are thankful for. This activity is similar to journaling and offers a therapeutic way for patients to work through some of the tough emotions they may be feeling during the holiday season.

- Hanukkah: It can be extremely important for Jewish families to celebrate their holiday. They should be encouraged to bring in a menorah, which for safety needs to be a nonflammable candelabra version. The nurse can ask to participate and listen to the blessings, play dreidel games, and help them to provide gifts to their children. This time of year is very meaningful for families culturally, and it can be extremely difficult to be in the hospital and away from family and friends. Staff need to pay close attention to a patient's psychosocial health during this time of year and patients' may require additional support measures to cope with the added grief and loss during this time.

- Christmas: For a large number of the American population, the Christmas holiday is one of the most difficult times to be confined to the hospital. The entire month of December tends to be a time when patients and families have traditions, and not being able to participate in those traditions causes on grief and depression in many antepartum patients. During this time of the year, it can be challenging for staff to continuously support the emotional health of patients, so the clinical team might bring in support staff early and frequently to support patients during this difficult time. There is good news however; there are lots of ways to bring some fun and cheer to the hospital during the Christmas holiday. Here is a far-from-complete list of ideas:

    o Encourage patients to decorate their room. Garland, Christmas lights, a stocking for them and their baby, and other decorations bring the holiday into their room and lessen the feel of being in a hospital.

    o Some patients bring in winter or Christmas blankets and pillowcases.

    o Many craft stores sell miniature artificial Christmas trees and miniature ornaments. Patients can have someone bring them one of these small trees for the corner of their hospital room and then spend time decorating it.

- o   Many patients have cell phones, tablets, and MP3 players. During the holiday season, they can download and play their favorite Christmas tunes in their room on their devices.

- o   Online Christmas shopping is a great way to pass the time and helps moms feel that they are contributing to this annual task.

- o   I know I personally love decorating sugar cookies every Christmas, so every year I take in the premade cookie kits to patients. Patients can decorate the cookies and enjoy them, or if they have other children, it provides a great activity that they can do together during a visit.

- o   Donations of craft supplies can allow patients to do Christmas crafts. This not only gives them an activity to do, but also may provide something they can give as a gift.

For bedside staff, managing and supporting families can be overwhelming. It can be a full-time job, and in best practice, it should be. However, many budgets and productivity standards restrict that reality from happening. For care coordination and family support to be a reality for patients and staff, the practices must be supported by leadership and accepted as a priority by all staff members practicing on the unit. If everyone working with high-risk patients understands the importance of these care practices and equally participates in providing a level of emotional support to families, it becomes a team effort and a cultural norm within a unit. This cultural norm provides a compassionate and healing environment for high-risk patients who will receive care to increase their chances of improved health outcomes for themselves and their at-risk infant.

PREPARING FOR THE NICU

Aside from focusing on the important physical and psychosocial care of women on bed rest during their antepartum admission and stay, care providers should capitalize on having the prime opportunity to help prepare families for a potential NICU journey. This NICU journey could be due to premature delivery, a known neonatal anomaly in which post-birth resuscitation is required to support the newborn, or a medical complication that was identified predelivery.

Regardless of the reason, if a NICU admission after birth is suspected, a neonatal consult should be ordered as soon as possible to allow ample time for the NICU team to visit the patient and family to develop a trusted relationship with them. The earlier in the antenatal stay a NICU consult can occur, the longer the team and patient can develop that relationship; as a result, the recommendation should be for care teams to obtain these consults as early as possible after antepartum admission. The longer a patient and provider team can interact, build trust, and discuss potential outcomes, the more likely they will be able to agree on resuscitation and postresuscitation care plan for the newborn that all parties feel comfortable with and are ethically and morally accepted by parents and providers alike.

Did you notice I am referring to these consults as neonatology consults or neonatology consults? I am referring to them that way very purposely because they are very different consults. Neonatology consults are likely what you can guess they are; they are a consult with a neonatologist. They are very focused on the medical components of care, and the neonatologist can discuss the specific diagnostic and analytic outcomes of infants born in similar situations. These consults are highly informative to families, especially those facing situations in which their child is at the cusp of viability and the "neonatologist's goal is to facilitate an informed, collaborative decision about whether life-sustaining therapies are in the best interest of this baby" (Schetter & Tanner, 2012, "Abstract" section).

A neonatal consult however is one that should be performed by a member of the NICU nursing team that can:

- Establish a more long-term relationship with the family: Think of how reassuring it would be for the family to meet a NICU staff member while on bed rest and then see that same familiar face later. They will have a sense of comfort seeing someone they already "know," and often, they have more trust in an entire team of strangers when they have met someone on that team prior to interacting with the others.

- Begin to prepare the family for what to expect about the NICU environment: The best way to do this is to give them a tour of the NICU. Be sure to ask when a good time is for the family and schedule the tour when it works for them. If a mother wants her significant other to be present, then be sure to accommodate that request. Take mom down in a wheelchair, or if she isn't stable enough for that, wheel her down in her hospital bed if the NICU is able to accommodate the bed. It is key to do everything you can to get the family down to see the unit with their own eyes prior to delivery. Being able to see, hear, smell, and experience the environment prior to visiting their child will help that first visit so much less anxiety provoking because they already know what the environment looks like. If you can't get mom to the unit, do your very best to describe it to her. Tell her what it looks like, how it is laid out, what sounds she will hear, who will be present, how she will be let in, where she will sit; give as much detail as possible. Better yet, work with your marketing team to create a tour video of your unit that can be hosted on your hospital website. That way, moms and families can take a virtual tour and see the unit, as can out-of-town family and friends who can't visit but are curious about the NICU.

- Talk them through who will be present at the delivery if the NICU care team is involved: It can be extremely terrifying to go into labor and have an entourage of people run into your room. Prepare the family so that when babies are in need of NICU care at delivery, it is very normal for the NICU team to attend for the safety of the infant. Hopefully after this discussion, they won't be alarmed when a nurse, practitioner, physician, and respiratory therapist or others come rushing in like in a late-night medical drama show.

- Describe to them about the admission process and what will happen immediately after delivery: Giving them some descriptive images of what they can expect helps alleviate some of the anxiety of the unknown. Of course, you cannot predict how the delivery and resuscitation will go, but you can give them typical resuscitation scenarios. Let them know, for example, where you plan to resuscitate the baby, who can be with you and the baby during the resuscitation, how you will communicate what is going on, and where you will take the baby once the baby is stabilized. Be sure to tell them that things could change in the moment, and if that is the case, the team will communicate with them; they should know that the baby's safety and best outcome is the goal.

- Share with them the visitation process of the NICU: This may include how to visit while mom is still a patient on the postpartum unit and is separated from her infant, how to visit when mom is discharged home, how many people can visit at one time, and what rules the unit has related to sibling visitation. Parents are going to immediately stress about being separated from their baby, so providing them with the ways they can be united with their infant will be seen as providing them power. Give them this power!

- Tell them how they will be able to "parent" in the unit: It shouldn't surprise you that every parent imagines the perfect pregnancy, the perfect baby, and their perfect discharge from the hospital after a perfect delivery. They are going to grieve the loss of all of this, and they will question how they will possibly be able to be a parent to a baby who will be in the constant care of complete strangers. Again, give them some power. Give them some education, knowledge, and comfort in knowing that parents are a primary caretaker in the unit. If that isn't a concept you, or your unit, embrace yet, then you better ensure you read every single page of this book! Families are the primary providers in a child's life. Staff are the supporters, educators, medication administrators, psychosocial supporters, and around-the-clock monitors for critically ill babies; they support the primary providers and model the behaviors parents will need to learn to take their children home and care for them in their own environment. Let me state that again:

  > Families are the primary providers in a child's life. Staff are the supporters, educators, medication administrators, psychosocial supporters, and around-the-clock monitors for critically ill babies; they support the primary providers and model the behaviors parents will need to learn to take their children home and care for them in their own environment!

- Give them information about what gestational age norms are and how parents are involved in the care of babies at each of those ages: Parents, unless they are neonatal providers themselves, do not have the incredible knowledge and expertise that NICU staff have. They don't know what is normal or not normal or what to expect at each gestational age. It's the staff's job to teach this to parents. If delivery is expected at 26 weeks, for example, the neonatal consult should cover what norms one typically sees at that gestational week.

- Describe how families are kept comfortable in the unit: Hopefully, you have a nice way to keep families comfortable in the NICU. If you do, tell them that! Most units are getting into single-room designs where there are comfortable and private spaces for every family. Sharing that can be very comforting for families to know. If you do not have a single-room unit design, or do not have private spaces where families can retreat to for respite, find ways to make the unit as comfortable as you can for families when they are in the unit with their baby or babies. Some examples of comfort improvements for units that are challenged with space may be purchasing comfortable bedside chairs, having bedside tables for personal items to be placed, having a space where parents can store personal food/snacks, a safe area where family can play with older siblings, providing tablets or computers for families that want to connect to the Internet for research or to update social media sites and make other updates based on the feedback and suggestions from patients themselves.

- Share with them what support services are provided to them in the unit: It's great to let them know if you have a family-support specialist, social work team, a parent library, educational videos, family events and activities, meal vouchers, gas vouchers, dedicated parking spaces for NICU families, support groups, and any other unique support service your unit provides. Letting families know that your unit cares about them as a family and will be there with ways to support them through their difficult time will mean a great deal to them. Knowing that they have some support waiting for them on the other side of this scary adventure typically helps decrease some of their anxiety.

- Describe what community resources are available: Sometimes, families have no idea that a NICU even existed until they arrive at the hospital, so they also have no idea that there are resources and support for them in their community. Let them know about parent groups, support groups, educational opportunities, classes, events, social media sites, or other local unique resources in your community.

- Be available to answer any questions they have: These neonatal consults should be ongoing throughout the antepartum stay, and families should be encouraged to write down all of their questions. Check in with them from time to time so that you answer these questions. Most families get on the Internet and find their own answers, but as you know, there can be some very scary and inaccurate information on the Internet. Let families know that while you understand they want to research and learn what they can, you want to help provide them with accurate and up-to-date education on their concerns and questions. Encourage them to write things down so that you can then discuss everything together.

- Introduce them to other parents through a peer-to-peer support program: Being able to talk to someone who has been through a similar situation can be an extremely therapeutic exercise for families. If a mom is placed on bed rest and needs an emergency rescue cerclage, for example, connecting her with someone else who has been through that same experience can help her no longer feel alone in that terrifying experience. Connecting her with another individual allows her to ask questions that only a patient who has experienced that situation can truly answer. Another example might be if a mom is going to deliver a child with a known gastroschisis, connecting her with a mother who previously delivered a baby with a gastroschisis will allow her to ask the questions she wants to ask another mother who has been through the same situation. (Note: Peer-to-peer mentor groups need to be set up and properly implemented in units prior to connecting parents to one another to ensure quality, confidentiality, and therapeutic response, and we will address the topic of peer-to-peer mentor groups later in the text.)

As can be seen, a neonatal consult can be much more inclusive and, in my opinion, is much more supportive of the family. Please don't think that I feel that neonatology consults aren't important because they are very much so. Both consults should happen and both play vital roles in helping prepare families for premature deliveries. However, I think it's the connection and the relationship that families can build with NICU nursing staff prior to an admission that can be so incredibly powerful. if NICU nursing staff can check in frequently with families who have a long antepartum stay, very close and trusting relationships can be formed; families have reported feeling much less stress, less anxiety, and more trust in the care team when their baby is finally born, which is something that we can't deny would be a benefit to all of our patients.

Fortunately for staff, these neonatology and neonatal consults also pave the way to begin the care-coordination efforts that benefit these families if they are indeed admitted to the NICU. The consults themselves establish family-supportive care, and in talking with the families and answering their questions, NICU staff begin to gain insight into the needs, disparities, and risk factors that will face the family and that need to be addressed prior to discharge. How many times have you heard that discharge begins at admission? Well, in this case, discharge begins prior to admission!

Unfortunately, not all NICU admissions can be planned and prepared for, so how do you prepare families for a preterm birth or NICU admission if you do not have time? What if mom and family arrive in labor and delivery in active and imminent labor and they are unable to stop the progression of her labor? What if baby and mom are in an emergent situation and baby has to be delivered quickly? Staff can still do a great deal to prepare a family, but it takes commitment and dedication at the organizational and the department level to make family support successful in these situations. In the midst of an unplanned premature delivery or a delivery emergency, a staff member needs to be assigned to be the family to be a support specialist who focus just on that family. Based on current practices and standard roles within the labor and delivery settings, there is typically someone always assigned as labor nurse, baby nurse, scrub tech, scribe, and other roles. If it is an even more complicated delivery, more skilled staff are brought in for safety and assigned their designated roles. It should be standard to bring in a family-support specialist during these high-risk delivery situations and this person's sole responsibility should be to focus on one thing: *SUPPORTING THE FAMILY*.

During the delivery, the family-support specialist can stay at the head of the bed with mom and support her using the following interventions:

- Describe in nonmedical language what the providers are saying out loud to one another.
- Answer questions the parents may have in the moment.

- Can explain procedures that are being performed to the mom and/or baby.
- Hold a hand, place a hand on a shoulder, get tissues, get a seat for the mother's support person (especially for the times when they look like they might pass out!), and safety direct family to the baby when they are allowed to get close.

Overall, the family-support person's primary goal should be to offer presence and talk through some of what they would have discussed predelivery if they would have had the opportunity. The family-support specialist should understand that families will likely not comprehend much of anything they say in that moment due to shock, disbelief, and fear. The support specialist can prepare families for next steps or next procedures before they occur, as best as possible. Any preparation is better than none.

Author's Personal Story

I have had the honor of meeting many women on bed rest and supporting them on their antepartum journey during my time as a family-support specialist. In fact, in that role one of my primary responsibilities was to establish a relationship with the bed-resting women who had received a neonatology consult. Once a neonatology consult had been ordered on a patient, I engaged with patients and their support systems and did my part to help prepare them for a potential NICU admission. I focused my efforts on helping prepare them for what to anticipate if their baby required a NICU stay, communicated with the NICU staff about the needs of the family once they came to the unit, began care-coordination efforts that could be initiated prior to delivery, and provided ongoing family support during the mother's hospital stay to help alleviate emotional and psychosocial distress for the family.

One of the patients I particularly remember was A.S., who was admitted to the labor and delivery unit with preterm labor at 22 0/7 weeks' gestation. She was G1, P0, pregnant with twin boys, had involved and supportive family members, and a very supportive and involved boyfriend and was told she would be in the hospital until she delivered. At 22 3/7 weeks' gestation, A.S. had an emergency cerclage placed and was prescribed very strict bed rest that excluded her from using the restroom. She faced the reality of using a bedpan and having sponge baths for the unforeseeable future and suddenly had to accept the fact that the hospital was now her temporary home.

I met with A.S. and her boyfriend a few days after her cerclage was placed and introduced myself as the NICU family-support specialist. They had previously met with our neonatologist and knew the grim statistics if her twins delivered in the next few days. I informed the two of them that I would be a point of contact for them throughout the hospitalization to answer any questions they had about the NICU and what to expect about the potential NICU journey ahead. I made sure they knew I was not another doctor (although I later learned they indeed thought I was the doctor) and that I would be collaborating with the neonatology team to help develop a supportive resuscitation plan when it came time for delivery. A.S. and her boyfriend were extremely sweet and

(continued)

(*continued*)

very open to talking with me, but because they were young teenagers, I was afraid that they were not grasping the severity of the situation.

I kept our initial meeting as a very informal and friendly visit and returned the next day with a planned agenda. I knew that it was going to be important to educate these young soon-to-be parents on the reality of what they were facing but in such a way that was both informative but not scary and overwhelming; a balance that is always extremely delicate and complicated. I entered the room with a bag full of goodies (let's be honest, who doesn't love gifts and freebies?) and one by one I went through what I have come to coin as my "bed-rest survival kit."

1. Journal and pen: When in a room for a long time, alone, an individual has plenty of time to think. Add the stressful situation of being faced with the unknowns of potential medical complications for your children, *lots* of questions and panic can come up. I like to give patients a journal and pen to keep at their bedside table, and I encourage them to write down every thought and question they have about their pending pregnancy and delivery so that when care providers visit, they have something to prompt discussion. Speaking from my own experience, I know that when physicians or nurses ask me on the spot if I have any questions I freeze up and always say no. But as soon as they leave the room, I immediately can think of questions I should have asked. So I ask patients to write everything down so that they have them right there.

2. "Watch Me Grow" board: Many women I have met on bed rest tell me "I'm sick of this. I just want to deliver and be done. My friend delivered at such and such gestation and her baby is fine." Have you heard that line? Of course, many preterm infants deliver and, because various interventions, do well. Yet we all know that every baby is different, so you can't promise that this baby will fare as well as their friend's. In fact, you can't promise that a term baby will not have complications at birth. So I have developed a "Watch Me Grow" board that helps parents visualize the reality of prematurity. The board houses three diapers; an extreme premature size, a premature size, and a newborn size. Beneath each diaper, the weight recommendation for each is shown; then I ask that if she were to deliver that day, which diaper would her baby fit into. When many realize that their baby would be wearing the extreme premature size, their mouths drop open and the realization hits them. They didn't even realize diapers were made that small. They can't even begin to imagine a baby being so small that it would fit into something that tiny. (Then when you tell them that sometimes the diaper has to be folded over to fit the baby, they become even more shocked.) This diaper board gives patients something tangible and visible to focus on, and over and over again, I hear that it is the one thing that motivates them to comply with their bed-rest orders when they want to give up because they can "see" what a difference growth in utero can make. When

(*continued*)

(continued)

you can educate them that every week, every day, and every minute they stay pregnant, their baby has a better chance of growing and fitting into a larger diaper, they feel like they can do something for their child. They feel empowered to make a difference! This board can be kept by their bed, on their windowsill, or anywhere in their room and kept as an education piece for family and visitors. Education is knowledge; knowledge is safety; and safety can lead to better outcomes.

3. Water bottle: Helping bed-rest mothers stay hydrated is important. Of course, you have to balance the physician orders if they place the patient on any type of fluid restriction, but giving mom a special water bottle that is different than the plain old hospital one is just more *fun* and makes drinking her water more exciting.

4. Customizable calendar: Keeping track of milestones is a wonderful way for bed-rest moms to stay on track, celebrate their accomplishments, and commemorate all of their milestones. Providing them with a calendar that they can customize, decorate, and fill in provides them with not only an activity to keep them busy while on bed rest, but also a record of what takes place while they are in the hospital. They can track who comes to visit, what tests they have done, what gestational milestones they hit, what big events occur, and anything else they feel is important to celebrate. Many staff encourage moms to cross out each day they continue to stay pregnant so that they can see how many days they were able to maintain their pregnancy and help provide a safe delivery for their baby. This is a fantastic idea! The more ways staff can find ways to encourage patients, the better.

5. Activities: There is only so much daytime TV one person can watch. Providing some activities is a good idea, so I tend to include adult coloring books and colored pencils (the pencils can also be used with the calendar), crossword puzzle books, and Sudoku books. Other hospitals I have worked with have included knitting needles and yard with "knitting for beginner" instructions, which I just love!

6. List of ways that friends/family can help: If patients have a support system, usually they want to help. The problem is that people don't know *how* to do so. I like to include a list of suggestions on how patients can ask friends and family to help while they are in the hospital. This provides them some ideas on how others might be able to support them if they too can't think of how to ask others for help.

By going through this kit, I was able to establish a relationship with A.S. and her boyfriend as an individual who was there to provide information, education, and support. In addition, I was able to provide a lot of very important basic information without them noticing. I informed them about the importance of writing down their questions, I educated them about prematurity norms and expectations, they learned about the importance each day staying pregnant can mean to their unborn children, they found out how much support

(continued)

(*continued*)

is available to them, and most important, they learned they were far from alone in what seemed like a very isolating and scary experience.

I continued to visit with A.S. at least twice a week for 8 weeks. During these weeks, I was able to slowly provide more and more education based on the questions and thoughts written in her journal; we were able to address each of her fears, frustrations, and concerns. I scheduled times that she and her various family members could tour the NICU, and they each got to physically see where the twins would be if they were in fact delivered early as anticipated. During the tours, A.S. was able to meet new staff members each time, become a little more familiar with the environment, hear the sounds of the various monitors and pumps, and see the equipment frequently used. Being physically in the unit gave her the opportunity to ask very specific questions without the stress of having her children already being in the unit and being the ones hooked up to all of the equipment, which, I believe, was the best way for her to learn about the unit and various machines, equipment, and people.

Because A.S. was a patient on our antepartum unit for 2 months, we had plenty of time to establish a relationship in which she felt comfortable asking questions and was able to advocate for what she wanted for both her and her children when it was time for delivery. She was able to participate in the resuscitation plan and knew ahead of time what to expect when it was time to deliver. For me, what was most beneficial is that during the 8 weeks I met with her, I was able to assess what needs her and her family were going to have after delivery, so I could relay that to the NICU team ahead of time. Having the ability to begin care coordination efforts before the delivery increases efficiencies and reduces the time it takes to provide care in the NICU setting.

A.S. ended up with a cesarean delivery at 30 5/7 weeks. Was she scared that day? Yes! But she went into the operation with the knowledge she wanted, the information she needed, surrounded by staff she felt comfortable with and trusted, which helped her feel less alone and anxious about the next phase of her journey.

Family Story

Maleah Sarafinchan shares her personal story of experiencing hospital bed rest and highlights what advice she wishes she would have been given when she faced her days lying flat in the hospital:

"August of 2016, my husband and I were excited for our kid-less date night. We got tickets to see the new Borne movie. Little did we know, that night was going to be the start to a life experience we will never forget. After the movie, which was amazing, I had a strong craving for Rice Krispies treats. Unfortunately, my bladder had another plan and before going to the store to cure my craving, we had to make a bathroom stop. Before

(*continued*)

(*continued*)

we had reached our destination, I turned to my husband, panicked because I had just peed on his car seat. Embarrassed to get out of the car and go inside to clean up, I got out slowly looking behind me to see what I had left behind. I was in shock and I had no idea what it was, but after having a few issues prior, I wasn't really concerned. I had too many false alarms, so I was not interested in going in and racking up another doctor bill. A few minutes later I stood there ready to go to store because I NEEDED those Rice Krispies treats! My husband refused to get them unless I called my doctor to make sure I didn't have to be seen. I gave in and called the doctor, and she demanded that I come in after hearing the description of the fluids (which I will spare you from). I got the 'I told you so look' from my husband as we sped to the hospital.

"When we arrived they did several tests, told us a million stories to all of the situations that we could be possibly facing, and by then we were terrified. After waiting a few hours, the doctor finally came in with results. 'Your water broke a while ago. What came out today was the last of it and there is nothing left for the baby to survive. You're going to be admitted so we can help as much as we can.' Everything happened so fast, and the next thing I knew, I was on an ambulance stretcher being placed in the back, zoning out to the sirens. This was my third child, and I had no idea what to expect. I was put on my second bed rest with this pregnancy at only 24 weeks; this time I wasn't allowed to go home. I was going to have to be on hospital bed rest attached to monitors and machines, IVs, and the whole works. I moved from room to room with panicking nurses thinking any moment was the moment as they were telling me how to sit, lay, turn, or flip while trying to figure out which position was right for my fighting baby. I was falsely prepped and delivered to the OR. I was given several steroids and had to be hooked up to magnesium sulfate two different times but felt like years. Eleven days later after battling nurses, machines, constantly watching the monitor numbers, missing other children, watching my husband pace every inch of the hospital room over and over, hardly sleeping, and obsessing over the worst possible outcome, the numbers on the screen kept dropping. I was rushed to the OR again, but this time I was prepped and ready for real. I was now 25 weeks and 3 days along in my pregnancy, which I knew had a horrible statistical survival rate. I was shaking uncontrollably, so the nurses covered me with warm, bright-white hospital blankets and compression devices on my legs; then the white curtain went up. It was time.

"I previously told my husband to distract me. I told him to talk, sing, or whatever he could do. He did amazing. His voice isn't the best, but he gave the nurses a good laugh. I make fun of him now because one thing he said in the OR was 'No wonder you wash your face every day. You don't have any blackheads.' That is all I remember. Then a rush came over … the baby, the miracle was out, weighing 1lb 9oz. They wrapped her in something that looked like a thick clear plastic bag, hooked her up to CPAP and rushed her away to the NICU. My husband stayed with her, and I got wheeled back to my room, back to bed rest, but I was told she was beautiful!

"The next day I got in a wheelchair and my husband pushed me to see our new miracle. I had never seen anything so small and fragile or more loved. My thoughts were scaring

(*continued*)

(*continued*)

me. She was in a box, connected to machines and wires; her skin was transparent; she didn't have eye lashes or eyebrows or fingernails, or toenails; half her face was under a mask; and she needed a special blue light to keep her warm. It made me feel like I wasn't enough or I couldn't do my job correctly as a mother. There are no words or emotion to describe what it's like seeing your baby like this. I was too scared to touch or hold her.

"We sat there and prayed. Getting wheeled back to my room, we stopped at the chapel and prayed some more. Although it is a terrifying experience, we were beyond blessed. Doctors moved my room again, but this time I got a family room where my husband had his own bed and my other kiddos could sleep over as well. This was definitely a mood booster. Showing the kids their new baby sister was hard because they were so concerned and had so many questions, but it helped me be stronger for them and for our miracle baby. When they went home later, I was able to get wheeled to have alone time with the baby. I held her for the first time and they called it 'kangaroo time' or skin-on-skin contact. Even though she was the size of her father's hand, just being able to have that touch and connection put me at peace. I was released from the hospital at day 16 then put on bed rest once again at home. That was the third bed-rest order with the same pregnancy by 26 weeks. Luckily for my family, we didn't live too far from the hospital; we were able to visit every day our daughter was in the NICU, which was 103 days. We didn't have any major complications in our journey, other than a few minor setbacks when our miracle was released to come home; she still needed oxygen and still needed to be protected more than most due to her immune system fighting harder than it should. Holidays, birthday parties, gatherings, and outings all became irrelevant for a while during that phase and it all eventually passed.

Looking back on the experience, what would have been the most helpful advice that I could have been given while on bed rest would have been:

- Pay attention to the meds you are getting. I had an older nurse give me half of my dosage her entire shift and I had no idea why I was in so much pain.

- Try hard not to stress about outside life right now. Focus on you and that baby. I was the worst at this. Having two other kiddos at home, a job to make sure I'd have when I was off leave, pets, a husband I didn't want to leave my side, holidays coming up, and school starting soon had a huge impact on my stress levels. Whatever it may be, you cannot control everything so let it go.

- Take help anytime it is offered, even if you don't normally do so. It has a huge impact on your stress levels, which will benefit you and that precious baby.

- Don't be afraid to speak up to doctors, nurses, or family if you don't like something, need to change something, the paperwork you have to fill out, even to the NICU visits. You have to make the best of your stay for you and the baby, and only you know what that consists of.

- Stay as positive as you can be!

(*continued*)

(*continued*)

- DO NOT Google the horror stories of your situation; it makes everything so much worse, and you are creating your own story, not living anyone else's.
- Sleep as much as you can.
- Encourage friends and family to visit as much as they can to help spirits stay up.
- Bring books, movies, crafts, puzzles, and food.
- Ask others to help with the other kiddos and with cleaning and caring for the home.
- See if a friend will create a GoFundMe account for your unique situation, which will help alleviate some stress for you and your family.
- Prepare the significant other to be prepared to always be on call. Everything happens so quickly.
- When there are other children in the family, talk with them that they may see their mom in pain (both physically and emotionally), but it will all be worth it when the family is all together!"

RECOMMENDATIONS/SUGGESTIONS FOR BEST PRACTICE

1. Integrate multidisciplinary professionals into the care team of antepartum patients to optimize the overall health and well-being of high-risk inpatients. Examples may include professionals such as physical therapists, dieticians, physiologists, and licensed clinical social workers.

2. Provide body pillows or other pregnancy positioning aids that assist in the comfort of patients who are confined to prolong bed rest.

3. Create policies and procedures that develop cultural norms addressing both the physical and psychosocial side effects experienced by patients on bed rest, and routinely prepare families for these expected side effects.

4. Encourage patients to make their hospital room more like home.

5. Order neonatology and neonatal consults as early as possible after an antenatal admission.

6. Have miniature refrigerators and microwaves for long-term antepartum patients to have in their rooms.

7. Provide "bed-rest survival kits" to patients.

8. Focus on ways to celebrate special days and events for and with patients.

9. Create and provide patients with a list of resources that are available to them within the hospital and community.

10. Equip patients with ideas on how friends and family can help while they are on bed rest.

11. Capitalize on the time women and their families are in the hospital to prepare them as much as possible for a potential NICU admission. Part of the education should include physical and virtual tour options of the unit.

12.   Have a supply of craft projects, some which are holiday specific, for antepartum patients to work on.

13.   If patient rooms have televisions with DVD players, create a unit collection where that patients can check out videos. If the rooms have smart televisions, consider purchasing a unit subscription to an online video service in which movies can be rented by patients in their rooms.

RECOMMENDED RESOURCES

Here are some helpful tools and resources that will support the success of implementing best practice recommendations to provide support of high-risk bed-rest patients and preparing them for a potential NICU admission.

First is a sample job description for a family-support specialist. The best practice recommendation is to have staff members hired into separate support roles, and they would ideally receive additional training and support to learn how to effectively care for families in crisis across the perinatal care continuum (Figure 2.1).

Our second resource is sample rack cards that can be extremely helpful to have available for bed-resting patients and their support network. These cards list ways that mom can survive bed rest, how her support person can help her survive bed rest, how friends and family can help with the hospitalization, and how other children can cope and stay connected to their mom while they are separated from her (Figure 2.2).

The third resource is an example of the "Watch Me Grow" board that was referenced during the author's personal story. This board can be purchased from Patient+Family Care (www.patientfamilycare.com), and hospitals can place diapers on the board and use it as a motivator for women to comply with bed-rest orders, as well as an educational piece for patients and their families (Figure 2.3).

Last is a quick reference sheet that can be easily reproduced for patients that provide a list of recommended websites and books that can provide education, information, support, and peer-to-peer connection while they are on bed rest. These resources are professional, reliable, and approved by providers as safe resources for patients (Figure 2.4).

Job Title: NICU Family-Support Specialist
Job Description

POSITION PURPOSE

The purpose of the NICU Family-Support Specialist is to have a dedicated staff member available in high-risk situations to provide consistent, continuous, and reliable services, including education and support to families within the antepartum, NICU, and postpartum units.

Figure 2.1 ■ Sample: Family support specialist job description.

ROLE AND RESPONSIBILITIES

- Assist in supporting the psychosocial health needs of antepartum patients during their hospitalization after neonatology consults have been obtained.
- Provide ongoing neonatal consults throughout the antenatal admission of high-risk patients.
- Provide education, information, and psychosocial support to antenatal patients and their families.
- Coordinate and provide tours of the NICU for antepartum patients and their families.
- Begin care coordination for antepartum patients in collaboration with the NICU team if a NICU admission is anticipated.
- Attend high-risk deliveries and stay close to the family throughout the entire delivery process to meet any needs they may have.
- Accompany new families during admission to the NICU.
- Support families who find themselves facing neonatal transport.
- Collaborate closely with case management, social work, psychology, and other care providers throughout the NICU journey to provide education and support and to connect families to support services.
- Plan and host family events.
- Participate in peer-to-peer mentor group recruitment, trainings, meetings, and events, as well as pair families with appropriate trained mentors.
- Maintain active involvement in the bereavement committee and support bereaved families.

QUALIFICATIONS AND EDUCATION REQUIREMENTS

A current staff member may be designated for this position, or the hospital may hire a new individual to fill this position.
- Master's degree in social work, education, nursing public health, or related field is preferred.
- Active license to practice as a registered nurse or social work is required.
- A total of 1 to 3 years of recent experience working in a level III NICU or pediatric unit is required.
- Basic knowledge of the psychosocial and medical issues that face antepartum and NICU families is required.
- Demonstrated ability to sensitively engage with parents and their support systems is required to provide compassionate and culturally sensitive support.

PREFERRED SKILLS

- Experience in planning and coordinating meetings and events
- Comfort in having difficult and emotional conversations with families in crisis
- Ability to teach to a variety of learning styles
- Flexibility, ability to prioritize tasks frequently, and ability to multitask with frequent interruptions
- Exposure to high-risk deliveries
- Strong communication skills

Figure 2.1 ■ Sample: Family support specialist job description. (*continued*)

**Surviving Bed Rest
for
Mom-to-Be**

- Read books; find others that you can start a book club with

- Journal about your experience; your fears, frustrations, goals, accomplishments and your emotions

- Mark your progress and milestones on a calendar; visually see your hard work is paying off

- Join an online support community

- If you are anticipating a premature delivery, read up on NICU and premature baby care

- Find someone to pamper you with a pedicure, manicure or massage

- Talk to your provider to see what exercises are safe for you to do and STAY ACTIVE

- Learn to knit, crochet or cross stitch and make a gift for your baby

- Throw a party each week when you make it to a new gestation, invite family, friends and staff to celebrate with you!

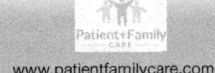

www.patientfamilycare.com

**Helping Mom Survive Bed Rest
for
Significant Other**

- Spend as much time with the mom-to-be as you can

- Surprise her with flowers or other small gifts to cheer her up and brighten up her room

- Check out some books on how to support bed resting mothers and begin reading up on what to expect

- Ask lots of questions so you are well informed of what is going on and what the care plan is

- Ask family and friends for help! They want to so don't be too proud to let others support you during this time

- Find family or friends who will help set up a meal calendar for you and your family

- Offer to purchase remaining baby items you may need

- Give mom-to-be a massage from time to time to help her relax

- Connect with other significant others who have experienced their partner being placed on bedrest. Find out what helped them

- Stay active and encourage mom-to-be to do her bedrest exercises

- Plan a date night! Get your favorite food, light candles (battery operated ones if you are in the hospital), pop some popcorn and watch a movie

- Help plan and attend celebrations to recognize each milestone and each new gestational week she is still pregnant

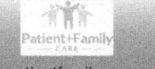

www.patientfamilycare.com

Figure 2.2 ■ Sample rack cards with bed-rest survival tips.

<table>
<tr><td>

**Helping Mom Survive Bed Rest
for
Family and Friends**

- Get her books to read and offer to start a book club

- Play board games or card games with her

- Plan a movie night and watch a movie together

- Help her get pampered with a pedicure, manicure and/ or massage

- Purchase a body pillow/pregnancy pillow to help her stay comfortable

- Offer to help with other children she may have

- Offer to help with household chores; garbage, mail, cleaning, laundry, cooking meals and caring for pets

- Prepare meals for her and her family: set up a meal calendar so others can help too

- Encourage her to journal and track her progress and milestones on a calendar

- Encourage her and help her stay positive. Watch for signs of depression and encourage her to talk to her doctor if she is experiencing emotional distress

- Keep her active and encourage her to keep up with safe bedrest exercises

- If she is in the hospital, take familiar things from home to help brighten up her room

- Throw her a party each week when she reaches a new gestation and let her know you are celebrating each milestone with her

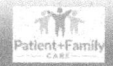
www.patientfamilycare.com

</td><td>

**Helping Mom Survive Bed Rest
for
Siblings**

- Spend as much time with your mom as you can

- Color or draw a picture for your mom

- Reed with or to your mom

- Write and illustrate a book for your mom and what you think it will be like to be a big brother/sister

- Make a list of all the fun things you want to teach the baby when they grow up

- Ask if there are books about becoming a big brother/ sister that you could read

- Play games with your mom

- Participate in fun art projects with your mom to make somethings special for the baby

- Ask if there are chores at home you could do to help your mom and your family

- Have a movie and popcorn night with mom and watch your favorite movie together

- Participate in any celebration your mom has to recognize her hard work, dedication and love for you and your soon-to-be new baby brother/sister

Note to Siblings: When your mom is on bedrest, it can be really hard for you to understand why she can't do the things she normally does. Be sure to talk to your mom or others family if you are feeling sad or upset. They can help you learn ways to better understand your emotions and fears.

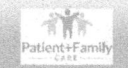
www.patientfamilycare.com

</td></tr>
</table>

Figure 2.2 ■ **Sample rack cards with bed-rest survival tips.** (*continued*)

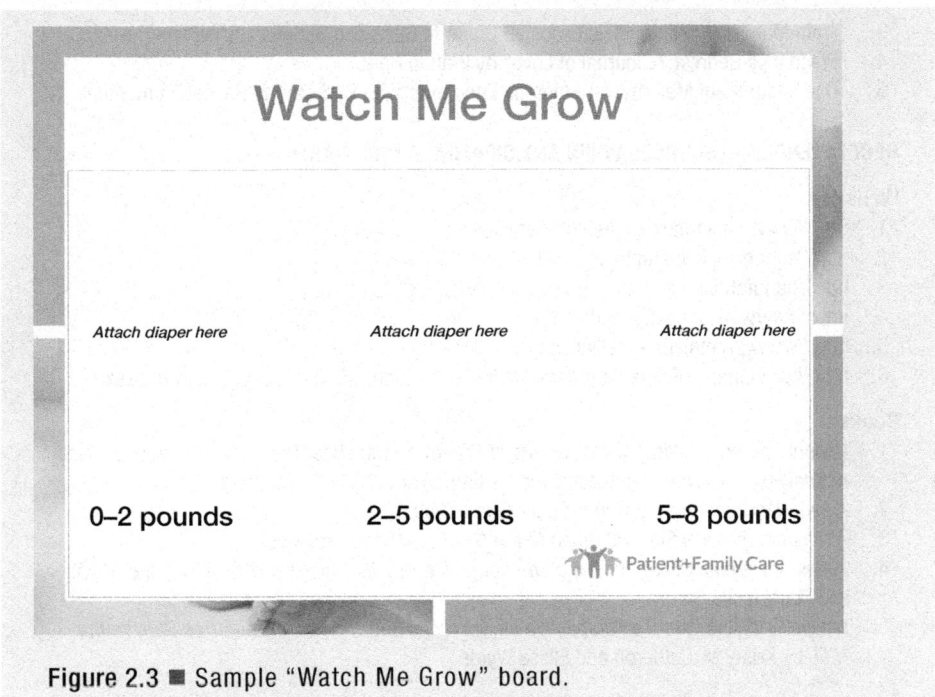

Figure 2.3 ■ Sample "Watch Me Grow" board.

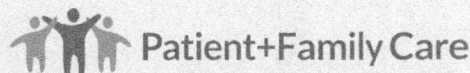

RECOMMENDED RESOURCES WHILE ON HOSPITAL BED REST:

Websites:
1. http://www.keepemcookin.com
2. http://www.patientfamilycare.com/high-risk-pregnancies
3. https://www.sidelines.org
4. https://mamasonbedrest.com
5. http://www.highriskhope.org
6. https://www.babycenter.com/pregnancy-bedrest
7. http://betterbedrest.org
8. http://www.parents.com/pregnancy/my-life/bed-rest
9. https://www.whattoexpect.com/pregnancy/bed-rest

Books:
1. *Surviving Pregnancy Bed Rest* by Kristina Seleshanko
2. *Days in Waiting: A Guide to Surviving Pregnancy Bedrest* by Mary Ann McCann

Figure 2.4 ■ Recommended resources: Hospital bed rest.

3. "From Mamas to Mamas: The Essential Guide to Surviving Bedrest" by Darline Turner
4. "Pregnancy Bedrest: A Journal of Love" by Wanda Hale
5. "One Recumbent Mommy: A Humorous Encounter with Bedrest" by Rachel Blumenthal

RECOMMENDED RESOURCES WHEN ANTICIPATING A NICU BABY:

Websites:
1. http://www.patientfamilycare.com/families
2. http://support4nicuparents.org
3. http://handtohold.org
4. https://www.nicuhelpinghands.org
5. http://www.preemieparentalliance.org
6. http://www.marchofdimes.org/complications/the-nicu-family-support-program.aspx

Books:
1. *Understanding the NICU: What Parents of Preemies and Other Hospitalized Newborns Need to Know* by The American Academy of Pediatrics and Jeanette Zaichkin
2. *A Parent's Guide to Surviving NICU* by Krystal Abbott
3. *A Preemie Parent's Survival Guide to the NICU* by Megan Grandinetti
4. *Intensive Parenting: Surviving the Emotional Journey through the NICU* by Deborah Davis and Mara Tesler Stein
5. *Mitchell's Gift: A Parent's Perspective on Surviving Life ... With a Premature Baby in the NICU* by Kristy M. Cameron and Elissa Wylde

Figure 2.4 ■ Recommended resources: Hospital bed rest. (*continued*)

Case-Based Learning

M, is a 34-year-old, G3, P0, who presented at 20 4/7 weeks with premature rupture of membranes. This pregnancy is her third via assistive reproduction. Both previous pregnancies resulted in early second-trimester losses. M, and her partner are excited to have carried the pregnancy further this time than previously.

M, is the primary income earner as a family law attorney in private practice. She is an athletic, marathon runner, who currently enjoys bike riding and yoga as her daily exercise.

M.'s partner is a web designer who works from home. They have been partnered for 6 years and plan to be married next month. M. is placed on bed rest with bathroom privileges and given latency antibiotics. When M. completes 24 0/7 weeks' gestation, you are alerted to an inpatient needing prenatal neonatal consultation. You arrive at M.'s room to find her working on her laptop on a conference call. You interrupt long enough for a brief introduction and to ask about a good time to return.

When you return at the appointed time, M. cheerfully greets you and begins to ask numerous questions about the chances of survival of her baby. Your review of

(*continued*)

(*continued*)

the medical record indicated that a neonatology consult was completed yesterday with both parents present.

QUESTIONS

1. What are the contextual elements of M.'s anticipatory guidance?
2. What factors may be affecting M.'s questions about her baby's condition?
3. What are your next steps?

ANSWERS

Many factors provide background understanding of M.'s situation. These include her support system(s), education, socioeconomic level, employment status, lifestyle, and medical history. The socioenvironmental stressors of bed rest and preterm birth may be exacerbated by the trauma of M.'s previous losses, impact of financial worries as the primary breadwinner, inability to exercise, and the resultant deconditioning, disruption of daily schedule (including sleep), loss of control, fear of the unknown (and unknowable), alteration of current (and future) life events, and worries related to the pregnancy, as well as the long-term impact on partnering and parenting.

Pregnancy puts women at risk for anxiety and depression; the incidence is increased in mothers of preterms and newborns requiring mechanical ventilation (Rogers, Kidokoro, Wallendorf, & Inder, 2013). M.'s previous losses and the fear of the unknown may contribute to greater risk of anxiety and/or depression. Postpartum mood disorder screening and follow-up are indicated (Hutti, Armstrong, Myers, & Hall, 2015; Kolte, Olsen, Mikkelsen, Christiansen, & Nielsen, 2015; Scheans, Mischel, Munson, & Bulaevskaya, 2016).

Several factors, such as stress, may make retention of information difficult for M. Chronic sleep loss during pregnancy is a determinant of stress; it impacts memory and contributes to depression and pregnancy outcomes (Horsch et al., 2017; Palagini et al., 2014).

The use of "plain language" is incumbent on us all, but we often fall short. It is important to remember that assessment of understanding is always needed, since education, income, or occupation ensure health literacy. Information may be forgotten if learned in a highly emotional state such as M.'s. As a member of the "millennial" age demographic, M. is likely used to accessing information via the Internet and seeking information from multiple sources (Hussey, Frazer, & Kopulos, 2016).

M.'s educational needs and understanding may be enhanced (while avoiding feeling patronized) by expecting that repetition will be needed. Try to use M.'s own terms. Provide visual and written materials as well as accurate websites. Review her retention of the information with the use of "teach back" methodology can be effective (Hussey et al., 2016; Stikes, Arterberry, & Logsdon, 2015).

(*continued*)

(*continued*)

REFERENCES

Horsch, A., Gilbert, L., Lanzi, S., Kang, J. S., Vial, Y., & Puder, J. (2017). Associations between maternal stress during pregnancy and obstetric and neonatal outcomes. *Psychoneuroendocrinology*, *83*, 28. doi:10.1016/j.psyneuen.2017.07.313

Hussey, L. C., Frazer, C., & Kopulos, M. I. (2016). Impact of health literacy levels in educating pregnant millennial women. *International Journal of Childbirth Education, 31*(3), 13–18. Retrieved from http://icea.org/wp-content/uploads/2015/12/CBEd-JUL-web-FINAL.pdf

Hutti, M. H., Armstrong, D. S., Myers, J. A., & Hall, L. A. (2015). Grief intensity, psychological well-being, and the intimate partner relationship in the subsequent pregnancy after a perinatal loss. *Journal of Obstetric, Gynecologic & Neonatal Nursing, 44*(1), 42–50. doi:10.1111/1552-6909.12539

Kolte, A. M., Olsen, L. R., Mikkelsen, E. M., Christiansen, O. B., & Nielsen, H. S. (2015). Depression and emotional stress is highly prevalent among women with recurrent pregnancy loss. *Human Reproduction, 30*(4), 777–782. doi:10.1093/humrep/dev014

Palagini, L., Gemignani, A., Banti, S., Manconi, M., Mauri, M., & Riemann, D. (2014). Chronic sleep loss during pregnancy as a determinant of stress: Impact on pregnancy outcome. *Sleep Medicine, 15*(8), 853–859. doi:10.1016/j.sleep.2014.02.013

Rogers, C., Kidokoro, H., Wallendorf, M., & Inder, T. (2013). Identifying mothers of very preterm infants at-risk for postpartum depression and anxiety before discharge. *Journal of Perinatology, 33*(3), 171–176. doi:10.1038/jp.2012.75

Scheans, P., Mischel, R., Munson, M., & Bulaevskaya, K. (2016). Postpartum mood disorders screening in the NICU. *Neonatal Network, 35*(4), 240–242. doi:10.1891/0730-0832.35.4.240

Stikes, R., Arterberry, K., & Logsdon, M. C. (2015). A nurse leadership project to improve health literacy on a maternal-infant unit. *Journal of Obstetric, Gynecologic & Neonatal Nursing, 44*(5), 665–676. doi:10.1111/1552-6909.12742

REFERENCES

Abu-Saad, K., & Fraser, D. (2010). Maternal nutrition and birth outcomes. *Epidemiologic Reviews, 32*(1), 5–25. doi:10.1093/epirev/mxq001

Durrance, C. P., & Guldi, M. (2015). Maternal bed rest and infant health. *American Journal of Health Economics, 1*(3), 345–373. doi:10.1162/AJHE_a_00021

Greer, I. A. (2012). Thrombosis in pregnancy: Updates in diagnosis and management. *Hematology, 2012*(1), 203–207. doi:10.1182/asheducation-2012.1.203

HCPro. (2012, November 27). Complications from immobility by body system. Retrieved from http://www.hcpro.com/LTC-286850-10704/Complications-from-immobility-by-body-system.html

Lewis, J. G. (2012, August 17). Turning trauma into story: The benefits of journaling. Retrieved from https://www.psychologytoday.com/blog/brain-babble/201208/turning-trauma-story-the-benefits -journaling

Maloni, J. A., Chance, B., Zhang, C., Betts, A. W., & Gange, S. J. (1993). Physical and psychosocial side effects of antepartum hospital bed rest. *Nursing Research, 42*(4), 202–203. doi:10.1097/00006199-199307000-00002

Masley, P. M., Havrilko, C., Mahnensmith, M. R., Aubert, M., & Jette, D. U. (2011). Physical therapist practice in the acute care setting: A qualitative study. *Physical Therapy, 91*(6), 906–919. doi:10.2522/ptj.20100296

Pacific College of Oriental Medicine. (n.d.). Massage for pregnancy & childbirth. Retrieved from http://www.pacificcollege.edu/news/blog/2015/01/13/massage-pregnancy-childbirth

Rubarth, L. B., Schoening, A. M., Cosimano, A., & Sandhurst, H. (2012). Women's experience of hospitalized bed rest during high-risk pregnancy. *Journal of Obstetric, Gynecologic and Neonatal Nursing, 41*(3), 398–407. doi:10.1111/j.1552-6909.2012.01349.x

Schetter, C. D., & Tanner, L. (2012). Anxiety, depression and stress in pregnancy: Implications for mothers, children, research, and practice. *Current Opinion in Psychiatry, 25*(2), 141–148. doi:10.1097/YCO.0b013e3283503680

van Ravesteyn, L. M., Lambregtse-van den Berg, M. P., Hoogendijk, W. J. G., & Kamperman, A. M. (2017). Interventions to treat mental disorders during pregnancy: A systematic review and multiple treatment meta-analysis. *PLOS ONE, 12*(3), e0173397. doi:10.1371/journal.pone.0173397

SUPPORTING FAMILIES DURING HIGH-RISK DELIVERIES

3

SUPPORTING THE PATIENT AND FAMILY DURING THE DELIVERY

Supporting women and families during labor is one of the pivotal roles of a labor and delivery nurse. In fact, when you talk to the majority of labor and delivery nurses, they will tell you that they go into this specialty because they recognize what a privilege it is to share in the experience of bringing a new life into the world. They have a desire to serve patients in that unforgettable experience and want to support that life-changing moment so that it is memorable, personal, safe, and everything that the family wants it to be. However, "labor support does not always occur because nurses tend to have coexisting responsibilities for more than one laboring woman, spend large amounts of time managing technology or keeping records, and begin or end shifts in the middle of women's labors. While providing labor support is an important component of nursing care, only 6.1% of nurses' time [is] spent in providing supportive care" (Barrett & Stark, 2010, para. 1).

This statistic is concerning on multiple levels but is most alarming because of the fact that the "experience of childbirth plays a major role in how first-time mothers will develop good self-esteem, positive feelings for the baby, an easier adjustment to motherhood role, and also future childbirth experiences. In order to provide better individual support to women during childbirth, the health care providers are required to put more focus on psychosocial aspects, but without neglecting medical safety" (Nilsson, Thorsell, Wahn, & Ekström, 2013, Introduction). How can providers place a high priority on supporting the psychosocial support of families during childbirth and delivery if only 6.1% of their time is available to provide such care? It is absolutely necessary to find the answer to this question, and as professionals, we have the obligation to address it as a top priority when it is known that there is a direct correlation on how the long-term health of mothers and infants fares based on how they are supported during this critical event in their lives.

Not only is it important for labor and delivery professionals to prioritize the psychosocial support of women and families during labor and delivery, but it is also essential for staff to place an even higher priority on the psychosocial support for women and families facing a high-risk delivery. Families delivering a premature infant or a child with a known illness or life-altering complication are going to face much higher rates of stress during the delivery period. Parents living these experiences are sensing the excitement of getting ready to meet their new child while being troubled about whether or not their child will survive long after birth or be born alive at all. Caregivers must recognize and acknowledge this unique stress, and arranging the appropriate staffing to support families in these situations is one of the most critical interventions labor and delivery professionals can provide.

In some high-risk delivery situations, families will head into the delivery with some preparation. Antepartum patients who have been on bed rest or were diagnosed with a high-risk pregnancy were likely given some indication that the delivery may come early or could be medically complex. These families have hopefully already developed a relationship with trusted medical personnel who will be with them in the delivery room (regardless of whether it is a vaginal or cesarean delivery) and will have slightly less anxiety due to the support they were given prior to the delivery. In addition, studies have "found that childbirth information received by mothers during antenatal period influences their sense of control and empowerment during labor and delivery" (Iravani, Zarean, Janghorbani, & Bahrami, 2015, Discussions), which also aids in the reduction of stress at the time of delivery.

In these situations, support from staff should be focused on the needs of the family and should provide ongoing, understandable, and accurate information about what is going on in the moment. In an ideal situation, the family-support specialist assigned to care for the delivering family would have already established a relationship with them prior during a neonatal consult and would be able to build on the established relationship and known education previously provided. What tends to be of utmost importance for the family-support specialist in these situations is to recognize that during high-risk deliveries, staff frequently tend to move very quickly, which can be overwhelming and stressful for families. They see the rush in everyone's movements and the focus of their attention and easily pick up on the severity of the situation. In addition, when the health of a mother and/or infant are at risk during a delivery, the number of attending staff increases exponentially, and families are often frightened at the sight of numerous additional strangers running into the room or rushing toward the operating room to prepare for their delivery. Staff who are assigned as the family-support specialist can reduce a family's stress in these times by calmly talking them step-by-step through the development of events, being available to answer questions, and explaining who is responding to the delivery and describing their specific role.

Regrettably, not all families are given the opportunity to be prepared prior to the emergent situation. These situations are even more stressful for both families and staff because emotions run high, outcomes are unknown, and it can be very difficult for staff to know what to say to families. Nurses want to make patients feel better, and sometimes there is nothing that can be said or be done that will make them feel better. In these times, "emotional support [should be] directed toward activities such as continuous presence, positive reassurance and praise" (Barrett & Stark, 2010, p. 13). Simply allowing families to feel, as well as assuring them that their confusion and grief about the loss of their perfect pregnancy and delivery can be some of the most effective support one can provide. Again, being present to guide a family through the medical complexities of what is occurring in the rushed moments, being available to answer questions, and providing honest information about the condition of both mom and baby should be the priority of the family-support specialist during these high-risk deliveries.

In all high-risk deliveries, whether or not families have warning, staff members should advocate for the mother and family to maintain as much control over the situation as possible. When the health of a mother or unborn child is at risk and an emergency delivery is required, birth plans often are tossed aside by medical professionals. As many labor and delivery providers know, birth plans are often very sacred to families, and "when expectations are altered, the care providers and support team become vitally important in helping to negotiate changes [to] foster a positive birth experience" (Cook & Loomis, 2012, p. 159). As previously mentioned, positive birth experiences lead to better health outcomes for both mom and baby, so it is incredibly important for staff to focus on providing the best experience possible for families, even when the situation is far from ideal or deviates from a family's desired plan.

How specifically can labor and delivery staff support families during a high-risk delivery to turn a stressful, overwhelming, and potentially devastating situation into a positive birth experience? Believe it or not, staff can perform many interventions to provide a lasting positive impact on families, and they are interventions that are easy and inexpensive and can be provided by any staff member who would be assigned to support families:

- Define *family*: *Family* is defined by the patient and should include anyone who is a support to her. If the patient has an entire room full of people who are important and provide comfort to her—they are family. If the patient is alone and has no one with her, then staff has to step in and provide that safety net of support. Patients cope through the stressful delivery and the postpartum stay more successfully if they have the comfort of their support networks, so allowing them to be surrounded by their support should be allowed and encouraged by labor and delivery unit policies.

- Prioritize safety: In medical emergencies, safety always has to remain a priority. With that in mind, the previous intervention may have to be altered in situations if the safety of the mother, infant, or staff could be compromised. However, the decision to limit the number of family members must be highly scrutinized to determine whether it is truly due to safety concerns or to the inconvenience created for staff. If family presence is compromising patient or staff safety, staff needs to have a compassionate and empathetic conversation with the patient and family members about the need to limit the number of family present. Staff must keep in mind that these family members are a comfort to patients in one of the most terrifying and frightening times of their lives and that separating them increases stress and anxiety. Providing an explanation that the primary goal is to keep mom and baby as safe as possible hopefully encourages cooperation and ensures that they will be reunited as soon as possible. When deliveries occur in an operating room, policies usually preclude more than one support person from accompanying the mother. This practice automatically eliminates the issue of multiple family members. However, in high-risk situations, the number of support people allowed in the operating room with the mother should be reconsidered. At minimum, two support individuals should be allowed. This change in practice serves two purposes:

- A mother going into a high-risk delivery in the operating room is typically sad, is worried, and experiences anxiety because of the full loss of control. She also has feelings of hope, envisions the moment of her child's birth and wants more than just one person there to witness that moment. Most typically, a mom chooses to have her partner and her own mother with her.

- Mom's partner, who may be fearful not only about the outcome of the delivery, but also about the health of the mother, goes into to the operating room with added anxiety. Allowing an additional support person to go in with the couple provide as support person for them. It is critically important to provide equal support to both partners during the delivery because they are the pending parents and have psychosocial needs that must be addressed and supported during the delivery.

- Be culturally sensitive: Each patient and family approaches pregnancy, birth, and the journey into parenthood differently. "This must be encouraged and nurtured by staff who prepare clients for childbirth so that it is a safe and memorable experience for the family by listening, respecting preferences, recognizing differences and supporting choices" (Greene, 2007, "Diversity" section). Staff should be continually educated about the cultural norms of the primary populations in the area so that they feel confident and comfortable with the care patients will expect to receive. However, there is no way that staff can be expected to be the experts in knowing how every culture celebrates and honors birth, so interviewing patients and families regarding this should be routine at admission. The nurse should spend time finding out from the patients and their families what is most important to them in regard to their support network, pain control, diet and nutrition, and breastfeeding and postpartum practices; then the nurse should do whatever possible to honor their rituals and practices.

- Be emotionally present: Having the sole responsibility of focusing on the family allows staff to be present and assess the emotional, spiritual, and psychosocial needs from moment to moment. If fully present with a family, "nurses have a potential to alleviate existential and spiritual suffering through consoling presence. By connecting deeply with patients and their families, nurses have the possibility to affirm the patient's strength and facilitate their courage" (Tornøe, Danbolt, Kvigne, & Sørlie, 2014, "Conclusions" section) that will positively reflect on their memory of their time in nursing care.

- Provide accurate information: The nuances of the medical world are often foreign to the majority of patients and their families. This is true for stable medical situations, let alone high-risk and complicated situations. Parents are unprepared for the many decisions that they are likely going to have to make; without knowing what those decisions will ultimately mean for their child and their family, they are going to look to their providers to give them honest, accurate, and candid information. Parents have shared that they want to be given hope, even when hope is slim, but do not want to be given false hope.

- Take photos: Support individuals in healthy, term deliveries often start taking happy birth photos. Or in some cases, birth photographers are hired and capture the moment with both the mom and the support members in the shots together. When the delivery is high risk, especially when unplanned or rushed, families often are so distracted by fear that the last thing on their mind is a camera. In fact, I often hear from families that even if a camera crosses their mind, they can't imagine ever wanting to have a memory of this moment once they get through it. As research has shown in scenarios of bereavement and loss, photography is a very therapeutic memento for families and captures a part of their journey. Ask the family if they have a camera or even a cell phone and offer to take some photos for them. Capture images of the delivery, of mom and her support network together, and of the staff working hard together, as well as other important images that capture the moment. For example, the clock and mom's wristband tend to be photos parents cherish the most.

- Encourage family participation: Assist the family in being their own advocate and participating in as many aspects of their care and decision making that they can. In addition, find ways that mom and her support network can actively participate in the delivery process. In a vaginal delivery, for example, find ways support individuals can help mom cope during the delivery. Have them keep a cool wash cloth on her forehead, rub her back between contractions, count out loud during a contraction, massage her feet, breath with her to help aid in pain control and other interventions that mom feels would help her during her delivery.

- Don't neglect the support person: As mentioned previously, when partners are involved, don't neglect their needs during this stressful time. Often, staff focus so much of their time and effort on supporting and caring for the mom, partners suffer silently on the sidelines. These are, many times, the people I worry most about, not just in that moment, but also long term. These support individuals are worried about their child and their partner and often go undiagnosed with posttraumatic stress disorder from the event. Stay in tune with how they are doing and be sure to meet their needs as well. Check in with them often, offer them support, give them the same education and information you provide the mother, and treat the mom and support partner as a couple rather than individuals.

INCLUDING FAMILY IN NEONATAL RESUSCITATION

When a high-risk delivery results in the need for neonatal resuscitation, the ongoing support of families must remain a priority and absolutely should include the family. Many delivery rooms are designed for resuscitation to occur in the same room as the mother and family, and in these instances, family and their assigned staff member (the family-support specialist) should approach the resuscitation bed with the resuscitation team as soon as possible. The support specialist can provide ongoing education about what interventions are being provided to the infant and can answer questions the family may have about the resuscitation; in addition, the family is afforded the opportunity to witness the efforts being made to stabilize their child.

Years of research have been conducted on the risks and benefits of including families in the resuscitation of their children, and "the majority of parents believed that being there and being able to touch their child provided comfort to their child, and helped the parents to adjust in the event of the loss of the child" (Sawyer et al., 2015, "Introduction" section). Also, "standardized psychological examinations suggest that, compared with those not present, family members present during attempted resuscitations have less anxiety and depression and more constructive grieving behavior" (American Heart Association, n.d., para. 1), which are direct outcomes that healthcare professionals should aim to provide this fragile population.

With the abundant amount of research available that supports the presence of family at resuscitation, there still is no universal acceptance of this practice. There are multiple reasons as to why this is, including staff comfort levels of having family present, varied levels of experience among the resuscitation team, legal angst, staff fears that family presence negatively impacts the effectiveness of cardiopulmonary resuscitation, staff's unease about being watched in a critical situation, physical layout of the delivery and resuscitation environment, and past negative experiences with family presence. Staff also have shared that they fear that families may be negatively impacted if they witness their child being resuscitated and feel they are actually protecting parents if they exclude them from the situation.

The topic of family presence at resuscitation remains controversial, but with a desire to prioritize care to be family focused and most supportive, families should be offered the option to be present at resuscitations. Not only is this practice important for the psychosocial well-being of the family, but it also can provide families with the opportunity to stay involved in even the slightest ways, which can help them feel connected to their child. Although the condition of the newborn may be uncertain and fragile, finding ways for connection can be of utmost importance. In situations in which the child's life is uncertain, finding ways for parents to be involved can provide moments of parenting and a lifetime of comfort for that family.

I often get asked by teams what can a family member do during a resuscitation? I can tell you that a family member can do quite a bit if you have a supportive multidisciplinary team that is willing to genuinely accept how important it is to allow a parent to parent their child in that critical moment of their child's life. A few examples that could be considered may include the following:

- When a freshly warm blanket needs to be placed under or on top of the infant to protect their thermoregulation, allow the parent to place the blanket.

- Allow a family member to gently place a hand on the child's hand to provide comfort and psychologically feel that they are present for their child when the baby needs their family the most.

- If an overhead warmer is monitoring the infant's temperature, give a family member a temperature range to watch for and ask them to alert staff if the temperate drops below or rises above a specific number.

- If a diaper is placed under or on the infant, ask the family member to assist with placement.

- When the team is ready to weigh the infant, let the parent press the "weight baby" button on the scale.

- If measurements are taken, allow the family to be close enough to see the tape measure and have them to double check your measurements.

Whether these or other ideas are developed to include families during resuscitation, they all should be established and evolved within every labor and delivery setting to foster attachment and connection between parents and their children in the most critical of situations. It "is now well-accepted that pediatric care should be provided within the context of families, with parents considered essential partners in their children's care" (Curley et al., 2012, para. 1).

CARING FOR MOM AND BABY AS A DYAD DURING EMERGENCIES

When possible, keeping an infant and a mother together after birth is ideal. "Mothers and babies have a physiologic need to be together during the moments, hours and days following birth, and this time together significantly improves maternal and newborn outcomes" (Crenshaw, 2014, "Abstract" section). Although this practice is easily encouraged and adapted with healthy and term newborns, it should be regarded as an even higher priority when an infant's condition is critical. If infants and mothers are separated for resuscitation and the infant may not survive despite the most coordinated resuscitative efforts, can you even begin to imagine what the effects will be on that family for the rest of their lives?

As mentioned previously, many labor and delivery rooms are equipped to resuscitate neonates in the room with the family. Unfortunately, not all are, and mother and infant separation is potentially unavoidable. Medical equipment is available, including a mobile trolley, which was developed to avoid maternal–infant separation should the need for resuscitation arise immediately after birth. Hospitals with delivery rooms that are not set up to resuscitate infants should inquire and invest in a method that would in fact allow resuscitations to occur near the mother to eliminate separation. If separation is unavoidable, however, staff should decrease the time family is apart, and a support person should be allowed to accompany the infant to the adjoining resuscitation room. A key role for family-support specialist staff in this situation is to maintain ongoing communication with the mother so that she is continuously aware of what is going on with her child.

For units able to keep infants in the same room with mothers during the neonatal emergency, multiple setups are most frequently seen. The most common is to have resuscitation occur on an infant warmer at the foot of a mother's delivery bed. This allows the mother to witness the resuscitation and be present for the entire stabilization of her child. Unfortunately, mothers often cannot see anything that is occurring at the warmer because the resuscitation team surrounds the infant and is more focused diligently on stabilizing the newborn's physiological condition (which, of course, is the priority) than on being out of the mother's way. Other units place the infant warmer to the side of the mother's delivery bed, which allows for a little better viewing by the mother, yet the resuscitation team still surrounds the infant and still blocks her view. In fact, this setup is usually less than ideal because the infant team is in the way of the team caring for the postpartum mother.

Regardless of where the resuscitation warmer is, the key is to have it in the room to avoid separation. When deliveries occur in an operating room, mothers and infants typically are together; again, this configuration varies. Some operating rooms are equipped to resuscitate infants in the same operating room where the cesarean birth took place, whereas others require the infant to be taken to an adjoining resuscitation suite. Once again, alternative modalities would allow the resuscitation to take place near the mother and should be considered and trialed by the staff to eliminate the need to separate mothers and infants after birth.

What would be an even more ideal situation for the maternal–infant dyad in these emergent situations? Infant resuscitation on the mother's chest (in less emergent situations). Some neonatal resuscitation already occurs on mothers' chests and has for quite some time. However, can you imagine if even more resuscitations, and more critical resuscitations, occurred this way? What can you imagine the benefits would be to the mother, the baby, and the family? Of course, proper positive pressure ventilation (PPV) and chest compressions would be extremely difficult to perform adequately on a mother's chest, but imagine for just a moment the following scenario:

A premature infant that had clear fluids at delivery is immediately placed on the mother's chest. The team is able to warm, dry, and stimulate the infant, as well as perform any suctioning that is required. Overwhelming evidence emphasizes the "importance of improved prognosis in newborns allowed to undergo a smooth transition at birth by delaying cord clamping until ventilation (spontaneous or PPV) of the lungs is established" (Vali, Mathew, & Lakshminrusimha, 2015, Review—Fetal Circulation). This also provides time for the airway to be positioned and opened and the team to either assess for spontaneous respirations or to initiate PPV. If PPV is necessary, the cord can be cut and the infant placed on a nearby warmer that is prewarmed to reduce the risk of the infant developing hypothermia. Further resuscitative efforts can continue near the mother and family, and the infant's airway can then be stabilized. Once the airway is secure, either with a continuous positive airway pressure (CPAP) apparatus or an endotracheal tube connected to a transport ventilator, the infant could then be placed back on the mother's chest for ongoing resuscitation and stabilization. Intravenous lines could be placed, medications could be administered, and continuous fluids could begin infusion all while baby is lying safely on mom's chest. How many of you are hesitant and thinking I am the most unrealistic person in the world right now? I openly admit this is extremely unlikely and there are many, many risks involved with this idea. But if the care team can collaborate and the hospital environment is prioritized to keep families together to optimize the maternal and infant long-term health outcomes, I honestly think that these scenarios need to at least be put out there. I have to believe that there are teams out there that are brave enough to try this. Just consider how an infant's thermoregulation would stabilize if they were skin-to-skin with their mother during resuscitation? Think of how a mother would feel as a parent if she were physically a part of the most critical moments of her child's life? In fact, when you consider resuscitation in less resource-rich countries, a mother's chest is often

Benefits for Mom	Benefits for Baby
• Increased feelings of bonding and attachment to child • Improved breastfeeding success/breast milk production • Sense of providing parental support to their child • Reduced symptoms of depression • Decreased physiological stress in the postpartum period	• Improved thermoregulation • Improved cardiopulmonary stabilization • Comfort of immediately hearing mother's heartbeat • Potential reduced responses to pain

Figure 3.1 ■ Benefits when resuscitation occurs on the mother's chest.

the only way providers can reduce the risk of hypothermia in premature infants after delivery. It might be a futuristic goal, but there are many benefits to both moms and babies (Association of Women's Health, Obstetric and Neonatal Nurses [AWHONN], 2016). I think that this idea should at least be considered in the next reiterations of our neonatal resuscitation programs (Figure 3.1).

Some hospitals are setting the stage for best practice for caring for mom and baby as a dyad by no longer having NICUs. Instead, they are equipping each labor and delivery room with the necessary setup to care for a level III neonatal patient. This allows neonatal resuscitation to occur at the mother's bedside, followed by the beginning and continuation of neonatal care in the same room. It ends the traumatic separation experiences that most mothers face when their infants are whisked away to a NICU down the hall, on another floor of the hospital, or worse, transported to a completely different facility. Often, it takes hours or days before a mother is reunited with her child once the separation occurs. What a novel concept it is to deliver high-risk and premature infants in delivery rooms that also serve as their long-term potential NICU room, where parents will be welcome to be with their child 24/7.

Author's Personal Story

I met J.S. the morning of her delivery. I was asked by our attending neonatologist to accompany him to J.S.' room and provide a combined neonatology and neonatal consult. J.S. was going to have a cesarean delivery in 2 hours and was going to be giving birth to a child with a very rare form of achondroplasia. This was a diagnosis that she and her husband had been made aware of only weeks before. Until that point, everything about the pregnancy had been going well and was uneventful. The prognosis for this infant was very poor, and the obstetrical team caring for J.S. did not anticipate the child to be able to survive birth; if she did, they did not believe she would be able to live very long.

(continued)

(*continued*)

The neonatologist and I walked into the room, where I anticipated meeting a family that would be somber and subdued. I was greeted by a group of people who were smiling and laughing. This entire family was there actually glowing in a way, and J.S. was lying in her hospital bed being held by her husband and seemed to have this peace about her. As the neonatologist and I introduced ourselves and what our roles would be in the upcoming delivery, we learned that this close-knit family was extremely grounded in their Christian faith and they were ready and prepared to accept whatever plan God had for them and their child. I remember being in awe of this family's strength, and during our time with them, I was given the incredible opportunity to find out how we could personalize the upcoming experience for them to truly honor their beliefs and their religious heritage.

As the assigned family support person, I had the sole responsibility of helping this family create a supportive delivery plan for their upcoming high-risk delivery. What I remember most about the creation of this plan was that not only was this family involved in developing the plan, but they also prayed each step of the way hand in hand and asked God for guidance and peace for each tough decision that had to be made. What was agreed on in the end is that J.S. would enter the operating room suite with her very best friends, who happened to be a married couple. This couple would stay at the head of the operating table with J.S. and guide her in prayer throughout the delivery. This decision was made to accommodate the desire for the baby to be accompanied by J.S.' husband (the baby's father) into the resuscitation suite after delivery. Unfortunately, the department she was delivering in was undergoing construction and the operating room in the labor and delivery unit did not support the space to resuscitate an infant. There was a window between the operating room and an adjoining resuscitation suite that was opened so that the team could communicate with one another and J.S. and her husband could talk to one another during the delivery, despite the slight separation.

When it was time for the delivery, J.S. and her friends were brought into the operating room. Their positive moods were still present, yet I definitely could sense a higher level of stress within each of them. The anesthesiologist working the case greeted the three of them as they entered, and then he walked over to the stereo. He hooked up an MP3 player, and before I knew it, the room was filled with Chris Tomlin music and J.S. and her friends were singing along and became lost in worship. I later learned that when the anesthesiologist spent time meeting the patient and her family, he too took the time to find out what was most important to them; when he learned how critical their faith was in carrying them through this emotional day, he asked if they had any music they would request to have playing during the birth of their beautiful daughter.

I had the extreme honor that day of supporting J.S. and her family through one of the most emotionally filled days of their lives. I stood at the head of the bed with the two support people, and between verses of their favorite songs, I provided them every update I could on how the surgical procedure was going and when delivery was close. At the moment of delivery, the entire operating room went silent. Of course, it wasn't—the music continued, there were monitors and alarms sounding, suction was quickly collecting fluid

(*continued*)

(*continued*)

next to me, and there was a whole team of staff in the room that had to have been making some sound. Yet it was as if we all were holding our breath just to see whether this little precious baby girl would take one of her own. In reality, it was likely only seconds, but it felt like minutes as we all stood there staring and waiting.

Then we heard a cry.

The silence was broken, and everyone hustled into action as they went into full resuscitation mode. Dad was right there at the resuscitation warmer ready to be with his daughter, and as I looked at J.S., she was beaming with joy. She and her support team were overwhelmed with happiness and almost in unison they proclaimed, "God said yes." I congratulated J.S. and informed her that her daughter had been taken over to the resuscitation suite. As we had discussed previously, my role was going to shift from being with J.S. during the delivery to going and being with her husband during the resuscitation, if the situation got to that point. I would then go back and forth between the resuscitation suite and the operating room to alternate providing support and information to dad and updates on what was going on to mom.

I very happily can say that the resuscitation went unbelievably well, and the little girl beat all odds that day. She fared far better than anyone anticipated. Even more remarkable, she not only fared better that day, but she had a much smoother NICU course than anyone imagined. She was discharged home and is thriving today as a happy, healthy, and energetic young lady.

Family Story

Colin Morrison shares his personal story of what it was like to become a father after an emergency cesarean section was performed unexpectedly at the birth of his first son.

"It's an amazing thing to learn you are going to be a father. The wave of emotions rushes over you quickly. As a school teacher on summer break, most mornings in July involved my wife waking up leisurely and doing a little bit of work in the nursery along with doing her best to take care of herself and the little nugget insider of her. The morning of July 31 was quite a bit different than most mornings in July. Stephanie woke up with some abnormal stomach pain, so we called the doctor, and he recommended we go to the hospital. I selfishly asked her if I could take a quick shower so that I could head straight to work after we went to the hospital. Ha!

"Little did I know I wouldn't be going to work that day.

"We got the results from the first test they performed, and it showed that she had high levels of protein in her urine. If you combine that along with high blood pressure and swelling feet, I learned it meant she had developed preeclampsia. The triage nurse said, 'You probably won't be leaving the hospital without the baby.' What she didn't know is how

(*continued*)

(*continued*)

much of a fighter my wife is, and after bed rest was prescribed, day by day, her symptoms improved. We continued to talk about 'going home' until the morning of August 6. Stephanie knew something just wasn't right, and before we knew it, the doctor who was attending that day got some bad news from the lab work and told us, 'It's baby time.'

'It's baby time' meant an emergency C-section because Stephanie had developed HELLP syndrome. Getting the baby out right then and there was the only thing that would save Stephanie's life. Her liver enzymes were extremely elevated, her blood platelets were really low, and her blood pressure was off the charts. Needless to say, we were scared and there was nothing we could do. We were at the mercy of the people taking care of us. Everything happened so fast. I am not sure if I had time to be scared at the time, but in hindsight, I know I certainly was. I have always appreciated more information versus too-little information, and I would say that I personally could have used a little bit more information in that instance because I didn't really know what was going on and I wasn't really aware how serious it all was. The staff overall was great though and remained very calm, which encouraged me to remain calm as well because freaking out wouldn't have helped the situation at all. I could tell that the OB was starting to get concerned because she ordered the tests STAT and it was taking a longer time than I think she expected. The anesthesiologist came in and introduced himself but didn't really give us that much information. I remember they finally got the tests back that they needed and quickly wheeled Steph into the OR. One of the nurses asked me to wait in the hallway outside so that I could be there to help with Jackson when he came out.

"Because it was an emergency surgery, I could not be in the operating room with Steph and the team. I therefore had to anxiously wait across the hall for them to take the baby out. I remember standing there in the hallway thinking, 'Isn't there a better place that I could wait? Isn't there anyone who can tell me more about what is going on and what is going to happen?' I was definitely freaked out at that time and remember feeling pretty lonely standing out there waiting. I wasn't sure of the proper protocol for that moment because I obviously had never been in a situation like that before. The explanation I was given about what was going on was very short and to the point. It seemed to be an all-hands-on-deck situation, so perhaps there wasn't anyone who could have stayed with me.

"Jackson William Morrison came into this world at 4:25 p.m. on August 6. I remember seeing him for the first time as they whisked him into the room I was in. He looked like a normal little baby, just a bit small considering he was born at 33 weeks. In hindsight, I guess 3 pounds 15 ounces is more than 'a bit small.'

"The next 10 minutes involved the doctors and nurses calmly taking vitals and letting me cut the umbilical cord. I was scared, nervous, and unsure about what was going on. The team was so professional and the neonatologist was so calm, as was the rest of the support staff. Honestly, having a nurse grab my phone and start taking pictures of these moments is something I will never forget and has had a huge impact on me. I never would have thought that we should take pictures of that moment, but I am so thankful we did.

(*continued*)

(*continued*)

The nurse happened to catch me in a video tearing up and getting emotional (something I don't typically do very easily). I find myself going back and revisiting those pictures and that video to reminisce on that time, only to bring back that wave of emotions all over again, which actually is pretty therapeutic. Each of the nurses was fantastic, making light jokes about the situation, which really helped me remain calm also. For example, one of the nurses guessed how long Jackson was and she nailed it. We all laughed at her which was great for the moment. I remember the respiratory therapist being pretty quiet. He was calm but didn't say much, so I wasn't sure of his role. Perhaps that is just his personality, but I do remember that. He would whisper to the neonatologist and then the doctor would relay his message to me. I don't remember there being a resuscitation but perhaps I was just naive that it was going on. I did cut the cord, which I thought was really cool, and even was able to pose for a cheesy picture that commemorated that moment.

"I remember one of the nurses mentioning to us while we were on bed rest that if the baby came soon, we might have to spend a little time in the NICU. That didn't even register to me because, again, we thought we were going to be able to head home after some time. The respiratory therapist who was tending to Jackson in his first few moments of life found that he was having trouble breathing. At that point, the doctor came over to me and said that they were going to have to take Jackson to the NICU to help get him breathing right. He asked me if I had any questions. 'Sure. When will we be able to go home?' His response made my jaw hit the floor. 'Typically, NICU babies go home around their due date.' It was right then when I remembered that his due date was September 23 and I quickly calculated that meant about 7 MORE weeks in the hospital. So much for the birth plan we had developed. So much for our brief 'normal' stay in the hospital followed by the obligatory Welcome Home, Baby Boy sign over our front door. So much for finishing the nursery together. So much for a lot of things we had planned. Hello new reality and hello NICU.

Jackson needed help breathing. They had given Stephanie two rounds of steroid shots to help Jackson's lungs develop in womb, but it wasn't enough when he was born. He was put on a CPAP Machine which is this really scary mask that helps force air into his lungs. I didn't really know what to expect, but I do think that the staff tried to prepare me for it. It was scary to see him like that and knowing how important it is for humans to breathe, I thought a lot about the prognosis which could have gone a million ways at that point. Combine that with an IV for his nutrients and more monitors and wires than I could count, he wasn't exactly the 'cordless baby' we had in mind. Even holding him was a challenge, but we were determined to do so because we wanted him to know we loved him.

The next 5 weeks in the NICU involved us taking each day at a time. Slowly but surely, Jackson fought his way to a point where he was healthy enough to come home. There were many, many milestones that he reached while in the NICU and each one was a little celebration: Milestones such as being moved off the CPAP machine and onto a nasal cannula, going from the incubator into a regular crib, being put on a feeding tube and eventually having that removed, taking his first bath, and learning to breastfeed. All of these things led to him coming home after 34 days in the most amazing place in the world.

(*continued*)

(*continued*)

Fast forward 2 years to pregnancy number two. We were hesitant to try again after the experience we had with Jackson. After numerous tests and visits with doctors, we decided that having a second baby is what was best for our family. At 38 weeks, Stephanie delivered a healthy baby boy via C-section. Carter Lion got to come home after 3 days in the hospital. We were finally one of those parents who got to go straight home. Everything at home was fantastic until we got the call from our pediatrician. 'Get Carter to the NICU as fast and safely as possible; they have a bed waiting for him.' Carter was born with slightly elevated bilirubin levels. Apparently, those levels had spiked and it was discovered when we had taken him to the doctor for his first visit.

That was the most harrowing drive ever across town to the hospital. I was followed up by the most bittersweet reunion you could imagine. Hi, Dr. Hello, Nurse. It's good? Seeing you again. Carter checked into the NICU at 4 days old and was immediately placed under the bilirubin lights. His levels were at a point where if they would have stayed there, he could have developed brain damage. Slowly but surely, the lights worked and his health improved. We avoided a full blood transfusion but did have to get 'topped off' with some healthy blood. After 8 days in the NICU, it was Carter's turn to come home. The doctors never have figured out what happened to Carter, but it just goes to show you there is a lot to learn still about pregnancy and birthing healthy babies."

RECOMMENDATIONS/SUGGESTIONS FOR BEST PRACTICE

1. Assign a family-support specialist to stay with families during high-risk deliveries.

2. Allow patients to define who their family is.

3. Change existing policies that address the number of support people who are welcome to accompany a mother during her delivery. When considering the operating room setting, allow up to a minimum of two support people to accompany a mother during high-risk deliveries.

4. Staff should obtain ongoing education on cultural sensitivities related to birth practices of their community population. Because staff cannot be expected to be experts in all cultures and religious beliefs, it should become normal practice at admission to ask all patients how staff can respect cultural and spiritual beliefs.

5. Staff should encourage and/or take photos for families during high-risk deliveries to help capture special moments that will become special mementos later on.

6. Families should always be welcomed to be present for infant resuscitations.

7. Staff should involve family in moments of resuscitation.

8. Maternal–infant separation should be avoided when possible, even in the event of neonatal emergencies.

9. In future building plans/expansions, create labor and delivery rooms that also serve the purpose of a NICU room so that families can deliver and then stay with their child during neonatal care.

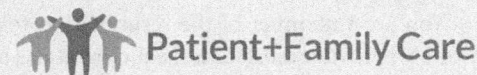

Patient+Family Care

Websites:
1. https://www.aap.org/en-us/continuing-medical-education/life-support/NRP/Pages/NRP.aspx
2. https://www.cdc.gov/reproductivehealth/maternalinfanthealth/pqc-states.html
    a.   https://www.cpqcc.org/sites/default/files/DRToolkitUpdateFinal5-18-11.pdf
3. https://www.acog.org/Clinical-Guidance-and-Publications/Committee-Opinions/Committee-on-Health-Care-for-Underserved-Women/Health-Care-Systems-for-Underserved-Women
4. http://www.nationalperinatal.org/transculturalresources
5. https://www.nih.gov/institutes-nih/nih-office-director/office-communications-public-liaison/clear-communication/cultural-respect
6. http://www.healthpei.ca/nursingeducation/index.php3?number=1044324&lang=E
7. https://www.nurse.com/ce/cultural-competency

Books:
1. *Pocket Guide to Culturally Sensitive Health Care* by Barbara Stuart
2. *Maternal-Newborn Nursing: The Critical Components of Nursing Care* by Roberta Durham and Linda Chapman
3. *The Gift of Birth: Discerning God's Presence During Childbirth* by Susan Windley-Daoust
4. *Nursing Leadership for Patient-Centered Care: Authenticity, Presence, Intuition, Expertise* by Harriet Forman
5. *Healing Presence: The Essence of Nursing,* Second Edition, by JoEllen Goertz Koerner

Figure 3.2 ■ Recommended resources for staff to increase professional knowledge and competence in supporting families in high-risk delivery situations.

RECOMMENDED RESOURCES

Several websites and books may be of particular interest to professionals who are looking to provide additional resources and information on cultural sensitivity in their practice and ways to be more mindful about being present for patients (Figure 3.2).

Case-Based Learning

B. is a 24-year-old, G2, P1, at 38 6/7 weeks' gestation with an uncomplicated prenatal course. She has been laboring naturally (as desired in her birth plan) for 6 hours when she feels a gush of fluid, which is noted to be grossly bloody. Fetal heart tones show a deceleration to 50 beats per minute. An emergency Cesarean delivery is planned under general anesthesia. B.'s husband has just left for their nearby home to retrieve a forgotten item. The anesthesia provider is en route from another part of the hospital.

(continued)

(continued)

You are a member of the resuscitation team, the first to arrive in the operating room, where the resuscitation equipment has been readied. B. is sobbing loudly while she is being prepped for surgery. At delivery, B.'s baby is depressed and requires full resuscitation, including chest compressions and epinephrine administration. Baby's father arrives at 10 minutes of life. He is pale and shaking as he approaches the open warmer.

QUESTIONS

1. What are the contextual elements of B.'s emotional state just prior to surgery?
2. What are your thoughts about how to support her?
3. What interventions might provide support to dad?
4. What are your next steps?

ANSWERS

B. may be feeling alone, frightened, and vulnerable. She could be feeling a total loss of control and powerlessness over the events transpiring around her. After months of planning, her dream of the perfect delivery and baby is being upended, and she may already be grieving the loss.

Support for B. includes allowing her to feel and express her emotions. Use plain language to explain what is happening and why. In cases in which mom is awake, adjusting the resuscitation equipment so that she can see what's happening can be reassuring. When possible, provide for initial care at the bedside to enable the parents to be involved in the first moments of their baby's life and to touch their baby during stabilization (Sawyer et al., 2015).

When dad arrives, support him by being by his side, carefully explaining what is happening, and answering questions about mom and baby. This is an event that healthcare staff have experience with and practice for; we know the lingo and the algorithm. Not so for dad—it is unexpected and terrifying; he is watching two of the people he loves most in the world undergo emergency procedures. That is not to say that he should not be with his family during this emergency—quite the contrary. Family-witnessed resuscitation is beneficial and may reduce feelings of distress for parents. Jabre et al. (2013) reported that symptoms of distress were present for up to a year after the event and were higher in family members who did not witness the resuscitation compared with those who did. Having a staff member providing plain-language explanations of what is happening and reassuring parents that there is nothing they could have done to prevent this can help with this traumatic experience (Sawyer et al., 2015).

Calling the nursing supervisor, the chaplain, or a nearby family member to be with dad are options to consider if the perinatal and neonatal teams are occupied.

Parents experience positive and negative impacts from their experiences in the NICU (Janvier et al., 2016). Being thrown into an unexpectedly high-stakes experience

(continued)

(*continued*)

in an intimidating environment leads to feeling powerless and uninformed. Bonding is disrupted; parents may be afraid to handle their small or ill newborn. In addition to strong staff support, many parents benefit from exposure to other families who have been through similar experiences and have felt the roller coaster of emotions that can be part of a NICU stay (Hall, Ryan, Beatty & Grubbs, 2015).

Unexpected poor perinatal or neonatal outcomes and/or loss can have a lasting effect on nurses, who can be so affected that they are "second victims." This can lead to posttraumatic stress, depression, burnout, symptoms of pain and loss, and lifelong memories of the event. Self-care for staff who are involved in cases with unexpected outcomes includes resiliency training and attention to work-life balance (Hall, Cross, et al., 2015; Puia, Lewis, & Beck, 2013).

REFERENCES

Hall, S. L., Cross, J., Selix, N. W., Patterson, C., Segre, L., Chuffo-Siewert, R., ... Martin, M. L. (2015). Recommendations for enhancing psychosocial support of NICU parents through staff education and support. *Journal of Perinatology*, 35, S29–S36. doi:10.1038/jp.2015.147

Hall, S. L., Ryan, D. J., Beatty, J., & Grubbs, L. (2015). Recommendations for peer-to-peer support for NICU parents. *Journal of Perinatology*, 35(Suppl. 1), S9–S13. doi:10.1038/jp.2015.143

Jabre, P., Belpomme, V., Azoulay, E., Jacob, L., Bertrand, L., Lapostolle, F., ... Adnet, F. (2013). Family presence during cardiopulmonary resuscitation. *New England Journal of Medicine*, 368(11), 1008–1018. doi:10.1056/NEJMoa1203366

Janvier, A., Lantos, J., Aschner, J., Barrington, K., Batton, B., Batton, D., ... Spitzer, A. R. (2016). Stronger and more vulnerable: A balanced view of the impacts of the NICU experience on parents. *Pediatrics*, 138(3), e20160655. doi:10.1542/peds.2016-0655

Puia, D. M., Lewis, L., & Beck, C. T. (2013). Experiences of obstetric nurses who are present for a perinatal loss. *Journal of Obstetric, Gynecologic, & Neonatal Nursing*, 42(3), 321–331. doi:10.1111/1552-6909.12040

Sawyer, A., Ayers, S., Bertullies, S., Thomas, M., Weeks, A. D., Yoxall, C. W., & Duley, L. (2015). Providing immediate neonatal care and resuscitation at birth beside the mother: Parents' views, a qualitative study. *BMJ Open*, 5(9), e008495. doi:10.1136/bmjopen-2015-008495

REFERENCES

American Heart Association. (n.d.). Family presence during resuscitation. Retrieved from https://eccguidelines.heart.org/index.php/circulation/cpr-ecc-guidelines-2/part-12-pediatric-advanced-life-support/intra-arrest-care-updates/family-presence-during-resuscitation

Association of Women's Health, Obstetric and Neonatal Nurses. (2016). Immediate and sustained skin-to-skin contact for the healthy term newborn after birth: AWHONN practice brief number 5. *Nursing for Women's Health*, 20(6), 614–616. doi:10.1016/s1751-4851(16)30331-2

Barrett, S. J., & Stark, M. A. (2010). Factors associated with labor support behaviors of nurses. *Journal of Perinatal Education*, 19(1), 12–18. doi:10.1624/105812410x481528

Cook, K., & Loomis, C. (2012). The impact of choice and control on women's childbirth experiences. *Journal of Perinatal Education*, 21(3), 158–168. doi:10.1891/1058-1243.21.3.158

Crenshaw, J. T. (2014). Healthy birth practice #6: Keep mother and baby together—It's best for mother, baby, and breastfeeding. *Journal of Perinatal Education, 23*(4), 211–217. doi:10.1891/1058-1243.23.4.211

Curley, M. A., Meyer, E. C., Scoppettuolo, L. A., McGann, E. A., Trainor, B. P., Rachwal, C. M., & Hickey, P. A. (2012). Parent presence during invasive procedures and resuscitation. *American Journal of Respiratory and Critical Care Medicine, 186*(11), 1133–1139. doi:10.1164/rccm.201205-0915OC

Greene, M. J. (2007). Strategies for incorporating cultural competence into childbirth education curriculum. *Journal of Perinatal Education, 16*(2), 33–37. doi:10.1624/105812407X191489

Iravani, M., Zarean, E., Janghorbani, M., & Bahrami, M. (2015). Women's needs and expectations during normal labor and delivery. *Journal of Education and Health Promotion, 4,* 6. doi:10.4103/2277-9531.151885

Nilsson, L., Thorsell, T., Wahn, E. H., & Ekström, A. (2013). Factors influencing positive birth experiences of first-time mothers. *Nursing Research and Practice, 2013*, 1–6. doi:10.1155/2013/349124

Sawyer, A., Ayers, S., Bertullies, S., Thomas, M., Weeks, A. D., Yoxall, C. W., & Duley, L. (2015). Providing immediate neonatal care and resuscitation at birth beside the mother: Parents' views, a qualitative study. *BMJ Open, 5*(9), e008495. doi:10.1136/bmjopen-2015-008495

Tornøe, K. A., Danbolt, L. J., Kvigne, K., & Sørlie, V. (2014). The power of consoling presence—hospice nurses' lived experience with spiritual and existential care for the dying. *BMC Nursing, 13*(1), 25. doi:10.1186/1472-6955-13-25

Vali, P., Mathew, B., & Lakshminrusimha, S. (2015, January 22). Neonatal resuscitation: evolving strategies. *Maternal Health, Neonatology and Perinatology, 1*(1), 4. Retrieved from https://mhnpjournal.biomedcentral.com/articles/10.1186/s40748-014-0003-0

SUPPORTING FAMILIES WHEN BOTH MOM AND BABY BECOME ILL

CARING FOR MOM AND BABY AS A DYAD DURING EMERGENCIES

When possible, keeping an infant and a mother together after birth is ideal. As stated in the previous chapter, "mothers and babies have a physiologic need to be together during the moments, hours and days following birth, and this time together significantly improves maternal and newborn outcomes" (Crenshaw, 2014, "Abstract" section). Although this practice is easily encouraged and adapted in healthy and normal deliveries, when mom and/or baby become ill the general practice is to separate the dyad to safely care for the critically ill patients in specialized units. These specialized units have trained staff that know how to properly care for the complex medical conditions of an ill postpartum mother or fragile newborn, the proper equipment that is necessary to treat the age-adjusted illnesses, and the correct supplies that assist the trained staff to provide the best care possible to the respective patients. Although these specialized units offer incredible, much needed, and often life-saving care for patients, they also separate the infant and mother during the most critical hours after delivery.

The golden hour, which is the first hour immediately following birth, gained awareness in the perinatal space after the World Health Organization and the United Nations Children's Fund created a joint statement in 1989 to support the initiation and continuation of breastfeeding. The Ten Steps to Successful Breastfeeding (n.d.) were developed as an initiative at this time as well, and one of the 10 steps includes "plac[ing] babies in uninterrupted skin-to-skin contact with their mothers immediately following birth for at least an hour" (Pound & Unger, 2012, Table 2) to optimize the successful initiation and duration of successful breastfeeding. However, the benefits of skin-to-skin contact and uninterrupted mother–infant time in the immediate postdelivery period goes far beyond the optimization of nutritional support in the newborn. "Being skin to skin with mother protects the newborn from the well-documented negative effects of separation, supports optimal brain development and facilitates attachment, which promotes the infant's self-regulation over time" (Phillips, 2013, "Abstract" section). In addition, "skin-to-skin contact improves physiologic stability for both mother and baby in the vulnerable period immediately after birth, increases maternal attachment behaviors, protects against the negative effects of maternal–infant separation [and] supports optimal infant brain development" (Phillips, 2013). When clinicians are faced with a high-risk situation in which both the mother and the infant are physiologically unstable, would this knowledge not help make the case that keeping mothers and infants together should be a priority?

In October of 2017, British Colombia's CBC News reported that Teck Acute Care Center would house North America's first NICU where mother and child would receive medical care in the same room, from the same nurse. This type of care delivery unit design will eliminate families being separated when babies are ill because neonatal care occurs in the same room as a mother's postpartum care. Although this is going to be a game changer for neonatal, maternal, and family-centered care, I would argue we could still do much better. I am not minimizing the incredible impact this will have and how wonderful it is that units are taking such drastic steps to implement change to support the psychosocial support of families, but I do believe we should consider combining adult ICUs with NICUs to fully support the most vulnerable of patients and families. Consider this concept for just a moment: a critically ill mother and a critically ill infant next to one another in the same ICU, receiving care from the same staff. What would that do for families?

When we stop to consider the impact that a critically ill mother and infant have on a family, there is an insurmountable new host of issues that families face. Not only do families inherit the worries and stressors that all NICU families face, but they also now face an entirely new set of issues that come with the worries of a mother being in an ICU concurrently. Families have to learn all of the equipment and rules of the NICU while also learning the culture and environment of an adult ICU. Families are meeting the team members caring for their new sweet baby while engaging in intense conversations with various specialists with expertise in caring for adults. The NICU and ICU are often geographically separated within the hospital, so families frequently have to travel back and forth between the two and have to share their time between the two units. This time sharing is grueling because families feel torn spending time with either patient. When they are with baby, they feel guilty they aren't with mom; when they are with mom, they feel guilty they aren't with baby. Support individuals and families who find themselves experiencing double the stress, double the anxiety, and double the trauma.

First and foremost, it is incredibly important for staff in both units to recognize the unique stressors of dual-ICU families and find the best possible ways to address them. Psychosocial support must be a top priority when caring for families who are separated between two units and two critical situations. The families in a dual-ICU situation is at higher risk for posttraumatic stress disorder, and it is critical to know that "following a stay in intensive care, 1 in 10 patients develop symptoms of PTSD. It is one of the most common and most distressing, yet least talked about, problems associated with intensive care medicine" (Wake & Kitchiner, 2013, "Not Only War Veterans" section). Full psychosocial support of these families should be considered, and interventions should be offered, depending on the individual needs of each family. Assessment of these needs should be conducted frequently, and every effort should be made to meet those needs while the families are still within the hospital system so that accessibility with limited barriers can be achieved. Examples may include providing families' access to clergy or spiritual care support, social workers, psychology, care mangers, referrals to outpatient behavioral health, referrals to psychiatry, and even access to local amenities to meet basic needs such as food and personal hygiene while at the hospital. According to Shorofi, Jannati, Moghaddam, and Yazdani-Charati (2016, "Discussion" section), "meeting the needs of patient's families can also develop their trust in the health care team, increase their satisfaction with hospital care and help them cope with the stressful situation. Not only patients but also family members should be the center of attention in the current critical care environment."

However, to fully support the psychosocial and emotional health of families, it is not enough to just address the stressors within the psychosocial realm, but units need to work together closely and collaboratively to change policy, procedure, and common practice to also support the practical domain. Changes in the physical and practical domain at the same time affords changes that promote families to be connected and find ways to bond, which will then lead to supportive measures that provide families the emotional support that they need to endure their journey. In a dream world, the ICU and NICU would become the same unit, but it is unlikely that we will see this level of intentional change in the near future. However, many practices can be implemented to bring about important and invaluable change for families in other ways through collaborative relationships between the two units.

Communication between the two units is a pivotal and vital component to improving care for the dual-ICU family. Patient report should be given to the oncoming nurse of the alternate unit so that each department is prepared to support the family. When a family shows up to visit their baby in the neonatal unit, they should not be burdened with the responsibility of having to inform the medical team of the latest update of the mother and what important milestones are occurring that day. Consider the increased stress it would place on a family if they were in the adult ICU and the staff were not aware that their infant was being taken to surgery that afternoon at a specific time and the adult team had planned to have the mothers' intubation trial occur at the same hour. Just as baby care in the NICU should be coordinated with a family's schedule, maternal and neonatal care should be scheduled between the two units to accommodate the family's schedule as best as possible. Communication could be even more improved if bedside report for both patients could be given at one bedside and with the family present. For example, the family could be at the mother's bedside for shift change, and the NICU nurse could be present for that report to not only hear the mother's report for themselves, but also to provide the report and update about the baby's latest condition. Overall, the main priority and goal should be to increase communication and scheduling collaboration between the two units with the family at the center.

Breastfeeding and nutritional decisions are very emotionally charged topics for new families, and when mother and infant are separated, providers in the ICU and NICU units can do a great deal to support the feeding desires of families. To begin, if families wish to exclusively provide breast milk to their infant, the neonatal unit should have donor milk available as an alternative, at least until feeding is established. Gavage feedings, finger feedings, or other alternative methods of feedings to avoid introducing bottles should be supported until the teams have time to assess the medical condition of the mother and determine when she may recover and be able to put the baby to breast. Offering donor milk and alternate methods of feeding provides the psychosocial and emotional support the family may need while adjusting to the possible need for a new feeding plan. Simultaneously, lactation support should be provided to the mother, no matter how ill she is, in the ICU. Staff or family members can assist the mother in initiating breast pumping on a schedule, and her milk can be delivered to the NICU for the baby if the medications she is receiving are not contraindicated in breastfeeding. If the medications that mom is receiving are contraindicated for breastfeeding, the milk can be pumped and dumped until her milk is safe to use; this establishes her milk supply if there is an anticipated recovery.

Finding ways to enhance bonding and connections among mom, family, and baby during geographical separation is also a fundamental priority any NICU should have as strategic family-centered care goals. The separation when mom is ill and in the hospital should amplify the significance of this priority. Neonatal staff can do many things to help improve the connection between baby and family during separation, including, but not limited to, the following:

- Provide ways that the families can Skype, Facetime, or videoconference from the ICU. This will allow mom to see her baby, and when families are with mom in the ICU, they can see the baby together.

- Trade scented blankets between mom and baby daily. Family or nursing staff can take a blanket that mom has been holding or was laying against her and a blanket that baby has been swaddled in to the other unit so that baby and mom can be comforted by each other's scent during their separation.

- Print photographs and post them next to mom's and baby's bedsides. Take lots of them! This not only personalizes the space, which will bring a sense of comfort, but it will allow the family to see mom and baby when they are with the other and bring a sense of family despite the separation. For a mother, having updated photographs of her baby provides an additional layer of support and often can aid as a motivator to participate in difficult recovery therapy.

- Provide families with a journal and encourage them to write in it each day, recording milestones, stories, updates, and so forth. Just putting their thoughts and feelings into words can be very healing. In fact, "expressive writing results in significant improvements in [long]-term physical health outcomes such as illness-related visits to the doctor, blood pressure, lung function, liver function and number of days in the hospital. Expressive writing has also produced significant benefits in a number of measures of immune system functioning" (Baikie & Wilhelm, 2005, "Objectively Assessed Outcomes" section). Some studies have also reported improvements "for emotional health outcomes including mood/affect, psychological well-being, depressive symptoms before examinations and post-traumatic intrusion and avoidance symptoms" (Baikie & Wilhelm, 2005, "Objectively Assessed Outcomes" section).

During this incredibly stressful time for families, supporting the physical and emotional health of family members is incredibly important, and staff in both the adult and the neonatal units should recognize that "members of critically ill patients often experience increased incidence of physical and mental health issues" (Day, Haj-Bakri, Lubchansky, & Mehta, 2013, p. R91). "The unfortunate reality is that family members of critically ill patients often experience increased incidence of physical and mental health issues, and are unlikely to prioritize their own needs" (Day et al., 2013, p. R91). With two family members already ill and at risk for long-term complications, family members should be encouraged to be proactive and mitigate risk for their own long-term health complications that can be caused from stress and anxiety. According to Bressert (2016, para. 2), "recently, much has been reported about stress and its relationship to other health problems, such as heart disease, blood pressure and depression. Stress also has been linked to suppression of the immune system, increasing your chances of becoming ill or altering the course of an illness if you already have one." The last thing a dual-ICU family needs is to find themselves dealing with their own health concerns due to stress, anxiety, and tension, which could be lessened if their psychosocial needs were supported by staff.

An easy way to support families during this time is to educate them on the importance of self care practices and to provide them with a tool that will provide a care strategy that includes five aspects of care that are necessary to heal (Mosher, 2017). Although numerous tools are available, one that is easy to use, is easy to replicate, and was developed for use in mothers needing to heal from postpartum mood and anxiety disorders is the N.U.R.S.E. Self Care Program. N.U.R.S.E. is an acronym for nourishment, understanding, rest/relaxation, spirituality, and exercise. "These five properties help individuals focus on behavior changes that will improve both their physical and emotional health and provide a foundation on which to build a fully customized tailored plan to help parents manage both their physical and emotional health" (Mosher, 2017, "Education During Hospitalization" section). It is best to encourage families to set personal goals, on a weekly basis, at minimum, so that their personal health remains a focus, enabling them to continue to cope with the stressors of dealing with two critically ill family members (Figure 4.1).

As one can see, many things need to be considered to support the emotional and psychosocial health of families who find themselves with both an ill mother and an ill infant after delivery, but if the work is done, the rewards it can provide to families make every ounce of effort on the part of staff worth it. Going back to the previous concept I asked you to consider, in which an ICU would care for both a mother and an infant next to one another, can you now imagine what that level of care would do for a family? In all honesty, most people would hear the idea of an ICU where mothers and infants were cared for together and would immediately say that the amount of work that it would take to make that happen would be too great and the hurdles too insurmountable to even begin to tackle. Yet when you look at all of the work and collaboration that it takes to successfully and supportively care for families split between two units, it actually might be much easier to care for families if both patients were cared for together in a single space.

Name:_ Date: _ _ _/ _ _ _/ _ _ _

Directions: In each category, write one to three realistic goals that you want to focus on in the coming week(s) to help improve your physical and mental well-being and health

N Nourishment	1. 2. 3. _____
U Understanding	1. 2. 3. _____
R Rest/Relaxation	1. 2. 3. _____
S Spirituality	1. 2. 3. _____
E Exercise	1. 2. 3. _____

Patient+Family Care

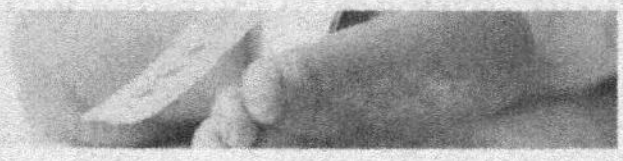

Figure 4.1 ■ N.U.R.S.E. Self Care Program.

N Nourishment	Getting proper nutrition is very important to help keep your body healthy. Be sure to eat at least three balanced meals each day, drink at least 8 ounces of water, take vitamins and medicine as directed by your doctor, avoid drugs and alcohol, avoid excessive caffeine, and find help with needs you may have (including, for example, cleaning, cooking, childcare).
U Understanding	Having the information and education you need to understand your child's and your own health and well-being is very important. Find a safe, accepting, and trusting place to ask questions, find books or other literature on specific topics, and journal your feelings.
R Rest/Relaxation	Your body needs rest and relaxation to heal, grow, and be healthy. Try to get at least 5 hours of uninterrupted sleep each day, customized to meeting the feeding care plan/needs of your child; practice healthy sleep hygiene practices; practice meditation and mindfulness; and find ways every day to do something that you find relaxing.
S Spirituality	Spirituality is not necessarily limited to organized religion needs, but it is a priority for you to find things that make you feel uplifted and joyful. This can be through connected relationships, solitude, appreciation of nature, participation in creative projects, or journaling.
E Exercise	Endorphins that are released with exercise are mood enhancers. You should try to get 20–60 minutes of physical activity per day, with the intensity based on your ability and doctors' recommendations. Try walking, jogging, yoga, water aerobics, or any other exercise routine that you enjoy doing.

Patient+Family Care

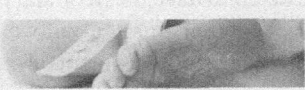
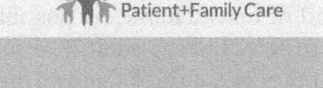

Figure 4.1 ■ N.U.R.S.E. Self Care Program. (*continued*)

CARING FOR FAMILIES WHEN MOM DOES NOT SURVIVE

In a best-case scenario, both mom and baby would receive the care they need to recover, would be reunited, and would be discharged in a timely matter and without long-term complications from their medical difficulties. Unfortunately, that is not always the case. Later in this book, we look at how staff can support families in the event of neonatal loss, but right now we are going to focus on the extremely important ways that staff can be prepared to help support families who have to endure the loss of a mother after the birth of a child.

"The most recent surveillance report shows that the 1998–2005 U.S. pregnancy-related mortality ratio was 14.5 deaths per 100,000 live births" (Creanga et al., 2015, p. 5), a number that is increasing in the country, so dealing with maternal death is an unfortunate reality many perinatal and neonatal nurses must face alongside families. What should have been some of the happiest days of the lives of these families suddenly turns into one of tragedy and immense sadness. Nurses and care providers find themselves having to step in and become bereavement specialists who need to realize "providing compassionate [end of life] care that is appropriate and in accordance with the patient's wishes is an essential component of nursing care" (Hebert, Moore, & Rooney, 2011, final para.). Care providers, while dealing with their own emotions regarding the loss, must prioritize focus on how to honor the life and death of a mother in the context of this newly formed and newly shattered family while taking into consideration how to honor the family's cultural, religious, and personal rituals.

Multidisciplinary teams should collaborate to provide the most comprehensive support possible to families who experience maternal loss. Social services, spiritual care, psychology, and other supportive disciplines should all be called together to attend a case conference with the family as soon as possible after the death. This allows important information about arrangements to be shared and initial steps to be made to start postmortem care. Each hospital needs to refer to its own internal policies and procedures related to postmortem care, but what should occur with the death of a mother is for every effort to be made to bring the family together before the body is ushered to the morgue and/or funeral home. All possible measures should be taken to have the neonatal patient transferred to the adult ICU so that the family can be together to say goodbye to the mother as a unified family. During this sacred time, families should be encouraged to participate in the following:

- Placing baby skin-to-skin with mother (with warming blankets to maintain proper thermoregulation for the infant).

- Obtaining bereavement photography with infant and mother and with the family together.

- Inviting spiritual leaders to be present with them during this time to lead the family in prayer/time for reflection.

- Inviting family and friends to come and be with the family to pay their respects and say goodbye, making adjustments to the standard number of visitors that are usually allowed into the ICU at a given time.

Staff can, and should, also participate in some of this time with the family to help capture memories that might not otherwise be captured for the family. This may include things such as the following:

- Getting locks of mom's hair for family members
- Getting handprints/fingerprints of mom
- Making plaster molds of mom's hands
- Providing the family with resources to support services

During the entire end-of-life and postmortem care process, collaboration between the adult ICU and NICU must be coordinated in such a way that families feel supported and cared for. After the death of a mother and even in the time leading up to the death, "provider communications and relationships are central to the processes of meeting the clinical needs of family members" (Steinhauser, Voils, Bosworth, & Tulsky, 2014, "Significance of Results" section). Family members surveyed about their experience of losing a loved one in the ICU have shared the importance of being included in communications, and they feel their experience is most affected by how the staff attends to their needs. Once again, all of these needs could be met much easier and provided in a timelier fashion if mom and baby were being cared for in a single-unit design.

Author's Personal Story

I came to work in the NICU one day and received report on the four patients I would be caring for that shift. I learned that one of the patients I would be responsible for was this adorable little boy that had been born at 30 weeks and 3 days and that his mother had become very ill due to preeclampsia and HELLP syndrome. Little H.M. had been delivered via emergency cesarean section, had Apgar scores of 3, 6, and 8 and was relatively stable on continuous positive airway pressure (CPAP). The full report was broken down more like this:

Gest Age/ Days Old	30 3/7 1
Neurological	Appropriate for gestational age
Respiratory	CPAP 5, 80% FiO$_2$, target sat range 90%–95%, breath sounds clear, mild substernal retractions, chest x-ray done
Cardiac	HR: 148–150, grade II systolic murmur
GI/GU	WDL Donor milk; cue-based feedings

(continued)

(*continued*)

Skin	WDL
IV	UVC/UAC
Labs/ Meds	CBC and culture pending, CBG q8hr NS, vitamin K and erythromycin given
Social History	Infertility history with family. Mom was G4, dP1, IVF with this pregnancy, hx of a 3 previous pregnancy losses one at 8 wk/14 wk/12 wk, respectively. Family lives 3 hours away and mom/dad were here on an anniversary weekend when she got sick and came in. She was on bed rest for several days while they were trying to manage her condition, but she continued to decline and became more acutely ill. Emergent C-section performed, and mom is in ICU intubated. Dad—J.M. Mom—A.M.

I immediately asked the nurse going off shift how J.M. (dad) was doing, and she said he appeared very withdrawn and quiet. He comes to the unit for short periods, doesn't say much, and declines any questions. J.M.'s mother and father would be arriving that afternoon, and she thought having his family around for support would really help. I also asked how A.M. (mom) was doing, and unfortunately, she had not received an update during the night. From what she had heard just after delivery, A.M. was really sick, intubated, and on lots of pressers, and her laboratory results showed gravely low platelets. As soon as I received full report on all four patients, I contacted the charge nurse of that shift and asked if she could reassess the assignment workload. I felt that all four patients were adequately paired together on the basis of care needs, but that I felt my workload would be difficult to manage if I were going to be able to adequately support the family who was experiencing a dual-ICU experience that day. Thankfully, there was flexibility with our staffing, and she was able to adjust the assignment. My workload was reduced to only two of the original four patients.

After providing handoff to a coworker, I immediately started on my routine first round of care. The second patient I had that day was a patient I knew well because I had been assigned as her primary nurse for many weeks prior. I was cued into her needs and her family's needs, and because of our established relationship, caring for their family was something I felt extremely comfortable with, so I was confident that I would be able to advance in many aspects of both the physical and psychosocial aspects of their care over the next 12 hours. With little H.M., I knew the shift would not be as easy. I had not met the family, we did not have an established relationship, and I could only imagine that they were facing indescribable levels of stress and fear. My heart ached for what they must all be going through. I was anxious to meet them and assess their current state so that I could determine what goals we could set together for the day.

(continued)

I performed my assessment and first round of care on my first patient, and her family was in the room for the morning. This family was very actively engaged and was very capable of managing the care independently. I performed their daughter's assessment and shared with them my findings, and we talked through the day's care goals together. Just as I was finishing up documenting her cares, H.M.'s dad came into the unit and approached his son's bedside. He appeared very tired with dark circles under his eyes and had a blank stare as he looked at his son. I calmly approached him and offered a tall chair so that he could sit next to his son and possibly be more comfortable. I pulled up a second chair and asked if it were okay if I sat and talked with him for a few minutes. He didn't respond, so I gently placed a hand on his shoulder, and it was at that moment that he even seemed to realize I was in the room with him. He apologized and said he didn't realize I was there. I could tell that this father was extremely stressed and overwhelmed and likely had not had any sleep, or if he had, it was not of the desired quality. I asked him how he was doing and what I could do for him. He wanted to know how his son was doing, and thankfully, I was able to give him a very positive report.

I sat with J.M. and, in the simplest terms I could use, gave a full systems report on his son. I explained all of the equipment and tubes that he was hooked up to and told him all of the great progress he had made since birth. I assured J.M. that I was sharing a lot of information and that it is really common for parents to not remember much of anything nurses share so that I would expect we would be talking about the same information again later. I encouraged him to ask questions along the way and as often as he wanted. I took the opportunity to ask J.M. about A.M. He became teary and said that he really didn't know. He said that the nurses and doctors constantly came into her room and did things to her and to machines but didn't tell him what they were doing or why. He said that often people didn't even introduce themselves when they came in, so he wasn't even sure who they all were. He felt invisible and as if his wife was just a case in a bed and not the amazing woman and now mother she was. He told me he was so scared and didn't know what to do or what he should be doing. I sat with J.M., let him talk through his feelings and fears, and did all I could to assure him that everything he was experiencing was normal and he was doing a fabulous job.

I offered and asked if he would like me to accompany him to the ICU to find out an update on A.M.'s condition so that, together, we could make a plan for the day on how he could manage time between mom and baby, how we could make a plan with his family arriving, and how we could plan time in the day for him and maybe even mom to hold H.M. skin-to-skin. He looked at me as if I was the craziest person on earth because how could a sick mother who was in an ICU hold her baby? I gently placed my hand on his shoulder again and told him I absolutely could not promise anything but that, if it were possible, I would love to help get mom and baby together. He wasn't aware of this, but in the past, I had been able to coordinate bringing NICU babies down to the adult ICU when moms were really sick. It took quite a bit of coordination and a *lot* of discussion with the neonatologist and hospitalist on service,

(continued)

(*continued*)

but I eventually was able to make it happen. With supportive physicians, nurses, and respiratory therapists, our teams were successfully collaborative and prioritized the family's needs in those critical situations and went outside our normal hospital policies to bring families together when they needed to be the most. With safety being a top priority, we took every precaution and had all hands on deck to ensure that the transport was well equipped and staffed, and we had great success! J.M. also didn't realize that the neonatologist and the hospitalist working this particular day were both incredible advocates of family support, and I was confident they would be supportive of this request if mom was stable enough.

After requesting that a coworker monitor my assigned patients for a little while, J.M. and I went down to the ICU together. We were able to find A.M.'s nurse, who shared that A.M. was suffering an ongoing severe headache and uncontrolled vomiting and had lost vision in her left eye that they hoped was not going to be permanent; they were still struggling to control her blood pressure. The goal for the day shift was to continue working on lowering her blood pressure, find a way to manage her nausea, keep her hydrated, and start total parenteral nutrition so that they could maintain nutritional support. I asked Tonya, the nurse, if she was aware that mom had wanted to exclusively breastfeed her baby, and Tonya said she had heard that but wasn't sure what they would be able to do about that since mom wasn't in labor and delivery. I politely informed her that we would be happy to coordinate that with her team and that I could have lactation come down. Tonya was open to that and said she would be willing to call down if I gave her the phone number. I gladly shared the number and while she was in the room, she called lactation and requested they come down when they could to help her with A.M.'s lactation needs, since she was unfamiliar with that type of care.

I continued to talk to Tonya and shared with her report on H.M. and asked if she felt comfortable with me talking to the hospitalist about maybe coming down with H.M. later in the afternoon, based on mom's condition. She told me that she had heard about babies coming down to the ICU before but had never seen it for herself yet, but if the doctor felt comfortable with it she would be happy to support that as well. I shared with her my past experiences and how I like to coordinate the visit with myself, her, and the respiratory therapy and that it would be great to even put baby skin-to-skin with mom. This is when Tonya looked at me like I was crazy. I saw her glance over at J.M. to see if he heard me and I could have sworn they shared a moment together where they both thought they were witnessing a crazy nurse in their presence. Tonya reluctantly said okay and walked out of the room for what I suspect was to get out before she got much more involved in what she thought was an impossibility for the day.

I left J.M. in the unit with mom and told him he could come back or call the unit anytime, but that if I hadn't seen or heard from him in 3 hours, I would come back to the ICU and check in. I performed the next set of rounds and just before I was getting ready to go to the ICU, J.M. arrived back in the unit. He came with his parents, who had just arrived at the hospital and were anxious to meet their new grandchild. I spent

(*continued*)

(*continued*)

a little time with them, sharing information about H.M.'s condition and the equipment, tubes, wires, and gestational age norms, and I asked which one of them was going to hold H.M.? Again, J.M. looked at me like I was crazy and asked if it was safe to do that. I spent time talking to him about how resilient babies are; I told him that even though H.M. is little and was born early, it is very safe to hold him and that it's really important to hold him. We talked about skin-to-skin care and its many benefits for both baby and parents (especially for mom); if he wanted to try, we could spend an hour or so participating in that if H.M. tolerated it. I shared with J.M. and his parents that H.M. had already been weaned down on his oxygen to room air and that we were going to trial him off of CPAP, so putting him skin-to-skin would be really helpful. Reluctantly, J.M. agreed and after we got him comfortable in a recliner and H.M. comfortably on his chest, I excused myself to allow private family time. I went and retrieved our unit's camera and returned a while later and offered to take a family photograph for them. I printed a few copies, immediately providing them with a keepsake; I also printed a copy to place next to H.M.'s crib, which brought a smile to J.M.'s face. H.M. did so well that he spent 1½ hours on his father's chest before returning to his Isolette. When he returned, respiratory therapy placed him on nasal cannula to see if he was ready to be off CPAP.

I walked back to the ICU with J.M. and his parents to talk with Tonya and see how A.M. was doing. She was still sick and had not made much progress during the day, but her vomiting was slowing down, which was a great improvement. I spoke with the hospitalist, and he felt that with the amount of time she was throwing up, it likely would be best to wait until tomorrow to attempt skin-to-skin contact. The neonatologist and I both agreed, but I still felt it was important to bring this family together. During the next round of care, we decided to coordinate a visit. I talked with the charge nurse of the ICU and asked if we could allow additional visitors temporarily that afternoon when I brought the baby down so that the family could be together. Once she agreed with that arrangement, I returned to the NICU and began coordination with respiratory therapy and the NICU charge nurse. Because both the respiratory therapist and I would be out of the unit, we found proper coverage for our responsibilities and began preparing the transport equipment. We set a transport Isolette to begin warming, found a portable oxygen tank, obtained a portable cardiorespiratory monitor, and prepared the chart documents that would need to go with us. I made sure I had the unit camera because I wanted to ensure we captured the first family photos.

Just as it was time to begin the next set of care, the neonatologist performed an assessment to ensure that H.M. was stable and ready for the trip to the ICU. We set off to the other side of the hospital and made it to the adult ICU without incident. When we arrived, Tonya had made room next to mom's bed for the Isolette and the respiratory therapists and I plugged all the equipment in and made sure everything was set up properly to care for H.M. in case he needed anything while we were there. A.M. seemed to light up immediately and as I looked over at her, I noticed a breast pump on her side table.

(*continued*)

(*continued*)

I asked Tonya how the lactation visit went, and she smiled and was excited to report that not only had lactation come down and initiated pumping with mom, but that 3 hours later, Tonya herself assisted mom in pumping; they had syringes of colostrum saved in the fridge. Tonya also told me that the pumping schedule was now included in the care plan and that it was also written on mom's white board so that everyone would know when she was due for her next pumping.

Mom was not going to be able to participate in skin-to-skin just yet, but we determined that if baby were swaddled and someone was close by, she could hold him, and if she felt like she were going to get sick, the baby could quickly be held by someone else. I waited to perform H.M.'s assessment and care until we were all in the ICU so that A.M. could watch and listen to the assessment while J.M. performed the care. A.M. loved watching him change his first diaper. I was able to take a photo of that for them and H.M. peed all over J.M. just before he could get the new diaper closed in time. I snapped a photo just in time to get that in action and J.M.'s face was priceless. After I helped get everyone cleaned up and H.M. swaddled up nicely, I had J.M. hand him to mom and I assisted them in positioning the baby near mom's chest so that she could see him and so that dad could have his hands supporting them both safely. It was a beautiful moment. Even though A.M. was incredibly ill, in that moment she looked happy and as if she could forget that she was in a health crisis of her own. J.M. was able to have both his wife and child together in his arms. The photo was priceless, and it was one that we printed and put next to both A.M. and H.M.'s beds that evening.

After an hour, it was time to return to the NICU, and as difficult as it was to separate the family, they were incredibly grateful for the time they had together. I explained to them that these visits were not something that could be done every day or every shift, but that we would arrange it every time we could. I assured A.M. that when she was more stable, we would arrange for skin-to-skin care. J.M. caught me just before I was leaving that shift and thanked me. He said that he has never been more scared in all his life and that he really didn't know if his wife or baby were going to live; he didn't think he would ever see them together. Just having that time together that day meant more to him than I would ever know and that having a team take the time to invest in his family like that, as a *family*, was exactly what he needed to get through the rest of this journey.

A.M. continued to recover slowly, and after 6 days, she was discharged from the ICU with returned eyesight and the ability to go home. H.M. was taken to the ICU two other times during those days, and in one of those visits, he was placed skin-to-skin for 6 hours. The hospitalist shared with me later that he felt as if it was only after the 6-hour direct maternal–infant contact that A.M. finally turned the corner. As J.M. told me later, he felt as if the first family visit gave him the confidence to face the journey ahead because he had his family together to fight for. He didn't feel lost and torn apart like he did initially. After hearing those two testimonies, I have made it a priority to unite families as soon as possible, no matter how sick mom or baby are after delivery.

Family Story

Dustin Fargher, a NICU graduate father of a previous 26-weeker, shares his story about being with his wife Amber when she was 26 weeks pregnant and was initially admitted to the hospital in preterm labor. Her stay quickly escalated into a medical emergency.

"I guess I'll start our story when my wife Amber was admitted to the hospital in November 2010. Amber was 26 weeks pregnant when we got to the hospital; we stayed there for a few days to try and keep Lily inside of her for as long as possible. Amber had developed a rare complication called HELLP syndrome (hemolysis, elevated liver enzymes, low platelet count); the cure was to take the baby out of the mother. However, with Lily being so premature, the doctors wanted Lily to stay in for as long as possible to develop as much as she could; it was certainly a catch-22 situation.

"On November 20, Amber's liver was about to burst, and the doctors had to do an emergency C-section to get Lily out and hope to save Amber's life. The doctors had already told us that the chances of saving Lily were slim to none, and at this point and there wasn't much hope for Amber either. When the doctors took Amber to prepare her for surgery, they gave me scrubs to come in after they had started and be by her side during the surgery. What the doctors told me and did not tell Amber was that they did not expect Amber to leave the operating room and were going to only try and save Lily. I was to say my goodbyes at that time. It was the first time in that hospital's history that they had already prepped the morgue before they started surgery because there was no expectation for Amber to survive. Amber's platelet count was at 17,000 microliters, and the human body has an average of 150,000–450,000 platelets normally. Platelets help clot the blood when flesh is cut (like in surgery), and since Amber virtually didn't have any, the doctors said she would simply bleed out and there wouldn't be any way for them to stop the bleeding.

"When we were still in the regular hospital room waiting endlessly for Lily to hurry up and grow and waiting to see how far Amber could make it before she couldn't take it anymore, the nurses started rushing around quickly getting her ready for the operating room in the middle of the night. At that point, we still didn't know the extent of how bad Amber's condition was; I just knew that she was in really bad shape. I finally did get one nurse to tell me that her liver was about to explode and if they would have left her for 30 more minutes, she would die. That scared me, but I felt the doctors knew what to do, and I wanted to stay out of their way while still being with Amber for support.

"Everything was moving so fast. It felt like Walmart on Black Friday: Chaos! The doctors grabbed Amber quickly and rushed her away to the operating room. One nurse threw me scrubs and told me to put them on ASAP and follow them to the operating room. When I got to the doors of the operating room, they wouldn't let me in because they were prepping Amber. The nurse told me I had to wait there for the doctor and that he would probably let me in before long, then she left. Waiting for the doctor felt like an eternity!!! I was waiting alone in the hallway, and the doctor finally came out to explain what was happening and what to expect while they were working on her. He explained that Amber would not survive the surgery as soon as they started to cut because of her platelet count being so low and

(continued)

(*continued*)

that Lily was their only focus to keep alive and that Lily had a very slim chance. On the way in, the doctor told me that it was imperative to not talk to Amber about her condition because it could complicate the surgery and that I was also to say goodbye. I wish we had had more information before the operating room to know what to expect and be more prepared. I also wish someone could have stayed with me in the hallway to explain what was happening better or even just for support. It was hard being alone and not knowing any information. It would have given me a chance to process what was happening.

"While I was in the operating room watching Amber's surgery, the doctors kept a very open line of communication between each other and myself and let me know what was happening throughout the process. One doctor even pulled me aside to show me Amber's uterus on a platter and where the placenta grew into it. After they pulled Lily out and got her into the other room with the incubator for resuscitation, the doctor told me directly that he didn't know how Amber was still alive, but because she was, they would sew her up quickly and x-ray her later for tools that may have been accidently left inside.

"Without going into too much detail of the surgery, I watched the doctors bring Lily into this world at 1 lb 6 oz. They immediately took her into the next room and started to revive her in the incubator. After 10 minutes, and on the doctor's final try, he managed to get her first breath. Meanwhile, Amber was a bloody mess, but, by the grace of God, was still alive. The doctors told me they didn't know why or how she wasn't dead, but it was definitely an unexplained miracle, 'an enigma.' They put a rush on putting Amber back together and hoped for the best. Lily was 3½ months early, and even though Amber was at 26 weeks, they said Lily was the size of a 24-week baby because the placenta grew into Amber's uterus and Lily wasn't getting fed properly.

"For me, nearly losing my wife and my daughter at the same time was very difficult; in fact, it was the most difficult thing I've ever had to go through in my life. In the moment, I was more concerned for Amber. I knew Lily only had a small chance to live, but Amber is my wife and meant more to me. She is the love of my life, and I would have been completely devastated and crushed if I had lost her. I feel that I should share how I felt with others more because there could be people that relate to how I felt and might need assurance that it's okay or normal, like having postpartum depression. When Lily was born, I resented her for nearly killing my wife. I also didn't have the connection that most parents have with their babies because she was not at home with us for the first several months and we didn't know from day to day if she would survive. So, I kept my distance emotionally with her and built a wall against her for several years. It actually took until about age six to truly feel a real connection with her, the kind of connection most parents have right away with their child. I feel ashamed talking about it, but it is the truth, and maybe other people out there have similar feelings.

"I wish we had a staff member that could have been there to help us through everything step by step. There wasn't a regular nurse or staff member that did that with us, but I feel they did a wonderful job communicating from one unit to the other during recovery. During the operation, I could be only with Amber. Lily was too delicate for me to be

(*continued*)

(*continued*)

with her at first. Once Lily was stable enough, they allowed me to look at her through the incubator. I stayed mainly with Amber during recovery, and when we had opportunities to visit Lily, Amber and I would go together to see her. The staff was very helpful in getting us in to visit Lily; however, I remember being turned down from seeing her quite a few times because of her fragile condition. That was really hard to deal with because we just wanted to see our baby girl and we couldn't. Sometimes I would hold it against certain nurses because one nurse would say 'No, you can't see her,' but another would say 'Sure, no problem.' That got really frustrating.

"One of the hardest parts of this process for me was not creating the first initial bond with our new baby. We had to wait until she was stable enough to be touched, and we could only touch her through the incubator. We had to wait several weeks before even placing our hand on her through the incubator. No holding, snuggling, and bonding was extremely hard for us and so was constantly not knowing if our baby was going to live today or the next. Hope and faith were our only options!

"I think the staff gave us several ways of trying to connect with Lily; I don't know if there were any more things we could have tried, but we did try everything they showed us, which was helpful. I feel that if there was a better way for the staff to help us connect with Lily, it would be to periodically ask us if we wanted to see her when she was stable and ready, instead of our constantly asking if we could see her over and over. It felt like we were always the ones pushing to connect with Lily rather than the nurses pushing for us to connect with her. That would have been a nice way to support us.

"About a month or so after Lily was born, Amber was finally recovering well, and Lily was showing signs of progress also. Amber and I have a blended family. I have two daughters (Megan and Madison) from a previous marriage, and Amber has a son (Cameron) from a previous marriage; we had Lily together. Our three older kids all get along and are smart siblings. They are 6, 7, and 9 years older than Lily. They were all too excited for Lily to be born and in my opinion, dealt with the whole situation very well. Lily's older siblings were very patient and hopeful throughout the process. They couldn't wait to see Lily and eventually hold her. It wasn't until the end of Lily's stay at the NICU that her siblings were able to get involved and hold her. They all did wonderfully with her, very careful and cautious. Lily's older brother Cameron was especially protective with her and would even caution the doctor or nurses as they checked on Lily. Of course, they now fight like cats and dogs!

"It's really hard to say if the staff could have done anymore to help connect the siblings. I think they did a fantastic job! Cameron spent a little more time with Lily than the other two siblings and was exceptionally protective of her, but by the time Cameron, Megan, and Madison could see her, hold her, and connect with her, Lily was close to coming home. The siblings really didn't spend that much time in the NICU while Lily was there. They did do a great job helping with her after Lily came home though. They all love her very much!

"We took Lily home on oxygen in March 2011. That was a happy day for all of us! There were other obstacles we would have to face once we got her home. Twice over the

(*continued*)

(*continued*)

next 10 to 14 days, we had to resuscitate Lily ourselves. The second time, I clocked it for 12 minutes before we brought her back to life. At that point we decided to give her back to the NICU. She stayed in the NICU for another 2 weeks. While she was there, the doctors figured out that Lily was suffocating herself to keep from drowning because of her extreme reflux. Once that was fixed, she was good to come home to stay.

"Lily is currently 6 years old and has no serious physical, mental, or emotional problems at all. She takes a pill for low thyroid and she looks about 2 years younger than she is, very petite, but she is strong and full of life and laughter. She resides in Hawaii now and is thriving here very much. She will be in first grade this year.

"I honestly don't know if there are ways of improving the process we went through or better ways of helping families cope with the trauma of this kind of situation. Every family is different and has different needs or expectations. One thing that stands out to me was, whether doctor or nurse, there were some with a pessimistic point of view and others with an optimistic point of view. I completely understand the pessimistic point of view because the constant loss of babies or babies with major issues must be extremely hard to deal with, so to not give parents hope and then see that hope crushed might seem to be an easier way to go. On the other hand, I believe that parents are looking for hope and expecting it from the doctor or nurse, and sometimes it takes that to just get through the day. For us, we had a close-knit family and church that supported us through thick and thin. Friends, family, and people from our church regularly came by the hospital to help in any way they could, and most of them simply offered their prayers. I'm so grateful to everyone for that! I feel really sad for the people that don't have the same support we had; I think the amount of hope they have is minimized and I believe you need that hope to keep going day after day. Eventually, everything does get better, and it always works out for the best!

"We owe a great deal of gratitude to the hospital, the doctors, and all the nurses and staff that were a part of keeping my wife and daughter alive. We feel that we have made some long-lasting friendships with one of the doctors and a couple of nurses as well, and we will be forever grateful for their service, kindness, and professional skill."

RECOMMENDATIONS/SUGGESTIONS FOR BEST PRACTICE

1. Develop ways to keep mom and baby together after delivery, despite needing ICU- and NICU-level care.

2. Assess dual-ICU families for posttraumatic stress disorder.

3. Provide all families in NICU, but especially dual-ICU families, with access to supportive services such as social work, spiritual care, clergy, psychology, behavioral health, and care management.

4. Implement ways to develop consistent communication between the ICU and NICU staff.

5. Offer patient report for both mom and baby at one patient bedside with the family present.

6. Embed lactation support in the ICU care.

7. Have donor milk available to offer exclusive human milk diets to NICU babies whose mothers are in the ICU and wish to exclusively breastfeed.

8. Allow alternate feeding methods, other than bottles, for families who wish to exclusively breastfeed, if mom will recover.

9. Introduce the N.U.R.S.E. Self Care Program to families to encourage self-care.

10. Allow Skype or Facetime between families who are separated.

11. Offer Scent Dolls or Scent Blankets to switch between baby and mom when both are in intensive care.

12. Provide dual-ICU families with journals and encourage journaling of experience and journey.

13. Take photographs for families and/or encourage photography.

14. For maternal bereavement:

    a. Provide family photography.

    b. Allow additional visitors.

    c. Encourage spiritual leaders to be present.

    d. Obtain keepsakes (handprints, fingerprints, lock of hair, hand mold).

    e. Keep baby and mom together with family

RECOMMENDED RESOURCES

Several websites, journals, products, and tools can be helpful for staff when looking for ways to support families when they are in dual-ICU situations or when a mother does not survive after the delivery of her child (Figure 4.2).

For hospitals that wish to implement a scented-heart program, in which both mom and baby trade off scented items, easy instructions can be provided to volunteers who wish to make fabric hearts and donate them to the hospital. It is important to find someone at the hospital who will be willing to be the contact to receive the hearts, initially wash the hearts, and then put them into the unit for use. Here is a sample template letter and pattern (Figure 4.3).

For hospitals that do not yet have a policy in place for using human donor milk in the NICU, it can be helpful to look at a sample policy and patient consent form, in addition to looking at the recommended websites (Figure 4.4).

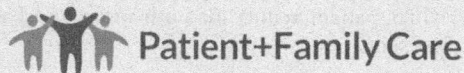

General Support:

1. https://www.hmbana.org
2. https://www.hmbana.org/locations
3. https://www.milkbank.org/using-donor-milk-in-the-nicu
4. http://www.prolacta.com/implementing-donor-milk-in-the-nicu
5. http://nwhjournal.org/article/S1751-4851(15)30669-3/fulltext
6. https://www.prolacta.com/Data/Sites/14/media/PDF/implementing-donor-milk-in-the-nicuvcc.pdf
7. https://www.ncbi.nlm.nih.gov/pmc/articles/PMC3663453
8. http://www.jognn.org/article/S0884-2175(17)30140-5/fulltext
9. https://www.caringbridge.org
10. http://share.marchofdimes.org
11. https://www.everymothercounts.org

Maternal Bereavement:

1. https://www.afesupport.org/get-support
2. http://www.sad.scot.nhs.uk/bereavement/maternal-death
3. http://www.seminperinat.com/article/S0146-0005(11)00162-5/fulltext
4. https://griefwatch.com
5. https://www.griefshare.org
6. https://opentohope.com
7. http://www.bereavementservices.org/app/files/public/5842/RTS-Trainings-overview-brochure.pdf

See products and tools for bereavement products

Products/Tools:

1. http://loveybabyproducts.com/research-behind-lovey-heart-scent
2. http://www.ltkeepsakes.com
3. http://www.funeral-urn.com/fingerprint-cremation-jewelry-and-thumbprint-memorial-jewelry.aspx
4. http://www.jewelrythatmatters.com
5. https://www.cremationsolutions.com/fingerprint-jewelry
6. http://www.cafepress.com/+fingerprint+jewelry
7. Search Amazon.com for Luna Bean Keepsake Hands DIY Plaster casting kit
8. Search Pinterest/Etsy for memorial/bereavement gifts

Figure 4.2 ■ Recommended resources to support dual-ICU families/bereaved maternal families.

Patient+Family Care

Project Contact: _____   Phone/Email: _____

Mailing Address: _____
_____
_____

Description:
One heart is given to the new NICU mom and one is given to the new baby. One heart is placed under the baby and the other heart is given to the mom to place next to her skin. Each heart absorbs the scent of the "wearer."

When mom comes to visit the baby, she exchanges her heart for her baby's heart, thus sharing the most wonderful smells in the world—mom and baby.

When mom is home and without her newborn, she inhales the beautiful scent of her child, and baby can sleep while being comforted by the scent of mom.

These little bits of love can be made out of any soft fabric—flannel or cotton scraps.

Instructions:
1. Trace the heart on the fold of the fabric. Cut.
2. Sew two hearts together—right sides together—using a ¼-inch hem. Leave a 1½-inch gap in the seam.
3. At the base of the heart as well as the top of the dip in the heart, stop the machine, make the turn, and continue sewing.
4. Turn inside out.
5. Clip both the dip and the base of the heart so that they turn and lay flat nicely. Be careful not to clip the seam.
6. Hand or machine stitch the opening.

Once you get a good number of these collected, please mail to the above address.

Figure 4.3 ■ NICU scented hearts.

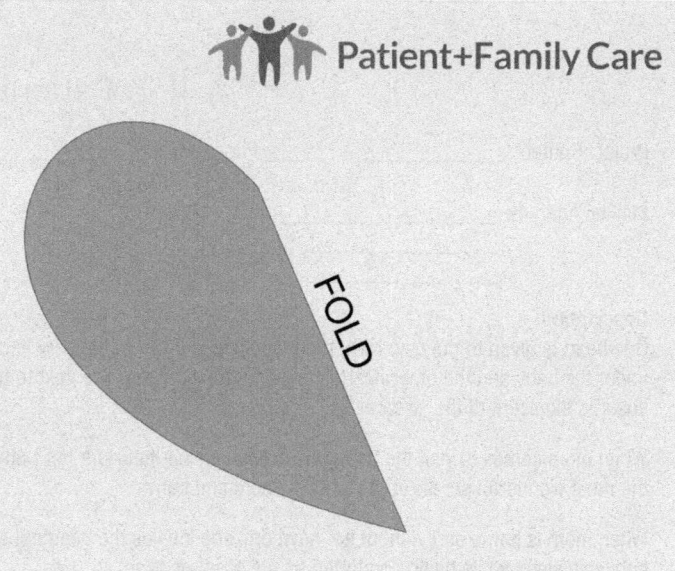

Figure 4.3 ■ NICU scented hearts. (*continued*)

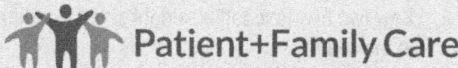

In the absence of your own breast milk, your infant's healthcare team recommends and will prescribe heat-processed, donor human milk for your infant if your infant meets one of these criteria:

   ✓ Birth weight less than 1,500 grams
   ✓ Your child having had some type of bowel injury such as necrotizing enterocolitis (NEC) or gastroschisis
   ✓ Your physician having requested to use donor milk for other reasons that he/she feels potentially adds further health benefits for your infant

Donor milk will generally be provided until mother's milk volume becomes sufficient or your infant reaches 32 to 34 weeks' gestation, at which point your infant will be switched to the appropriate standard infant formula in the absence of mother's milk.

In the absence of the infant's own mother's milk, donor milk offers many of the benefits of human milk for the infant, including the following:
• Infection-fighting factors
• Reduced incidence of NEC, a severe inflammatory bowel condition in premature infants

Figure 4.4 ■ Consent for use of donor milk in the special care nursery.

NEC, necrotizing enterocolitis.

- Active growth and developmental hormones
- Improved digestion
- Ideal nutrition

Donor milk banks receive milk from lactating mothers who have been carefully screened for health behaviors and communicable diseases, including AIDS, hepatitis B, hepatitis C, and syphilis. In addition, they must not smoke, drink, or take any medications regularly.

Donor milk is transported to the milk bank frozen. The milk from several donors is pooled together after thawing and then heat-treated to kill any bacteria or viruses. The milk is processed and then refrozen. The milk is sent to hospitals only after it has tested to ensure the absence of dangerous viruses and bacteria. Although every precaution is taken, there is a very small chance that an infectious agent may nevertheless be transmitted to your child by the milk, and your child could become sick. Please discuss any concerns you have regarding the use of donor human milk with your baby's healthcare team.

My baby's physician/nurse practitioner has described the need for donor human milk for my baby and has told me about the potential risks and expected benefits, as well as other methods of nutrition available and their risks and benefits. My physician/nurse practitioner has given me the chance to ask questions about the use of donor human milk, and all of my questions have been answered to my satisfaction.

I accept the use of donor human milk for my child:

Signature of Guardian:	**Date:**
Signature of Witness:	**Date:**

I understand that the use of cow's milk–based formulas may increase my child's risk of infection, intestinal complications, or allergies but decline the use of donor human milk for my child.

Signature of Guardian:	**Date:**
Signature of Witness:	**Date:**

Figure 4.4 ■ Consent for use of donor milk in the special care nursery. (*continued*)

Case-Based Learning

J. is a 29-year-old, G3, P3, who is 12 hours post–repeat C-section for a baby boy at 39 0/7 weeks' gestation. At 6 hours postpartum, J. complained of shortness of breath and collapsed in bed, witnessed only by her husband. The rapid response team was called immediately after J.'s husband calling out for the RN. J. progressed into full cardiac arrest, received

(*continued*)

(*continued*)

advanced life support procedures, and was transferred to the adult medical ICU on a ventilator with suspicion of venous thromboembolism versus anaphylaxis of pregnancy.

L. has been J.'s husband of 10 years, and he is father of their three children, aged 6, 3, and newborn. He is 32 years old and is a construction worker. The baby has been transferred to the nursery as a border baby while his mother is in intensive care. You come on shift and enter the nursery to complete your initial shift assessment on baby. The baby is in the crib next to dad, who does not make eye contact or move when you approach. When you introduce yourself, he mumbles and continues to stare into space. You ask for an update on his wife, baby's mom, and he slowly stands and walks out of the nursery.

You receive an update from the charge nurse that baby's mom is thought to have sustained a devastating neurological insult. The ICU team believes that she is likely brain dead, and a decision will need to be made about withdrawal of support.

QUESTIONS

1. What are the contextual elements of L.'s emotional state?
2. What are your thoughts of how to support him?
3. What are your next steps?

ANSWERS

It's no surprise that there is a significant impact on family members during and after a loved one's ICU hospitalization. Up to half experience acute stress, posttraumatic stress, anxiety, and depression. Many components, such as stressful (sometimes literally life and death) decision making and the burden of caregiving to the surviving family members, are at play (Davidson et al., 2017). L. is engulfed in this very scenario— suddenly, shockingly, he must care for and make life-altering decisions for his dying wife while bonding with a newborn and caring for two young children. In addition to fear and anxiety, L. could feel guilty about his role in the pregnancy that has harmed his wife, as well as feelings of inadequacy in his ability to protect his wife and family and anxiety about the future of his family. Withdrawal is a common response to being emotionally overwhelmed, and fear of asking questions permeates the parent experience in ICU (Lyndon, Wisner, Holschuh, Fagan, & Franck, 2017). A surviving parent can be preoccupied with, or stalled, in grief, making the absence of the deceased parent felt more profoundly across the family. L. must engage with his own grief so that he can attend to his children's grief-related and developmental needs (Werner-Lin & Biank, 2013).

Family involvement in ICUs is described by Olding et al. (2016) as having five components: presence, having needs being met/being supported, communication, decision making, and contributing to care. An initial step toward development of a caring relationship might be to help identify L.'s social and spiritual support system. Another step is to promote L.'s presence by supporting him with communication,

(*continued*)

(*continued*)

help with information gathering, and participation in decision making (Davidson & Zisook, 2017). Explore the broader sociocultural processes that shape L.'s ability to be involved. He may exhibit withdrawal from interaction and bonding with the baby. He may have multiple concerns about finances, time away from work, childcare, and support of grieving extended family members and friends.

This is a good case to illustrate the benefit of a care coordinator for communication facilitation, consultation with social work, and consultation with the palliative care team. A bioethics consultation may be provided, if needed, to clarify value-related conflict, and help decrease moral distress among ICU staff (Denney-Koelsch et al., 2016; Marty & Carter, 2017). As a patient advocate, facilitate baby "visiting" mom in the ICU. Lactation support may be requested for expressing milk for feeding, for preventing breast engorgement, and potentially breastfeeding, if possible (Crozier, 2017). Be prepared to provide reassurance that baby being skin-to-skin is not only good for baby, but also contributes warm memories for the family. Facilitate photographs of mom and baby, as well as the whole family together.

REFERENCES

Crozier, T. M. (2017, April). General care of the pregnant patient in the intensive care unit. *Seminars in Respiratory and Critical Care Medicine, 38*(2), 208–217. doi:10.1055/s-0037-1600905

Davidson, J. E., Aslakson, R. A., Long, A. C., Puntillo, K. A., Kross, E. K., Hart, J., & Netzer, G. (2017). Guidelines for family-centered care in the neonatal, pediatric, and adult ICU. *Critical Care Medicine, 45*(1), 103–128. doi:10.1097/CCM.0000000000002169

Davidson, J. E., & Zisook, S. (2017). Implementing family-centered care through facilitated sensemaking. *AACN Advanced Critical Care, 28*(2), 200–209. doi:10.4037/aacnacc2017102

Denney-Koelsch, E., Black, B. P., Côté-Arsenault, D., Wool, C., Kim, S., & Kavanaugh, K. (2016). A survey of perinatal palliative care programs in the United States: Structure, processes, and outcomes. *Journal of Palliative Medicine, 19*(10), 1080–1086. doi:10.1089/jpm.2015.0536

Lyndon, A., Wisner, K., Holschuh, C., Fagan, K. M., & Franck, L. S. (2017). Parents' perspectives on navigating the work of speaking up in the NICU, *Journal of Obstetric, Gynecologic & Neonatal Nursing, 46*(5), 716–726. doi:10.1016/j.jogn.2017.06.009

Marty, C. M., & Carter, B. S. (2017, September). Ethics and palliative care in the perinatal world. *Seminars in Fetal & Neonatal Medicine, 23*(1), 35–38. doi:10.1016/j.siny.2017.09.001

Olding, M., McMillan, S. E., Reeves, S., Schmitt, M. H., Puntillo, K., & Kitto, S. (2016). Patient and family involvement in adult critical and intensive care settings: A scoping review. *Health Expectations, 19*(6), 1183–1202. doi:10.1111/hex.12402

Werner-Lin, A., & Biank, N. M. (2013). Holding parents so they can hold their children: Grief work with surviving spouses to support parentally bereaved children. *OMEGA-Journal of Death and Dying, 66*(1), 1–16. doi:10.2190/OM.66.1.a

REFERENCES

Baikie, K. A., & Wilhelm, K. (2005). Emotional and physical health benefits of expressive writing. *Advances in Psychiatric Treatment, 11*(5), 338–346. doi:10.1192/apt.11.5.338

Bressert, S. (2016). The impact of stress. *Psych Central.* Retrieved from https://psychcentral.com/lib/the-impact-of-stress

CBC News. (2017, September 30). Vancouver hospital launches new kind of neonatal intensive care unit. Retrieved from http://www.cbc.ca/beta/news/canada/british-columbia/neonatal-intensive-care-unit-1.4310322

Creanga, A. A., Berg, C. J., Syverson, C., Seed, K., Bruce, F. C., & Callaghan, W. M. (2015). Pregnancy-related mortality in the United States, 2006–2010. *Obstetrics & Gynecology, 125*(1), 5–12. doi:10.1097/AOG.0000000000000564

Crenshaw, J. T. (2014). Healthy birth practice #6: Keep mother and baby together—It's best for mother, baby, and breastfeeding. *Journal of Perinatal Education, 23*(4), 211–217. doi:10.1891/1058-1243.23.4.211

Day, A., Haj-Bakri, S., Lubchansky, S., & Mehta, S. (2013). Sleep, anxiety and fatigue in family members of patients admitted to the intensive care unit: A questionnaire study. *Critical Care, 17*(3), R91. doi:10.1186/cc12736

Hebert, K., Moore, H., & Rooney, J. (2011). The nurse advocate in end-of-life care. *Ochsner Journal, 11*(4), 325–329. Retrieved from https://www.ncbi.nlm.nih.gov/pmc/articles/MPC3241064

Mosher, S. (2017). Comprehensive NICU parental education: Beyond baby basics. *Neonatal Network, 36*(1), 18–25. doi:10.1891/0730-0832.36.1.18

Phillips, R. (2013). The sacred hour: Uninterrupted skin-to-skin contact immediately after birth. *Newborn and Infant Nursing Reviews, 13*(2), 67–72. doi:10.1053/j.nainr.2013.04.001

Pound, C., & Unger, S. (2012). The baby-friendly initiative: Protecting, promoting and supporting breastfeeding. *Paediatrics & Child Health, 17*(6), 317–321. doi:10.1093/pch/17.6.317

Shorofi, S. A., Jannati, Y., Moghaddam, H. R., & Yazdani-Charati, J. (2016). Psychosocial needs of families of intensive care patients: Perceptions of nurses and families. *Nigerian Medical Journal, 57*(1), 10–18. doi:10.4103/0300-1652.180557

Steinhauser, K. E., Voils, C. I., Bosworth, H., & Tulsky, J. A. (2014). What constitutes quality of family experience at the end of life? Perspectives from family members of patients who died in the hospital. *Palliative & Supportive Care, 13*(4), 945–952. doi:10.1017/S1478951514000807

Ten steps to successful breastfeeding. (n.d.). Retrieved from https://www.unicef.org/newsline/tensps.htm

Wake, S., & Kitchiner, D. (2013). Post-traumatic stress disorder after intensive care. British Medical Journal, 346, f3232. doi:10.1136/bmj.f3232

SUPPORTING PATIENTS AND FAMILIES IN THE NICU

NICU ADMISSION

5

SUPPORTING THE PATIENT AND FAMILY DURING A NICU ADMISSION

Regardless of whether or not parents have time to anticipate a NICU admission for their child, the actual admission to the neonatal unit is inevitably a stressful and overwhelming time for families. Although care teams can provide a best-guess scenario of how they believe the admission will go and what the medical state of an infant will be, no one has a crystal ball to predict the exact outcome; therefore, the NICU admission is an entire course of unknowns. The parents of these infants "experience high levels of distress, including increased anxiety, depression, and trauma symptoms, as compared to parents of healthy infants" (Obeidat, Bond, & Callister, 2009, para. 4).

To assist in decreasing the levels of stress a parent experiences, a parent and a support person should be encouraged to accompany the infant to the NICU for admission. However, it is imperative that staff understand that when parents are present, a staff member, such as a family support specialist, should be assigned to be with the family members throughout the duration of their admission. This is because other NICU staff is busy and focused on initializing the medical stability of the infant. Assessing the neurological, respiratory, cardiovascular, digestive, integumentary, renal, muscular, endocrine, lymphatic, reproductive, and skeletal systems and intervening with noninvasive and medical techniques to stabilize the patient are the primary role of the medical team, and their focus should not deviate from caring for the baby. Typically, one infant has a team supporting it medically at admission, and that team can consist of a nurse, practitioner, physician, respiratory therapist, nursing assistant, phlebotomist, x-ray technician, and pharmacist. When you consider a parent looking at this large group of people surrounding one small infant, it can seem very overwhelming. If the condition of the infant is critical, the care team tends to move quickly and there is usually a lot of action and talking between everyone, which can increase the anxiety and level of stress for the parents. Parents have shared in numerous studies that they feel most supported when staff stay with them and have "the ability to understand another person's situation on the basis of the feeling of empathy, which means being emotionally responsive to the other person's needs without judging or criticizing them. Responding with empathy and compassion makes health care meaningful" (Wigert, Blom, & Bry, 2014, "Discussion" section).

Staff, to fully support a parent, should do their best to first meet a parent before the admission, if possible. This allows the staff and family to establish a relationship before the stressful delivery and admission time. If this is not possible, introductions should come from the assigned support staff as soon as possible so that the parents can be supported through the admission process. During this process, a family support specialist role should be to do the following:

- Remain with the family to offer support from the moment of delivery until the infant is fully admitted and stabilized.

- Be available to answer questions regarding the up-to-date information about the baby's condition.

- Translate any medical information and answer questions about procedures, tests, medications, and equipment.

- Introduce team members that come and go during the admission process.

- If mom is unable to be in the NICU immediately, go back and forth between NICU and mom's room (or to be the one to communicate with mom's nurse) to provide frequent updates about the baby's condition.

- Orient the family to the neonatal unit, including the following:
  - Handwashing policy
  - Ways to access/enter the unit
  - The baby's location within the unit

- Assess the family for what the members' needs might be (e.g., do they need water, something to eat, tissue, a chair to sit, a private space, help in contacting other family).

- Assist in capturing photographs for the family. It is great when a unit has a digital camera with instant print so that support staff can be allowed to capture images during the admission and then print a few photos for them to make colorful crib cards to take back to mom's room. When mom is ill, these initial photos are especially important and cherished. During the admission, support staff should also encourage the family to use personal cameras or phones to capture images so that other family members not present can see many of the "firsts" that are occurring. If the family is struggling in this moment, staff should offer to take a camera or phone of the families to take photos for them.

Both the family support specialist and medical staff can do a great deal to support families during the admission process by including family during the initial stabilization and admission. Allowing families to be an active member in the care team at this initial stage is incredibly important and, as stated by Lee and O'Brien (2014, para. 2), "integration of parents into their infant's care begins at admission." Parents often feel out of control and as if they aren't their child's parent because when their child requires neonatal care, they are unable to participate in many of the typical parenting responsibilities immediately after delivery. Both the medical team and support staff member can assist families in feeling more included and more a part of the child's care team by participating in the resuscitation and the admission. Parental tasks and responsibilities may include, but are not limited to, the following:

- Cutting and trimming the umbilical cord
- Taking an axillary temperature to compare it to an integumentary-recorded bed temperature
- Putting on and changing a diaper
- Gently holding a hand during painful procedures
- Providing containment
- Talking to the infant or praying over the infant if religious practices support prayer
- Providing the initial bath
- Pressing "weigh" on a scale so that they can participate in weighing their baby

EDUCATION AND INFORMATION SHARING

When it comes to sharing information and education with families during the admission, staff needs to realize that they are often in a state of shock and are so overwhelmed that they do not retain much of the information that they are given. The NICU is typically and often a foreign setting for families, and even those who have had tours before delivery, the environment becomes particularly stressful once they find their child in it. Staff "benefit from assuming that most of the information shared during this initial time period will likely need further reinforcement and repeating once parents are more apt to comprehend what they are being told. During times of stress and trauma, it can be very difficult for individuals to truly grasp and understand all of the information they are receiving, and that unfortunately can lead to even more stress and anxiety" (Mosher, 2017, "NICU Admission" section). The positive news for staff is that they can help alleviate some of the parental stress if they provide education and information that is broken down into easy-to-digest pieces.

The easiest way to break information down for families is to consider dividing it into two main areas of focus: basic unit information and medical information. It is important to focus on these two areas at admission because families need to be aware of the basics from the earliest stage possible. Staff need to assess a family for how they best learn before providing the education, document that learning style, then begin educating them on topics early and frequently for both the parents and all of their support individuals. Educating support individuals is vitally important because those folks not only serve as a second set of ears for the family, but also can help the family digest the information and reiterate the information later if the family has questions.

The information and education shared with families should be articulated in a message and language that families can understand, so if interpreters are needed, all effort should be made to include one. If an in-person interpreter is unavailable, then the second-best option is to have an on-screen interpreter through a medical service, followed by a speaker phone. Often, family members are pulled in to interpret, yet this should never be used in medical situations unless it is truly an emergency. Family members are experiencing the emotions and trauma of the event and should not be expected to take on the added responsibility of translating important medical conversations in a crisis situation. In addition, it can be impossible for the medical team to know just how much information they understand and what they are actually translating to the family.

Information should be tailored to each family and "when formulating how to best communicate with families, staff needs to assess the family's level of literacy" (Mosher, 2017, "NICU Admission" section). Figure 5.1 is a list of topics that are recommended to cover with families during admission, but the list is far from inclusive. It is meant to provide a starting point to get staff thinking about the types of important starting topics to discuss with families at admission.

Having an admission checklist with these topics written out and taped to the baby's bedside can be a helpful way to ensure that all admission information is shared with the family, and it provides families with a reminder of what information they have heard and what information they can ask staff to either repeat or share an initial time (Figure 5.2).

Basic Unit Information	Medical Information

• Way finding—where the NICU is located and where baby is located within the unit
• Handwashing policy and infection-prevention policy
• Ways to access the NICU
• Visitation policy
• Introductions—who is who in the unit
• Room orientation
  ○ Room setup
  ○ Type of bed baby is in
  ○ Monitors
  ○ Pumps
  ○ Respiratory equipment
  ○ Communication board
• Ways to contact staff with questions
• Ways to be comfortable in the unit
• Resources and support available
  ○ Parent lounge
  ○ Parent library
	• Systems overview
	• Gestational age norms
	• Understanding of readings on the cardiopulmonary/respiratory monitor
	• Understanding of readings on the oxygen saturation monitor
	• Medications/IV drips that the patient is receiving and why
	• Feeding plans
	• Importance of early and frequent skin-to-skin care
	• Overall prognosis
	• Information specific to the baby's condition and medical diagnosis
	• Unpredictable nature of premature baby's medical stability (ups and downs of the NICU journey)

Figure 5.1 ■ Admission education topics.

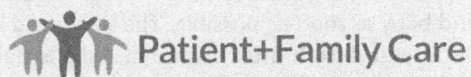 Patient+Family Care

Congratulations on the birth of your baby(ies)! We know the NICU can be an overwhelming and scary place, and there is a LOT to learn. We hope this checklist will help you know what information we feel is important to know in the first few days after admission and will provide you a visual way of keeping track of what you have and have not yet been taught by the staff.

IMPORTANT POINTS:

✓ This is only a guide! There may be more information the staff needs to share with you that is important.
✓ YOUR questions and priorities are equally important, so fill in the blank spaces so that we know what YOU want to hear about and learn.
✓ There is going to be a lot of information shared with you during this stressful time, so don't expect to remember everything. Even if it is checked off, ask staff to repeat information for you!

Unit Orientation Education	**Medical Information Education**
☐ Location of NICU	☐ Gestational age norms
☐ Baby's location in the unit	☐ Systems overview
☐ Handwashing/infection-prevention policy	☐ Understanding of readings on monitor
☐ Visitation policy	☐ Understanding of saturation parameters
☐ Room orientation	☐ Medication overview
○ Room setup	☐ IV overview
○ Bed types	☐ Feeding plan
○ Monitors	☐ Importance of early and frequent skin-to-skin practice
○ Pumps	☐ Overall prognosis
○ Respiratory equipment	☐ Specifics of condition/diagnosis
○ Communication board	☐ Unpredictability of premature babies (ups and downs of NICU journey)
☐ Ways to contact staff	☐
☐ Ways to be comfortable in the unit	☐
☐ Support resources available	☐
☐	☐
☐	
☐	

I have received the above information/education:

Signature of Parent:	Date:
Signature of Parent:	Date:

Figure 5.2 ■ Admission education family checklist.

One of the most important things to remember at NICU admission is to unite mom and baby as soon as possible. The safety and health of mom after delivery is crucial, and her medical team must ensure that she is stable after she gives birth, but as soon as she is determined to be stable, the postpartum medical team and the NICU team need to work together to coordinate her visit to the NICU to be with her child. Depending on the style and design of the NICU, it may be difficult to accommodate her if she needs to be transported in a wheelchair or bed, but all efforts should be made to make this visit happen. If there is space next to her baby's bedside, then mom should be wheeled down in her bed or in a wheelchair as soon as possible. When mom can be next to her baby, lactation specialist can visit her and initiate her first pumping there at the baby's bedside, which helps with lactation.

If a baby requires a higher level of care than a mom's delivering hospital can provide and requires transportation to a different hospital, staff will need to provide a different type of support to that family; we discuss how to support families that face neonatal transport in a later chapter.

Author's Personal Story

I was paged to attend the delivery of an infant at 30 2/7 weeks' gestation who was in acute distress. The mother had just arrived in triage, and the team noted late decelerations, an immediate cesarean was being performed. The neonatal resuscitation team rushed into the operating room alongside the mother's medical care team to prepare the warmer and equipment for the resuscitation, and I met the anxious father who was already dressed in his blue scrubs and pacing the hallway. The policy at this particular hospital is that the mother's support person must wait outside of the operating room until the anesthesiologist places the epidural/spinal and the operating team drapes and sterilizes the mother and field. Just before the initial cut, the father is then allowed to enter the operating room and is escorted to the head of the bed to be present for the delivery.

I introduced myself to B.A., and I wanted nothing more in that moment to have a magical wand that would somehow make this poor, nervous, soon-to-be-father less anxious. Not only was he pacing back and forth, but also every part of him was shaking, his knees, his hands, and even his voice, as he introduced himself back to me. I tried to distract him slightly by asking him simple questions like what his name was, what his wife's name was, if he knew if they were having a boy or girl, did they have a name picked out yet, what they did for a living, and other simple questions that did not require much thought at all. Nothing seemed to work. In fact, I felt like the more I tried talking to him the more anxious he got. His pacing got faster and his shaking more noticeable. I offered to go check on the progress in the operating room so that he would know how much longer the wait would be. He let out a big sigh and finally seemed to relax. That is what he needed to finally have some relief. He just wanted to know what was going on. Although his wife had been in the operating room for 10 minutes or so, to him it felt like it had been an hour. An update was what was going to bring him some respite.

(*continued*)

(*continued*)

I returned to B.A. within 2 minutes and was able to give him an update on how his wife was doing, how the team was doing, and how much longer it might be until he could go into the operating room and be with his wife. Typically, I am able to tell waiting fathers that things were going very well and that it will be only another minute or two. Unfortunately, in this situation, that was not the case. The anesthesiologist was having a very difficult time placing the spinal, and it was going to still be quite some time before he was going to be able to go in. B.A.'s wife was doing well though, and the team was monitoring the baby. The heart rate looked very reassuring, and so I was thankful I had good news to share behind what was news I knew he didn't want to hear.

The little bit of good news was enough to calm B.A. down, and I took my chances and started to ask him a few more questions. This time the distraction seemed to work and he not only answered them openly, but also started telling me all about the pregnancy, the nursery, their visits with a doula because his wife initially wanted a home birth so that she could have an all-natural delivery in which they were both fully present and involved in the entire process, their baby names, plans for work after the baby was born, and his thoughts about what they would do now that the baby was coming earlier than expected. It seemed to be therapeutic for him to just open up and talk about everything as we stood there in the hallway. It was his way of processing everything in that moment.

After 15 minutes, I went back into the operating room to see how things were going, and the anesthesia team had still not been able to successfully get a spinal into B.A.'s wife. The baby's heart tones were starting to become concerning again, so an emergency delivery was decided, and mom was going to be put under general anesthesia. For safety precautions, the policy at this hospital is that support individuals are not allowed to be present in the operating room when mothers are placed under general anesthesia. Because the medical team was now moving quickly to ensure the safety of both the mother and baby, it was up to me to go and update B.A.

After I shared with B.A. what was happened, his pacing immediately started back up again, and I noticed sweat beads forming on his forehead. I quickly gathered a cool washcloth from the empty room directly across from us, and I assured him that the delivery would be very quick and he could be with his baby immediately and then reunited with his wife as soon as possible. I asked him if he wanted to be involved in the delivery as much as possible or if he would like to watch and be updated as to what was going on. His pacing immediately stopped and he looked at me as if I was crazy. I repeated myself in case he didn't hear me, and then he asked me what I meant by his being involved in the delivery, since he wasn't going to even be present. I told him I would love to take him into the operating room hallway where he could watch the delivery from the window and see his baby being delivered. From there, he would see the time of birth and the first breath, be able to hear the first cry if there was one immediately, and see the neonatal team resuscitate and stabilize his infant in an adjoining resuscitation suite, where he could be right next to his baby and participate in some of the resuscitation. A slight smile showed up on his face and a tear formed and he just shook his head yes, speechless.

(*continued*)

(*continued*)

I led him into the operating room hallway and helped him properly gown up, and we watched as his precious little girl was delivered. The obstetrician held her up and showed her to her proud dad through the window and then handed her over to the resuscitation team. The team came through the operating room doors into the adjoining resuscitation suite, and I led B.A. into the suite and we approached the resuscitation warmer. I instructed dad that we could get close but needed to respect the space of the medical team so that they could safely stabilize his daughter. I calmly and quietly explained to B.A. what was going on, pointed out who was who, and pointed out the beautiful features of his daughter. The team was ready to weigh his daughter, so I asked if B.A. wanted to help. Helping merely meant pressing the "weigh baby" button, but his eyes lit up when he was asked. I asked if I could use his phone to take some photos, and he handed it over to me so fast it nearly slipped out of my hands.

B.A. pressed the button like only a proud new father could. As we waited to see the weight light up on the screen, the team began guessing the weight, and the neonatologist was only 2 oz off. B.A. was so impressed; I told him that when you have cared for babies for 24 years, you get really good at looking at a baby and knowing the weight. Because this family came in and so quickly went into the delivery, they did not have a chance to meet the NICU team prior. This was a perfect opportunity to start to give dad a little information about the team and what great experience they had.

B.A.'s baby girl was ready to have her cord trimmed, so once again I put dad to the task. Once he was up there and had his hands in there, I just kept him busy. The team was on one side of the bed and at the head of the bed, so we carefully stayed on the other side and I helped dad trim the cord, put on her first diaper, wipe her face and prepare her for the respiratory therapist to put on her continuous positive airway pressure (CPAP) nasal mask, and once the team was ready to head to the NICU, we walked alongside the transport Isolette and immediately started the admission education.

The Isolette stopped at the NICU double doors and waited for them to open and once they did, the team pushed the bed to the right and I asked B.A. to accompany me to the right. I told him it was really important for his daughter's safety and the safety of all the other babies in the unit that we wash our hands really well every time we come in. We walked over to the sinks and as I showed him how to properly scrub in, I shared with him the reasons why infection prevention is so important. I informed him that all visitors were required to wash their hands like this before they could enter the unit and that anyone at all that has any symptoms of illness are asked to stay out of the unit. I took the opportunity as we washed to explain to him that premature babies have immature immune systems and any germ that they catch can make them very sick. I also informed him that the handwashing and infection-prevention policy can be overwhelming. Many staff members would be reviewing it with him and all of his family and friends, so he didn't need to memorize it right then.

I showed B.A. how he could notify the staff that he had finished washing and was ready to enter the unit, and then together we walked through the halls to his daughter's

(*continued*)

(continued)

room. I pointed out the way finding that the unit had in place for families, which in this unit was a combination of animals and room numbers, but again I assured B.A. that staff would be reminding him again of all of this information later. We entered the room and I oriented B.A. to everything in the room. I showed him the following:

- Cardiorespiratory monitor, explaining what each of the colorful lines meant
- IV pump and the IV fluid that his daughter was receiving
- CPAP machine and how it was delivering respiratory support
- Oxygen saturation probe and how it monitored her oxygen levels
- The white board where daily information would be updated, and I asked him to help me update it for the first time. We entered his and mom's name, their contact phone numbers, baby's weight, baby's date of birth, and mom's room number. I filled in the staff information and informed him that every day he would be able to read this board to learn who was caring for his daughter and would see those staff member's phone numbers next to their names, so he could always contact someone if he had questions.

The neonatologist approached and wanted to give dad an update on his daughter's condition, so I took the opportunity to sneak off and grab the digital camera the unit had to take pictures for families. I returned to the room and took a close-up photo of baby A., and then when dad was available, I asked to take a picture of the two of them. Baby A. was stable and doing really well so I offered to provide them some time alone together and encouraged him to talk to her and gently hold her hand or provide her a hand hug. I told him I would return in a little while. I wanted to provide mom with an update and take her some photographs. I printed a few photos, glued them on some really cute scrapbook paper, wrote down the baby's date of birth and birth weight, and then walked down to find mom who was in recovery from her surgery. When I walked up to her gurney, she was just waking up from her anesthesia, so I arrived at the perfect time.

I was able to show her the pictures of her daughter and give her a full update of her medical condition. Because I had been present at the delivery, I was able to share every detail of the delivery, the resuscitation and stabilization, her husband's active engagement in the process, and the way that he hadn't left their daughter's side since she was born. Mom smiled and was so happy to hear that her husband and daughter were doing well, and she was even more excited to hear that he had put on a diaper because they hadn't made it to their birthing and newborn care class yet. I told her I would be sure to make sure he was present for the first meconium diaper and get pictures of that one for her, too. She gave a little chuckle and she went back to staring proudly at the photos, trying to decide whose features her daughter had. I talked with mom's nurse and told her that baby A. was in room 5 and that I was going back to make room for mom's hospital gurney. Mom's nurse assured me that they would come to the NICU after the recovery

(continued)

(continued)

room before taking mom to her postpartum room so that mom, dad, and baby could all be together.

I returned to the NICU and told B.A. that mom was recovering very well, was awake from the anesthesia, loved the pictures, and was thrilled to hear he had put on a diaper. He was originally happy to hear that his wife was doing well, but then promptly went back to being enthralled by his daughter, and I don't think he had any interest in listening to anything else I had to say. So, I didn't bother to tell him the plans and let it be a surprise that his wife was on her way down. Within 10 minutes, her bed was wheeled in, and B.A. looked up and appeared to be a little boy on Christmas morning. He was instantly so happy to start showing off his daughter to his wife.

After the family had some time together, I approached them with the camera and asked if I could place baby skin-to-skin on mom's chest since the respiratory therapist and assigned bedside nurse were available to assist at that time and that a first family photo would be wonderful to capture. They were ecstatic! As a healthcare team, we worked together to transfer baby A. over to mom, and instantly mom and baby both were content. I snapped a photo of the happy family and then allowed them some private time to be together while I went and grabbed an admission checklist.

When I returned later to the room with the admission checklist, it was so rewarding to see how much this checklist supported this couple. I shared the form with them and started to go over the topics, and B.A. would chime in and excitedly jump in to say he already learned about the handwashing policy. He would then tell his wife about it, and it was a wonderful teach-back moment for me to observe and a wonderful way for the information to be solidified for him as he taught his wife. He then wanted to check off learning about how to gain access to the unit, what the infection-prevention policy was, what the saturation parameters were for his daughter, and how to identify which staff members were caring for his daughter each day. His wife was so proud of all he had learned already, and he was certainly proud of all he already accomplished as a dad. In times when families can feel so out of control, this checklist provided a sense of great control for this family, and as the support specialist working with them, it was incredibly fulfilling to be able to offer them that type of support and inclusion in the admission process.

Family Story

Sheri Shelton shares her personal experience of having a high-risk pregnancy, losing one twin in utero before delivery, and visiting her surviving daughter in the NICU.

"I was excited to be carrying twins and enjoyed what I imagined was a fairly normal and predictable pregnancy. But at 24 weeks, I went in for a routine ultrasound and that is when everything changed. There was a problem identified on US in which both twin babies were not growing as they should, one more developed than the other. I was immediately

(continued)

(*continued*)

admitted to the hospital, and while I waited for the OB/GYN to come talk with me, I remember everything feeling like a tunnel, like I was staring right into headlights and time stood still. I was frozen. I was numb. The only thing I felt was confusion and disbelief. I just wanted someone to tell me my babies would be okay! That didn't happen. The doctor explained to me all of the physical disabilities and challenges a baby of 24 weeks could face, if delivered that night. From that terrifying moment to the day we actually left the NICU with our one baby girl, there were so many ups and downs. There are some things I remember as clear as a picture, but others are a bit fuzzy. I suppose that is the nature of experiencing this kind of trauma. One of life and loss.

"The doctor admitted me immediately to the perinatal ward on bed rest. I remained numb. I was in shock. But I knew I had to focus every bit of energy into my babies if they were going to have a chance. I could not read, talk on the phone, or go on the computer. My family was by my side. But I did not have visitors; I could not. The nurses came in every day, and they would add another day to the calendar of how many days I was pregnant. They would tell me, every single day I stayed pregnant mattered, and was so important for my babies. So my only focus, my only goal, was to add one more day on the calendar that my babies were growing inside of me. Day after day I visualized, I prayed, I talked to my babies. I honestly don't know how the time went by because I just lay there, doing everything in my power to keep my babies in, just one more day. Now, I don't remember when, but a new nurse came in to visit me. She didn't talk about 'one more day,' she was from the NICU. She introduced herself and was really sweet. She gave me information booklets and told me that I could have a tour of the NICU so I was familiar with it. I remember thinking, 'Why is she here? I won't be going to the NICU; my babies are going to make it to full term.' In my mind, babies that go to the NICU are babies that are sick—that may not survive. I honestly believed that wouldn't be our journey—that they would arrive full term and healthy. I had to believe that. So, I was nice to the nurse; she really was kind and seemed to know what she was talking about, but I ignored what she said and put the booklets in a drawer and completely forgot that she gave them to me.

"Ten days after my admission to the hospital, one of my twin baby girls passed away in utero. It was devastating. I went into what I can only describe as survival mode. I don't remember much from this period. I became even more focused, I visualized nutrition going to my baby and light surrounding her, and I talked to her, and I spent hours lying on my left side (as the doctors told me that was the best position), just breathing and praying. I don't remember how many more visits I got from the nurse from the NICU, but I continued to resist her information. In hindsight, I can see that it was fear—fear that if my baby had to go to the NICU, which meant I could lose her too. I felt a feeling that if I did as she said, and visited the NICU, that if I let that into my mind, then it was admitting defeat. That it was me letting my baby down. It would mean that I could possibly leave the hospital without any babies, that I might lose the one sweet precious girl that was fighting so hard to survive inside of me. So, I pushed that thought out of my mind and I

(*continued*)

(*continued*)

fought for her, and that meant I stayed as far away from any thought of the NICU that I could—until the day I was rushed into surgery for an emergency C-section and the day my daughter was admitted to the NICU at 29 weeks.

"My daughter's admittance to the NICU happened directly from surgery. I was put under general anesthetic for the C-section, and the last thing I remember were the doctors saying in a very fast, urgent tone that my baby's heart rate was dropping and my blood pressure was raising too high and we needed to do the surgery now! So I did not hear the first cry from my baby, I did not see her, I woke up in the recovery room, groggy, fuzzy, and then with an immediate panic inside. The very first thought in my mind was, 'Is my baby alive?' I remember hearing a nurse in the distance saying that I was waking up, but I couldn't make out too much. In the next instant a nurse was standing right beside me, talking to me. There was an immediate familiarity with her and it made me feel a sense of calm and comfort. I quickly recognized her; she was the nurse that kept visiting me in the hospital when I was on bed rest. She told me that my little girl was alive. She was 2 lb 4 oz, 13 inches long, and was quite a fighter. My little girl had something called a CPAP machine to help her remember to breathe (my interpretation), and the nurse took the time to explain it to me. I don't remember exactly what she said but the tone of her voice and her whole demeanor was kind, calm, and positive, so I felt like it was okay. The nurse handed me a picture of my newborn baby girl and told me she was being taken care of in the NICU. I was happy to know that the nurse who had cared enough to keep checking on me even when I was obviously not interested or open to her visits was the one that was taking care of my baby in her first few hours of life in the NICU. I will always be grateful for that moment. It was the moment that someone cared enough to be there right away to let me know my baby was alive and allow me to connect to her in the only way possible at that time. I didn't have to wait. I didn't have to wonder. There was someone there to support me and give me the information.

"I was taken up to the NICU right away, as soon as we could. I remember the trip to see my little girl for the first time. I was wheeled through the halls of the hospital lying on the bed from recovery because I still couldn't sit up. The halls seemed dark (even though I am sure being a hospital that they were lit up quite well). It may have been the fear that was welling up inside of me. Of course, I couldn't wait to see my baby for the first time, but if the truth be told, I was a bit scared too. Entering the NICU, it still seemed dark. The sounds of the monitors and the beeping were distracting and very hard to tune out. I was brought into the room where my baby lay. A yellow blanket was covering the Isolette. When the blanket was removed I could see that she was very vulnerable, lying in the middle of a large, plastic-covered crib. Her skin was so thin I could see her vessels. She had the CPAP machine that I saw in the picture. Looking at her I was so scared—scared for her, scared for me. Would I know what to do with such a fragile little baby? Would I hurt her? Would she be okay? But in the moment when I was allowed to reach my hand into the Isolette and touch her hand, everything was somehow okay. In that moment, I felt like a mother,

(*continued*)

(*continued*)

with a baby that really needed me. I am so thankful for being able to see and touch my baby as soon as I was able. The nurses were so good about making it seem normal somehow, making all the beeping and the cords and monitors and the fact that my baby looked like she was going to break if anyone touched her seem normal. And that made me feel like I could do it. On the way out of the room, I remember it being light, and another nurse sitting outside the room greeted me as if I was an old friend. I don't remember the rest of the ride back to the recovery room, or if I even went back to the recovery room. But I remember it being light. And I remember the smell of clean—I assume it was the hand sanitizer—because that smell became really familiar over the next couple of months. And when I remember my time in the NICU, I can still vaguely feel what I felt with that smell. I felt good. Because every time I smelled that, I was sanitizing my hands going into the NICU, which meant I got to hold my baby.

"The neonatologist that delivered my baby came to my room and told me that she came out crying and breathing on her own, that she didn't need to be intubated, which was not common for a baby that tiny. He called her a fighter. I was told the first few days were very crucial to allow her to be protected while we waited for a US (or CT scan?) of her head to make sure there was no bleeding. He was patient and kind and answered all of my questions.

"The next 2 months that my daughter had to stay in the NICU were difficult in a way that anyone could imagine having their baby in the hospital, fighting to survive and be healthy. But the feelings that have stayed with me from our time in the NICU, even though there was trauma, are feelings of comfort. I know that is only possible because the people that offered us so much support in the NICU *really* cared. They were always there for us and made all the difference."

RECOMMENDATIONS/SUGGESTIONS FOR BEST PRACTICE

1. Assign a family-support specialist to stay with families during NICU admissions.
2. Have a digital camera and instant printers available in the NICU.
3. Have in-person interpreters available in a patient's native language. If an in-person interpreter is not available, use on-screen or speakerphone options before using family members.
4. Have an admission education checklist available for staff and families.
5. Unite mom and baby as soon as possible after admission, even if mom needs to be wheeled to the NICU on her postpartum bed or in a wheelchair.

RECOMMENDED RESOURCES

Several websites and books may be of particular interest to professionals who are looking to provide additional resources and information on culturally sensitive care in their practice and ways to be more mindful about being present for patients (Figure 5.3).

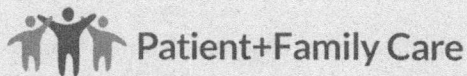 Patient+Family Care

Website Recommendations:
1. http://www.nationalperinatal.org/transculturalresources
2. http://support4nicuparents.org
3. https://preemieparentalliance.org/education
4. http://www.nationalperinatal.org/fantools
5. http://www.highriskhope.org
6. http://grahamsfoundation.org
7. https://www.nicuhelpinghands.org
8. http://nicufamiliesnw.org

Book Recommendations:
1. *Teaching Cultural Competency in Nursing and Health Care: Inquiry, Action and Innovation* by Marianne R. Jeffreys
2. *Cultural Competence in Health Care: A Practical Guide* by Anne Rundle and Maria Carvalho
3. *Building Cultural Competency: Innovative Activities and Models* by Kate Berardo
4. *Our NICU Journey: A NICU Journal for Tracking Daily NICU Activities for Your Baby in the NICU* by Trish Ringley
5. *Understanding the NICU: What Parents of Preemies and Other Hospitalized Newborns Need to Know* by the American Academy of Pediatrics and Jeanette Zaichkin
6. *Supporting Siblings and Their Families During Intensive Baby Care* by Linda Rector
7. *The Mindful Nurse: Using the Power of Mindfulness and Compassion to Help You Thrive in Your Work* by Carmel Sheridan

Figure 5.3 ■ Recommended resources for providing culturally sensitive care and being present for NICU families.

Case-Based Learning

P.R. is a first-time dad of P.R. Jr., just born at 31 weeks by urgent C-section for fetal indications. The pregnancy was complicated by preeclampsia and intrauterine growth restriction. P.R. is visibly shaking as he looks at his baby, who is tiny, but pink and breathing well on his own. While baby's mom recovers from the surgery, P.R. accompanies you to the NICU with his son.

QUESTIONS

1. In what ways might junior's dad react differently than his mom?

2. What are some interventions that might help P.R.?

(continued)

(*continued*)

ANSWERS

Fathers of babies in the NICU sometimes face slightly different issues than mothers. If the dad has paternity leave, he may be able to spend long amounts of time during the day with his newborn. However, sometimes dads are back to work sooner than moms, and end up spending less time in the NICU, and perhaps only in the evening. Their source of information may be secondhand from mom, and they may not have the same opportunities to ask questions of the attending medical staff.

Gender roles may be at play that affect family dynamics. Stress related to providing for a small, ill newborn may manifest in fathers as a strong, stoic exterior. They may not express fears or anxieties to avoid causing mom more stress. They may feel less important than mom and take a backseat to caring for the baby (Ireland, Khashu, Cescutti-Butler, van Teijlingen, & Hewitt-Taylor, 2016).

Postpartum depression can occur in fathers; they are at higher risk if mother is experiencing depression. Their symptoms may be different than mothers' due to the stigma and cultural norms. They may be tired, may not sleep well, may become irritable, and may lose the ability to concentrate. Substance abuse is another risk of paternal postpartum depression. Improvement in the recognition of paternal postpartum depression could result in improved support and treatment. More work is needed on this subject (Biebel & Alikhan, 2016).

As soon as possible, P.R. should be assisted in providing skin-to-skin care for his newborn. Kangaroo care is therapeutic not only for baby, but also for P.R. Per a report by Varela, Tessier, Tarabulsy, and Pierce (2017), while participating in skin-to-skin with their premature baby for the first time, fathers experienced a significant reduction in the physiological stress responses of lower blood pressure and cortisol levels. They concluded that enabling fathers to experience their first intimate contact with their newborn is an important NICU practice.

REFERENCES

Biebel, K., & Alikhan, S. (2016). Paternal postpartum depression. *Journal of Parent and Family Mental Health, 1*(1), 1. Retrieved from https://escholarship.umassmed.edu/parentandfamily/vol1/iss1/1

Ireland, J., Khashu, M., Cescutti-Butler, L., van Teijlingen, E., & Hewitt-Taylor, J. (2016). Experiences of fathers with babies admitted to neonatal care units: A review of the literature. *Journal of Neonatal Nursing, 22*(4), 171–176. doi:10.1016/j.jnn.2016.01.006

Varela, N., Tessier, R., Tarabulsy, G., & Pierce, T. (2017). Cortisol and blood pressure levels decreased in fathers during the first hour of skin-to-skin contact with their premature babies. *Acta Paediatrica, 107*(4), 628–632. doi:10.1111/apa.14184

REFERENCES

Lee, S. K., & O'Brien, K. (2014). Parents as primary caregivers in the neonatal intensive care unit. *Canadian Medical Association Journal, 186*(11), 845–847. doi:10.1503/cmaj.130818

Mosher, S. (2017). Comprehensive NICU parental education: Beyond baby basics. *Neonatal Network, 36*(1), 18–25. doi:10.1891/0730-0832.36.1.18

Obeidat, H. M., Bond, E. A., & Callister, L. C. (2009). The parental experience of having an infant in the newborn intensive care unit. *Journal of Perinatal Education, 18*(3), 23–29. doi:10.1624/105812409X461199

Wigert, H., Blom, M. D., & Bry, K. (2014). Parents' experiences of communication with neonatal intensive-care unit staff: An interview study. *BMC Pediatrics, 14*(1), 304. doi:10.1186/s12887-014-0304-5

SUPPORTING FAMILIES IN THE NICU

6

When families are in the NICU, "parents usually feel powerless and helpless; therefore, they may be more stressed and vulnerable to emotional difficulties than parents of full term babies" (Ionio et al., 2016, "Introduction" section). It is, therefore, incredibly important for staff to make it a priority to find ways to support families throughout the entire NICU stay to help reduce their stress and anxiety. One way that staff can reduce levels of worry and apprehension is through a unit culture of true family-centered developmental care. This type of philosophy "incorporates respect, information, choice, flexibility, empowerment, collaboration, and support into all levels of service delivery" (Cooper et al., 2007, "Introduction" section) and "incorporates the family fundamentally and consistently into the care of their baby, recognizing parents as important collaborative members of the NICU team and embracing their roles as facilitators of their baby's development" (Craig et al., 2015, "Summary" section). When parents are intimately involved in their child's care and feel empowered as a member of the care team, they feel more involved and included, which reduces their levels of anxiety and stress.

Sounds easy right? NICU staff should universally adopt family-centered developmental supportive care. Well, unfortunately although the concept of family-centered developmental care has been widely accepted and endorsed by many organizations, including the American Academy of Pediatrics, "gaps have been demonstrated between the goals of family-centered care and its actual practice" (Craig et al., 2015, "Background" section). Although there are many reasons for this, one of the primary reasons comes down to staff education. When looking at professional schools' curricula, there is very little emphasis placed on how to provide psychosocial support for patients and families, and staff are not prepared to handle the challenges of supporting NICU families who are in distress.

There are some ways that staff can receive education on family support topics and they include conferences, webinars, medical journals, unit-based education, and online education.

Conferences:

When looking at conferences for example, there is an annual Gravens Conference that is in collaboration with the March of Dimes. This conference is held every spring in Clearwater Beach, Florida, and the primary focus is always NICU Family Support topics due to the collaboration with the March of Dimes National NICU Family Support Program. Other National NICU nursing organizations also have NICU support topics presented at their annual conferences, so nurses can attend breakout sessions to hear specific topics that are of interest to them and that are focused on family developmental care practices.

Webinars:

Online webinars are available frequently and Dandle-LION is an organization that offers NICU Family Support topics fairly exclusively. The Family Advocacy Network, which is collaboration between The National Perinatal Association (NPA) and The Preemie Parent Alliance, is also another great option for finding quarterly webinar educational opportunities for family support topics. Taking time to search the Internet will provide additional opportunities for family-centered care webinars from various organizations.

Journals:

Reputable medical journals offer continuing education credits for professionals in many of their publications. Even if credits are not available, articles themselves provide wonderful up-to-date information and best practice recommendations. Professionals should be encouraged to spend time reading journals in their specialty field. A helpful way to encourage this practice is to have units and organizations purchase annual subscriptions to specialty journals that are delivered to the unit directly so that staff can read through the journals during breaks and meals in the lounge or break room.

Unit-Based Education:

Many NICU departments hold unit-based education opportunities for their staff throughout the year in which family-centered developmental care topics can be presented. These opportunities might include staff meetings, annual skills day, topic-specific online learning modules, simulation training, and even outside organization–sponsored training held on-site. For example, when purchased by an organization, the March of Dimes NICU Family Support Program offers staff training on-site for all staff who provide care to NICU families in the organization. Hand to Hold is another organization that offers a license program that hospitals can purchase, and when a hospital embeds its support program for families, it has staff training opportunities available to help educate on the importance of family support.

Online Education:

Online education has been around for quite some time, and many nurses use this technology to advance their careers and obtain higher degrees to further their education and knowledge. Unfortunately, there are few options for NICU-specific family-centered care courses. The Institute for Patient- and Family-Centered Care and the Institute for Healthcare Improvement both have some options for education, but they are not specific to the neonatal population. That has been the reality until very recently, however. Read on to see how this known gap is being addressed.

BRIDGING THE GAP FOR NICU PROFESSIONALS

As previously mentioned, "although attempts are made to educate NICU staff, many feel less than fully prepared to respond to parents' distress, meet their psychosocial needs and interact with them in ways that will enhance their coping both during their NICU stay and post-discharge" (Hall, Cross, et al., 2015, "Rationale" section). With this known issue, the NPA convened and facilitated a large workgroup of multidisciplinary professionals and NICU parents who were "experts by experience" and divided participants into six core teams. These teams focused on high-priority topics, including family-centered developmental care, peer-to-peer support, mental health professionals in the NICU, palliative and bereavement care, follow-up support, and staff education and support. Each team was then tasked to produce best practice recommendations on its particular topic for NICU families. What made this work so impressive was that the workgroup consisted of over 50 members representing 22 academic institutions and 29 organizations, including 19 professional groups and 10 parent groups.

The best practice recommendations were then published, and an extensive list of respectable professional and parent organizations subsequently indicated their support. These organizations include the Academy of Neonatal Nursing, American College of Nurse-Midwives, Council of International Neonatal Nurses, Marcé Society for Perinatal Mental Health, National Association of Neonatal Nurses, National Association of Pediatric Nurse Practitioners, National Association of Perinatal Social Workers, National Association of Neonatal Therapists, National Perinatal Association, Nurse-Family Partnership, Society for Maternal-Fetal Medicine, Transcultural Nursing Society, University of North Carolina at Chapel Hill Center for Maternal and Infant Health, Canadian Premature Babies Foundation, Eden's Garden, European Foundation for the Care of Newborn Infants, Graham's Foundation, Hand to Hold, Hope for HIE, NICU Helping Hands, Postpartum Support International, Preeclampsia Foundation, Preemie Parent Alliance, Preemie World, LLC, St John's Mercy NICU Parent Support, Tiny Miracles Foundation, and the Zoe Rose Memorial Foundation.

Once the recommendations were published, the NPA took the project a step further, acting on the belief that "staff education relating to the psychosocial needs of NICU families and methods of providing support should be provided to all NICU staff. 'All NICU staff' refers to all disciplines that interact with NICU families on any level" (Hall, Cross, et al., 2015, "Recommendations for Staff Education" section); they wanted to help educate on these published recommendations. To bring these recommendations to the forefront of professional education, the NPA partnered with Patient+Family Care and The Preemie Parent Alliance in 2017 to create a course that "defines standards for education and support for NICU staff that will enable them to feel sufficiently prepared to provide psychosocial care and support" (Hall, Cross, et al., 2015, "Rationale" section) to NICU families. The course, entitled "Caring for Babies and their Families: Providing Psychosocial Support in the NICU," can be found online at www.MyNICUNetwork.com.

My NICU Network is the result of a unique collaboration between perinatal professionals and NICU graduate parents; it is the first educational program for NICU staff that we know of that has been developed by a parent–professional partnership from start to finish. The educational course is customizable to allow individual NICUs to highlight areas that are most important to them, to provide an opportunity to include unit-specific policies and practices, and to include information on local community resources and parent support programs. Content is composed of written material, videos, audio clips, and over 80 downloadable resources and links to websites with related information. NICU professionals (nurses, physicians, social workers, psychologists) who complete the course, which engages learners through an interactive discussion board with both a NICU professional and a NICU graduate parent, receive eight continuing education credits. The course can also be embraced as a key driver of quality improvement projects within NICUs that are working to improve their delivery of comprehensive family support.

Online education has many benefits for staff in that the content can be completed at times that are convenient for the participant, can be worked on at any time of day or night for shift employees, is easy to access at work or at home, and allows students to revisit topics that are either of high interest to them or that they wish to gain further confidence with.

Organizations should place high priority on staff education, regardless of the method because "educating all staff and providing them with tools to better understand parents' needs, to provide culturally effective family-centered care and to enhance their communication skills can both decrease parents' risks to experience perinatal mood and anxiety disorders and increase parents' satisfaction with their NICU experience" (Hall, Cross, et al., 2015, "Summary" section).

NEONATAL INTENSIVE PARENTING UNIT

Once all staff are fully educated and ready to embrace family-centered developmental care, the next paradigm shift that should be a focus for units is to create what is being called a Neonatal Intensive Parenting Unit, or an NIPU. An NIPU is a very relationship-based culture in which "partnerships are based on the premise that intensive parenting should begin as soon as possible and be interrupted only when absolutely necessary" (Hall, Cross, et al., 2017, "Introduction" section). Dr. Hall and her colleagues identify that "research indicates the potentially better practices should lead to improved outcomes for NIPU babies, better mental health outcomes for their parents, and enhanced well-being of staff" (Hall, Hynan, et al., 2017, "Potentially Better Practices" section), which also equates to higher patient satisfaction scores, making organizations happier as well.

Within an NIPU, potentially better practices include the following:

1. Provide family support, including a consultation during an antepartum stay or as soon as a potential NICU stay is identified.

2. Provide a compassionate and culturally appropriate welcome into the NICU, including signage, limited medical terms, easy-to-understand written material, and parental access to their baby 24/7.

3. Treat parents as full partners of the care team.

4. Teach all staff about the fundamentals of family-centered developmental care.

5. Ensure that babies and parents are united as early and frequently as possible after delivery.

6. Provide services of neonatal therapies, including occupational therapy, physical therapy, and speech therapy to mentor parents on the importance of neuroprotective developmental care.

7. Educate parents on how to read and understand their baby's cues.

8. Provide parents with written and verbal information about the benefits of early and frequent skin-to-skin care.

9. Offer skin-to-skin care to all members of the family.

10. Provide parents information about swaddled bathing.

11. Increase the parent's engagement in all caregiving activities.

12. Offer various peer-to-peer support activities at various times of the day, with childcare and food free of charge.

13. Have a paid parent mentor coordinator on staff.

14. Include siblings as integral members of the family.

15. Include grandparents and extended family members as part of the family-support network.

16. Have a comfortable place within the unit so that families can seek respite away from their baby's bedside.

17. Have an educational library available for families where they can receive reliable educational information at their fingertips.

18. Have mental health professionals on staff and available for families (includes social workers, psychologists, and family-support specialists).

19. Screen all parents for postpartum depression and posttraumatic stress disorder and refer to professional support as needed.

20. Include family members as equal members of the multidisciplinary rounds team.

21. Hold shift change at the bedside and include family members in shift change report.

22. Include graduate family members in advisory councils that include unit policies and procedures.

It is extremely important to understand that "the NIPU is not a static system; it will be a dynamic, evolving place where new evidence-based better practice recommendations continue to be introduced and tested to determine what works best" (Hall, Hynan, et al., 2017, "Summary" section). Yet, as long as the unit gets started, the unit culture will begin and continue to develop and evolve to become one in which families feel like valued and supported members of the care team.

Figure 6.1 shows the six primary focus areas of what makes up the optimal NIPU, developed by Dr. Hall and her colleagues.

We have already discussed family-centered developmental care and staff education and support in this chapter, and later in this text, we look more closely at palliative and bereavement care, as well as postdischarge follow-up care. In the following paragraphs, we focus on the areas of peer-to-peer support and the availability of mental health professionals to NICU families.

Peer-to-peer support should be a substantial focus for any unit because "parents who receive peer support have been found to have increased confidence and well-being, problem-solving capacity and adaptive coping, perception of social support, self esteem and acceptance of their situation. Further, parents feel more empowered and interact with, nurture and care for their infants to a greater degree during more frequent visits to the hospital, leading to a shorter length of stay for their infants" (Hall, Ryan, Beatty, & Grubbs, 2015, "Introduction" section). Peer-to-peer mentors, whether they are paid or volunteer positions, should be trained to appropriately and compassionately share their experiences while creating a safe and nonjudgmental space for families in which they can share their fears and ask their questions. Support by peer mentors can be provided in many ways, including on the telephone, during social group events, in support group meetings, one-on-one in person meetings, or through an Internet platform.

That is not to say, however, that professional mental health support does not have its place in the NICU. As noted, numerous times, "research studies have documented elevated levels of emotional distress in parents during the hospitalization of their baby in a neonatal intensive care unit and thereafter" (Hynan, Steinberg, et al., 2015, "Background" section), and some families benefit from professional mental health support to cope with stress and emotional turmoil during the NICU journey. In fact, it is now recommended that "all NICUs with 20 or more beds [should] have at least one full-time master's level social worker

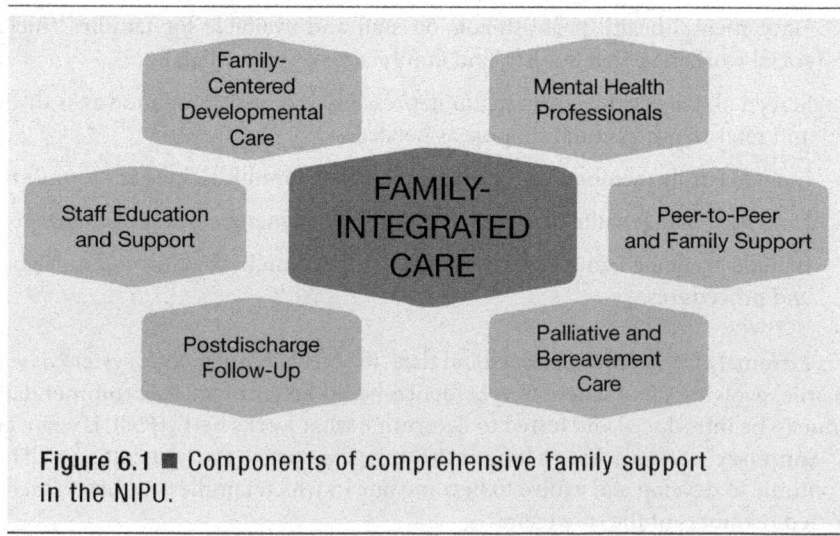

Figure 6.1 ■ Components of comprehensive family support in the NIPU.

and one full-time or part-time doctoral level psychologist embedded in the NICU staff. NICUs should also consider having full-time or part-time psychiatrists and psychiatric nurses on staff" (Hynan, Steinberg, et al., 2015, "Recommendations for NICU" section).

With layered levels of support, from bedside caregivers who are trained and educated on how to provide psychosocial support to NICU families, family-support specialists, social workers, peer-to-peer mentors, and psychologists, NICU families receive the appropriate level of emotional and mental health support they need when they need it to make their journey as positive and as stress free as possible. Each of these staff members has a unique role in supporting families. Yet there is one way these staff members can all help families in a unified way: encouraging families to participate in unit-sponsored activities and events because "we know that families cope so much better when they are able to connect with other families going through similar situations and when they can become a part of a community. Research is emerging as well showing the lifelong health benefits of infants who are brought up in a family whose parents are healthy both physically and emotionally" (Discenza, 2018, p. 146).

Some of the most popular peer-to-peer events include the following:

- Papa Pizza Night
  Dads get together to have pizza and mingle.

- Scrapbook Hour
  The unit prints pictures from the unit's digital camera and provides all the scrapbooks and materials. Parents come together for an hour and put together a scrapbook. This hour affords time for socialization and a time for a peer-to-peer mentor to facilitate discussion.

- Talk with a Doc
  A neonatologist spends an hour in which parents have an open discussion to freely ask questions.

- Sibling Saturday
  This is an event in which big brothers and sisters can participate in crafts and enjoy snacks while parents can mingle and meet one another.

- Walking Wednesday
  A fitness expert leads parents (and siblings) on a walk around campus for some light exercise and offers an opportunity for parents to meet one another in a casual manner.

- Massage Monday
  In a comfortable respite area on the unit, a massage therapist donates time, setting up the space with quiet music, flameless candles, healthy nonallergenic snacks, and fruit-infused water. Families are invited to relax together and rotate through 10-minute chair massages.

- Lactation Luncheon
  A lunch hour is hosted with a lactation specialist, and moms can have undivided attention from a lactation specialist and ask all the questions they have. They can

meet other moms during this time and find support among other women who are potentially struggling with the same lactation issues.

There are many other wonderful peer-to-peer support ideas, and when there is an opportunity for parents to connect with one another, "parental stress and anxiety, as well as depression, are all reduced. Peer support therefore offers a legitimate and unique form of assistance that is not typically met by the formal service system and one that cannot come from any other source" (Hall, Ryan, et al., 2015, "Abstract" section).

An additional layer of support NICU staff can provide families is to have an integrated self-care program embedded into the daily care plan for parents. As previously discussed, the N.U.R.S.E. Self Care Program is an "easy-to-follow, easy-to-teach, and easy-to-implement self care program [that] neonatal providers can feel confident providing that will foster optimal physical and emotional health for both infants and families not only in the immediate neonatal period, but also well into the future" (Mosher, 2017, para. 3). Because this program, and this topic, have already been presented and discussed, please refer to Chapter 4, Figure 4.1.

SIBLINGS IN THE NICU

"Just as it can sometimes be difficult for parents to feel like the baby's parents when the baby is hospitalized, it can also be difficult for siblings to feel like the baby's big brother or sister" (Rector, 2007, p. 30). Parents are dealing with their own stresses and anxiety, are frequently overwhelmed with information and emotions, and often do not know how to handle the emotions and questions that young siblings have. Staff in the neonatal unit need to be cognizant of the level of coping skills each family and each sibling has and realize that every child is going to handle the experience very uniquely and based on "their developmental level, maturity, temperament, past experiences, support systems, family dynamics, and cultural and religious beliefs" (Rector, 2007, p. 2).

Integrating siblings into the NICU family as an important member will help lessen the stress for families because staff will be providing some of the much-needed support and education to the siblings. When siblings arrive for the first visit, for example, they should be greeted as the big brother or sister and recognized as an important visitor in the baby's life. Parents are identified with an identification band, so siblings should also be banded with some type of big brother or big sister wristband. This not only makes them feel special, but also provides a priceless lifelong keepsake for that family. Many units provide siblings with welcome bags that often include the following:

- Sibling welcome book that talks about the NICU
- Coloring book
- Crayons
- Stuffed animal
- Crib card that they can decorate for the baby and hang up at the bedside

- Visitation certificate
- Picture frame craft to frame the first visitation photo that will be printed in the unit
- Disposable camera so that siblings can take their own photos
- Nonallergenic snack

When siblings are present in the unit, staff should include them in education and the baby's care as their age and maturity level allow. For example, siblings who are old enough should be encouraged to change diapers, take a temperature, help with swaddling, and even participate in skin-to-skin care. In fact, providing siblings with their own care checklist can be a magnificent way to help them feel empowered to partake in care and be a part of the family's care team. Participating in such activities provides an opportunity for "siblings [to] not only become acquainted with the baby but also begin a positive lifelong relationship with their new brother or sister" (Rector, 2007, p. 77).

Author's Personal Story

I met F.J. on the morning of his daughter's second day of life. I knew from my morning shift report that his daughter had been delivered the morning prior at a referring hospital at 26 2/7 weeks' gestation and was transferred to our NICU immediately after resuscitation and stabilization. F.J. accompanied the transport team in the helicopter and had been with his daughter throughout the day and a good portion of the night, before leaving to check in to the local Ronald McDonald house located on our hospital property. F.J.'s wife had delivered via C-section, so she was going to have to wait another day to come to the unit to reunite with her daughter.

F.J. was not present for morning bedside report, but the off-going nurse and I performed report at the bedside regardless, and I made sure we updated the dry erase board in the room with all of the names of the new care team members for the day, updated the date, and included my care goals. I performed the patient's assessment, completed all documentation, completed her feeding, and got her all tucked in nicely. Just as I walked into the hall, F.J. started to walk toward me. I did not recognize him, as I had not met him yet, but I had cared for my other patient many times in the past, so I knew by the process of elimination that this was her father. I introduced myself and took him into his daughter's room.

As I oriented him to the dry erase board and introduced the care team for the day, I made sure to inform him of what my particular goals were for the day. I then asked him what goals he had for the day. I was a little surprised to hear that his goal was to learn how to get his phone to stop buzzing. He shared with me that they recently moved to the West Coast from the East Coast, and all of his friends and family lived out of the area and were calling and texting him all night long wanting updates. He felt obligated

(*continued*)

(*continued*)

to respond to them, but he had gotten very little sleep because his phone was going off nonstop all night long as people were checking in. I wrote this as a goal on the board and assured him we would tackle the issue together that day and figure out a way to alleviate that stressor. I asked F.J. if he liked coffee and he said yes; I told him I would be back momentarily. We happened to have a respite area for families where coffee and tea were available for them during the day, and I went and grabbed a cup of coffee and a side of cream and sugar for him. He looked extremely tired, and I thought he might enjoy some caffeine to help wake him up.

Once I returned and he was enjoying his beverage, I updated him on his daughter's condition and how she did during the night. He made a comment that he wished his wife could see how great she was doing. I asked if she had seen her yet, and he said "no" with a little bit of sassiness to his voice. I sensed it was as if he felt I should know the answer to that question already. While I knew she had not physically seen her daughter yet, I wondered, however, if he had used his cell phone or if our unit tablet had been used to allow mom to connect and see her daughter. I explained this to F.J., and he said that she had not. He told me he never even thought about using their phones to video chat. I told him I would encourage him to do so, and if he wanted to do that during the next care time, I would love to participate in the conversation, walk both him and his wife through the assessment, and explain everything I was seeing and what everything meant.

An hour later, F.J. had his wife on the phone, and the three of us were talking and going through their daughter's head-to-toe assessment on their phone. It was a great way to connect with F.J.'s wife, despite our geographical separation. It was also a great way for the two of them to connect as a couple and her as a mother to her daughter. I spent 30 minutes talking with both F.J. and his wife in this manner, and it allowed us all to have time to get to know one another better and for me to answer any question that they had. One thing that was a distraction, however, was how many times F.J.'s phone buzzed with a phone call or a text.

As soon as we ended the conversation with F.J.'s wife, I sat F.J. down and started to address his concern for the day. I walked him through the suggestion of starting a social media site where he and his wife could post daily, hourly, or minute updates of their daughter's condition for all of their family and friends; those individuals could refer to the site for updates rather than calling him. I told him that he could use the hospital as the "bad guy" and tell them we do not allow cell phones in the unit if he felt that would deter people from bothering him. I informed him that many parents use Facebook, CaringBridge, or Share Your Story as platforms to create private pages to share with family and friends, and he immediately asked if I had a computer he could use. I escorted him to our family respite area, where we had the coffee and tea available, an educational lending library, couches and seats, nonallergenic snacks, and a computer where families could research medical information or post social medial updates like he was interested in doing.

(*continued*)

(*continued*)

Not long after I left F.J. in the respite area, he returned to his daughter's room with a smile. He felt very accomplished and informed me that he sent the link to every single person he knew. He was very grateful for the suggestion. He was also grateful for the bottle of water that was waiting for him and was surprised that I'd noticed he hadn't had anything to drink since his morning cup of coffee. I then sat him down and told him that it was really important for him to take care of himself. So often we hear that the best way to take care of others is to take care of ourselves first, but we often don't abide by that rule. I emphasized to him that having an extremely premature baby in the NICU is a stressful and overwhelming experience and that being healthy and well cared for was going to be key for him to be able to cope and to care for both his wife and daughter. I provided him with the N.U.R.S.E. tool, and together we created simple and very realistic goals for the first few days. I made a copy that we could place on the dry erase board so that other staff members could review it and encourage him along the way.

Later that afternoon, F.J. had to leave to go pick up his son from daycare, which closed at 6 p.m. He said that he was scared about what to tell his son about his sister. He knew his mom was having trouble, but they hadn't told him yet that she had the baby. He asked a lot of questions that morning before school, and he was very worried about his mom because she hadn't come home that night. He asked if I had any advice. I did, but I also knew I was not the best person to share that type of advice. He had 30 minutes before he had to leave, so I quickly called our social worker and our unit psychologist, and both came down to talk to F.J. The team spoke to him and provided him some wonderful ideas on how to talk to his son, and offered to be present at the first sibling visit, whenever he and his wife felt it was the right time to bring him in.

The first visit happened to be the following day when mom was discharged from the hospital and was able to come to the hospital for the first time herself. Her son had been acting out at daycare and the teacher called F.J. and asked him to come pick his son up from daycare for the rest of the day. So, F.J. went to pick him up and then picked up his wife from the hospital and aided in her discharge. As soon as all of the paperwork was signed, they were out of the door of that hospital and walking into the doors of ours.

I was honored to be working again that day, and was assigned to take care of baby J. I got to meet F.J.'s wife and son in person, and when the son arrived at the handwashing station, I started to show him how to properly wash his hands and why it was so important to keep our hands clean and free of germs. He cut me off mid-sentence, however, and decided to tell *me* how to properly wash my hands and why it was important to keep hands clean around small babies; he promptly and properly performed hand hygiene to the World Health Organization standards. I was quite impressed.

When we entered the unit, I verified both dad and mom's wrist band identification, and banded brother with a big brother band. I also handed him our Sibling Welcome packet. He was excited to get something, but I could tell he was more excited to meet his sister. When we entered the room, I had the digital camera ready to go so I could capture

(*continued*)

(*continued*)

photos of their first meeting. The lights were dimmed, and, unfortunately, when I took the first picture, the flash went off; F.J.'s son looked at me very sternly and in a loud whisper said, "Turn the flash off! That is too bright for my little baby sister!" I knew right then and there that this 6-year-old boy was going to be a very protective, very mature, and very loving big brother.

Over the next several months, the family was encouraged to participate in all aspects of care as they felt comfortable and as they were able. F.J. was the primary source of income for their family, so he returned to work several days after his daughter was born and came to visit in the evening after work, and his wife would visit during the day when their son was at school and after school daycare. They rarely came to visit together, except when the unit offered Sibling Saturday events or peer-to-peer events with free childcare. As mentioned previously, they recently had moved to the area, so they did not have family or friends to rely on to help with childcare. Both sets of grandparents had decided to wait and come when the baby had gone home so they could help more; therefore, these parents were on their own during this extremely stressful time. The social worker and family-support specialist helped them set up a Meal Train account, encouraged them to find a very inexpensive housekeeper who offered discounts to NICU families in the area, helped them with some financial aid applications, connected them with community resources, and even found transportation assistance for them when they wanted to leave the Ronald McDonald House and travel back home for a few days.

This family had a very small and fragile infant who needed meticulous medical care to survive. Yet they also required attentive psychosocial support to cope through their stressful journey, and with proper training and support, our NICU staff was able to provide that with ease very successfully.

Family Story

Up until this point, all of the family stories that have been shared have been quite positive and families have fond memories of how staff responded to their situations. It's important to know, however, that despite best intentions and best efforts by staff, the words and actions by providers are not always received well by families. Despite having goals to provide the best care, both medically and psychosocially, to families, not all families are going to feel that they received the best care by all providers. This chapter highlights some experiences that were less than amazing; I feel that these stories are really important for NICU staff to hear, not because I feel anyone did anything wrong, but because I think it is such a good reminder to us all that our words, our behaviors, and our actions affect every family so differently and that we need to be aware that our impact is lifelong on these families.

(*continued*)

(continued)

The first story is from Riki Court, who delivered a little boy at 27 weeks. What I love in her story is how she highlights how she learned to advocate for her baby through the support she received.

"My experience with the NICU was scary and wonderful all at the same time. My water broke at 22 weeks and I stayed at the hospital from that point on, until I delivered at 27 weeks. At the time I thought for sure I would never forget any details of my hospital stay or my NICU experience. I was wrong. Four years later and certain pieces of the puzzle are a little fuzzy at best. What I do remember is being talked to by many people over and over again about the probability of me delivering well before 38 weeks. I was told that anything before 24 weeks was more than likely not able to survive, and anything less than 32 weeks was going to be a real challenge for my baby boy. I was offered to go to the NICU a couple of times prior to delivering to see where my baby would be living, but in my mind that meant I was setting fate up and we would surely go there. I guess you could say like a jinx. I was given a couple of books. One in particular was about the weekly growth of the fetus. I remember reading that book and crying, and hoping, and then deep down determining that no matter what my baby would not just survive, but he would thrive! The power of positive thoughts and the love and support of my husband and family kept me from going insane.

"The night my son was born I remember having a C-section and when he was delivered there were no baby cries. All was quiet but the diligence of the doctors quietly communicating to one another. The doctor looked at my husband and asked him if he would like to follow them to the NICU. I knew it would be a while before I was done being put back together, and with the uncertainty of Isaiah's fate, I told him to go be with our son. He leaned down and kissed me, and then I was alone, except not. I was in a room full of strangers who had literally seen me from the inside out. I was wheeled back to my room shortly after, and there I waited for what seemed like forever. I can't tell you if Josh (my husband) was in my room when I arrived or if he came in shortly after. What I do remember is being told that as soon as my son was stable they would wheel me to the NICU to see my precious baby.

"The doctor came in and the look on his face had me extremely worried. He stated at this time Isaiah was really struggling and things were looking grim. He wanted to prepare us for the worst. After that, things were kind of a blur. Between the anxiety and the drugs from the C-section I was feeling pretty out of it. I know I had nurses come in and talk to me about what to expect when I went into the NICU. Finally, about 3 hours after delivery, the doctor came to my room and told my husband and me that Isaiah had finally stabilized. I was then informed that Isaiah weighed in at 1 lb 13 oz and barely measured 13 inches. He was on a breathing machine and would remain on it for a couple of days. He said it was a miracle that Isaiah pulled through, and the nurses agreed. I was told that when my water broke at 22 weeks, I lost a lot of amniotic fluid, and although my son was born at 27 weeks, his lungs were developed closer at the 23-week range. I was wheeled in my hospital bed down to my son's NICU room. I will never forget going

(continued)

(*continued*)

into this small, dimly lit room with machines everywhere. I wondered how my hospital bed would fit in his little room. I peered into his little incubator and through all the tubes and wires I saw the tiniest baby I had ever witnessed. The breathing ventilator machine he was attached to was so loud. In fact, I couldn't even hear my own sobbing over the ventilator. We took pictures and videos of our new baby, said our prayers, and then they wheeled me back to my room.

"Over the course of the next few days, I was introduced to the nurses on shift. They were warm and inviting to me. They explained what they were doing and why it was being done. I was told that there would come a time in the near future for me and my husband to help with his care. That would include baths, diaper, and clothes being changed. It all seemed so far away in the future as I hadn't even had a chance to hold my precious boy. It took nine long days before I was even offered to hold him. I had no idea what the protocol for holding something so tiny would be. I was afraid to ask and didn't want to seem selfish or controlling. On the ninth day I was struggling with my emotions. I remember feeling like such a failure for not doing what a woman is supposed to do. I wanted this baby, I planned for this baby, I changed my whole life (eating habits and daily exercise) to give this baby the best possible chance ever, and I still failed. The nurse on shift must have observed my demeanor. I had his little peephole open and I was slowly caressing his tiny translucent hand. She asked me so casually if I would like to hold my little guy. Yes, of course I did!

"For me, the lack of clarity of knowing what requirements were needed to have that first initial contact did not sit well with me. On the one hand, I was so grateful to finally hold him, on the other hand, I kept thinking what made today special? His stats were about the same as the last few previous days. Perhaps if I had been one of those demanding parents I would have gotten my way. I feel like I tried so hard not to be in the way or bothersome of the professionals who cared for my precious baby that I allowed my own needs to be neglected. I assumed when the time was right the opportunity to hold my child would be offered. I had heard of families who made the nurses lives difficult while caring for their preemies, questioning and arguing over the smallest of detail; I did not want to be *that* person. Sure, I asked questions. I was often asked how I felt about the procedures that were happening on a daily basis and the staff talked about the routine of care that would be given from day to day. I was asked on my opinion how I felt my child was being cared for, but I also respected the opinions of the nurses and doctors who saved my baby and didn't feel the need to second-guess them. I felt like they were competent caregivers, and I already had so much on my plate to worry about. Looking back and knowing what I know now, I wish I would have asked sooner if I could hold my baby.

"I was lucky enough to stay at the Ronald McDonald house on the same premises as that of the hospital. I had an advantage of being at the hospital with my baby every day for hours at a time. I made sure to make my presence known in the hospital by communicating with the nurses, doctors, therapists, and even the janitors. I took every opportunity to know when Isaiah's care team would be around and to talk to them and ask questions. I believe that by making myself available I was able to advocate for my tiny baby. Most

(*continued*)

(*continued*)

important, I believed in his care team. I trusted them. I allowed them to provide the care needed without interference because I knew that I alone could not save him. By putting my pride and fear aside and continually discussing the health of my child every day without antagonizing the professionals, I was able to stay informed. I think the biggest thing I stood firm on is having the hospital allow my daughter to be able to see her baby brother. The NICU has a firm policy of no small children in the rooms of the preemies. Understandably, preemies need a quiet and calm atmosphere. At the time my daughter was four, almost five. She was incredibly smart and mature for her age. She was so well behaved in the NICU. She was also one of the few children who got to be included through the whole experience. I talked to staff, managers, and supervisors about the importance of allowing her to be able to see her brother. We had no options for her other than to be with us at all times. We were staying two towns away just to be near our son full time, and not having our daughter with us was not an option. I am so thankful that Nevaeh was able to spend time with her baby brother in the NICU. She has a bond with her brother like I don't see often among siblings. I know that my children are close because she was able to be a part of her brother's NICU experience and to partake in his everyday hospital care. We did not shelter her from his condition because we did not know if he would survive and she loved her brother. She had a right to know about his progress.

"As a family we helped with Isaiah's care. Nevaeh, Josh, and myself gave him baths with the assistance of the nurses. I was encouraged to nurse him and have plenty of skin-to-skin contact with him. These moments are what a parent draws strength from. I often sat in his room listening quietly to Christian music, holding his tiny body next to mine and trying to convince myself that this was all going to be okay. Usually, I was able to stay optimistic. Picking out his outfits (once he was big enough to wear them), changing his diapers, feeding him, and taking family pictures with him brought a sense of normality to what was such a crazy and traumatizing situation. Evenings were always my favorite. The bedtime routine of bath time, feeding, and snuggles got me through the day. I was so fortunate to really have a relationship with Isaiah's nurses. And in the evenings, it was always a little easier to have a normal conversation with the men and women who looked over my sweet boy.

"Although my experience with the hospital staff was warm and nurturing, I cannot say the same for my husband. I am not sure what the stigma is with men at the hospital. I can honestly say that my husband bears the brunt of a lot of being overlooked as a parental figure. Often times, he wasn't acknowledged when we were together and talking to a health team about Isaiah's health and care. It took a while for the staff to warm up to him. It wasn't with all staff members but enough to make him feel uncomfortable and unwanted. I can't tell you if it had to do with his appearance (he has tattoos, shaved head, and a goatee) or perhaps it's because some men don't take an equal share in raising their children, but he was hurt and confused at first. I was determined to make him a part of whatever plan we decided to make and to not allow staff to undermine his concerns or his share of care with Isaiah. I tried to make it clear that *we* (my husband and I) would

(*continued*)

(continued)

discuss options and make decisions together. It was equally important for Josh to have a connection and bond with our son. Those small moments of care and cuddles are really all a parent has to look forward to when staying in the NICU. I realize that as the woman, it is my choice and everyone is concerned for the mother to have a strong connection with the child, but it is just as important for the father. I know I have the final say, since it's my body and all that jazz, but as a wife, life partner, and mother my decision affects my entire family. I strongly recommend a support group for dads. I was offered lots of venues to share my thoughts and feelings. I was very lucky to have such a strong family-support system. I often got together with some of the other mothers from the NICU. I had an outlet. I think in situations such as children being born sick and frail, it is important to not forget about the dads. Dads are expected to be strong and protective of their family, but in a circumstance where the dad cannot protect his child, then he too will feel vulnerable.

"Overall, I have a healthy son who is now 4½ years old. The 'what if 's' and 'wish I could have's' are over. I do not take for granted the care and attention that was given to him. I have nothing but the upmost admiration for the team that sought after my boy in his most critical time of need. We are so fortunate to have gone through this experience and come out the other side victorious. I am forever grateful to the staff who saved my son's life."

A second parent story is from Marianne Wolf who shares a story about being involved in rounds.

"My experience with the NICU all began on a weekend in the middle of July 2015. My little family of five took a road trip to Grandma's house in Utah. I was just short of 33 weeks and my pregnancy was healthy and uneventful. With the okay from my doctor we left California for a last family vacation before the baby was born. The drive was smooth sailing. and we made it 10 hours later. The next day was Sunday and we were getting ready for church. I bent down to pick up something and felt my pants get wet suddenly. This was odd and surprising, but with the task of getting three kids dressed and out the door, I quickly pushed the idea out of my mind. I mean, I'm pregnant right? Sometimes we leak. I didn't notice anything else for the rest of the day until we went on a family walk after dinner. I had only gotten in front of the neighbor's house when my pants felt wet again. I quickly ran inside and changed my clothes. I started to feel a bit nervous because this couldn't be happening on our vacation. I wanted to be sure my water had broken and the only way I could know for sure was using the bathroom and waiting to hear the trickle of water after I was done going. My fear was confirmed that night during our rousing family card game. I couldn't ignore it anymore. My water had broken; I was almost 33 weeks along, in a different state, and needed to go to the hospital. I told my family and they quickly jumped up and got a hospital bag ready for me. Side note: My family has experience. My sister's water broke with her fourth child when they were visiting out of state at 32 weeks. We all pitched in to care for her three kids while she was on bed rest at the hospital. At least I knew my kids were in great hands!

"My husband and I went to the hospital and went straight to Labor and Delivery and got admitted. Of course, the nurse had to verify that my membranes had ruptured, and

(continued)

(*continued*)

then of course the contractions began. They weren't going to stop my labor despite being 7 weeks early. Luckily, the contractions ended on their own, and I was moved to a room where the goal was to get me to 34 weeks. I was able to stay on bed rest the following week and had a scheduled C-section since my baby was breech.

"Spencer was born July 27, a late Monday night. I remember hearing my little baby boy cry as he was born and quickly passed into the NICU. He was 4 lb 15 oz and 18 inches long. I was able to see him briefly as the nurses wheeled my bed into the NICU after my surgery. He was perfect!

"I was able to see him again the following afternoon, and he had a feeding tube in his nose. I was able to nurse him and was encouraged to pump to get my milk supply going. My husband left me to tend to my three other kids and try to work. My job was to recover and see Spencer as much as I could. On Wednesday morning, I found Spencer connected to a lot more equipment. He was having trouble breathing and was put on CPAP. I was shocked, especially when there was no sign of his struggle the day before. I stayed with Spencer a lot that day and gave him lots of skin-to-skin time. I suddenly found myself watching his oxygen levels and heartbeat constantly. They fluctuated so much during the day. As the day progressed, Spencer's condition did not seem to be improving. The nurses were very kind and were quick to come to his aid when he seemed to struggle. I knew his condition was serious by all of the machines and attention he was getting, but I never felt afraid of possibly losing him.

"Thursday morning, I learned that his condition worsened in the night. When I arrived that morning, I learned that Spencer's breathing struggles had developed into a pneumothorax outside his left lung. The size of it and the pressure it was causing on other organs was a great concern. Early that morning, the doctor decided to put a chest tube into the top of his left side. I wasn't contacted about the procedure and learned it had happened only when I arrived. I believe the doctor had to act quickly and had finished the procedure only 30 minutes before I arrived. Had I been told, I'm sure it would have saved me from the shock I experienced and given me time to process what was happening. When I found Spencer, he was surrounded by more machines, was sedated, and had an additional band around his face to hold his mouth shut. I was told that putting the tube into Spencer had been more stressful on him because the doctor had to do the procedure before the pain medication had taken effect. He looked as helpless as I felt. I couldn't even hold him now with the chest tube. I wasn't upset that the doctor had acted without telling me. I felt very relieved that Spencer was in such good hands and really felt like all things were done for his best interest and care. I think my biggest struggle was processing the reality of Spencer's condition. But no one is ever prepared for these little surprises in life.

"Later that morning, Spencer's nurse approached me and informed me that the medical staff was gathering for Spencer's rounds meeting in a few minutes. She told me it was where I could listen and learn more about what was being done for Spencer, especially with the most recent procedure and pneumothorax. I had a few minutes to gather my thoughts and prepared myself to hear more of how serious Spencer's condition was. We met at the

(*continued*)

(*continued*)

nurses' station just outside of Spencer's room, since it was a centralized location to all of the patients. As I entered, the doctor approached me and introduced himself. He led me to a chair and introduced the members of the staff who were attending as they entered. I remember feeling relief and awe as I realized just how many people were here on Spencer's team. The doctor led the discussion and asked for a report from everyone in attendance. As I sat in the rounds and listened about the medication Spencer had, his nutrition, what the latest x-ray showed, occupational therapies, and concerns the nurses had, it was then that a new realization of Spencer's struggle came to me. The discussion continued to review Spencer's current state and what would happen that day to help him get better. The doctor turned and asked if I had any questions for the staff. I couldn't think of any as they had thoroughly explained what had been done and what needed to happen. He then excused the staff and asked me how I was doing. I told him that I was alright. And then he looked me squarely in the eye and said, 'Your little boy is very sick, but he's going to make it. He is our top priority.' I thanked him and returned to Spencer's room. The weight I felt was very heavy. This was a very serious situation. But I knew he was in great hands, the best care. I gave Spencer a kiss, took a deep breath, and left the NICU. I didn't feel like there was much I could do and I needed some time away to process. The long journey back to my hospital room was especially slow since I was finally walking the entire distance after my C-section and I did all I could to keep myself together. Once I got to my room, I sat down and turned on the TV for the first time since I had been staying at the hospital. After some lunch and a nap, I visited Spencer again and spent the rest of the evening at his side, much more comfortable with the machines and more aware of the care he was in.

"That was the only rounds meeting I attended during my NICU experience. I believe I was able to attend the meeting in the first place because I happened to be there at the right time. I was never told about rounds in the future. I'm sure it may have been that once I was discharged, I visited the hospital only to get a couple of feedings in. It may also have been that Spencer's health improved and we were moved to another NICU room. I did have meetings with the nurse over Spencer daily to hear what progress he made and what goals they were aiming for that day. Although I attended only one rounds meeting, I felt very much included in Spencer's care and am grateful I was able to meet the team that was going to help my baby get better. It was very humbling to see a team of professionals offer their concern and care for strangers and do all they could to help Spencer. I learned over the next 2 weeks what a big deal little victories are. He was able to get off all breathing machines a week after his delivery. Spencer left the NICU August 13th.

"In the end, we left California for a week-long vacation and came back 6 weeks later with a new baby. It was an exciting and stressful journey for our young family, but I am so grateful for the care Spencer received during his first few weeks of life. I know things happen for a reason and am grateful for the timing in Spencer's birth. Yes, it was inconvenient and a struggle being out of network and out of state, but I was surrounded by my family and the best care."

(*continued*)

(continued)

Maggie Fluck, who had an experience of her child being transported to another hospital, shares what that was like for her in addition to the added stress of being in the midst of lactating.

"Our daughter, Rachel, was born at 30 weeks. Only a few days before she was born did we find out she had duodenal atresia and Down syndrome. That was an emotional upheaval in itself, but she was also close to death at delivery because of a placental abruption and required a great deal of intervention to bring her back. She was born at our local level-three NICU hospital but needed to be transported to another hospital for her eventual surgery. Four days after her birth, the day of my discharge and the day my milk decided to come in, we walked into our house only to receive a call to immediately come back because they were packing Rachel up for transfer. I needed to pump, but I had no time. Back we went to the hospital, a 20-minute drive, to say goodbye to her and then back into our car to follow the ambulance for 45 minutes to the next hospital. Upon getting to the new hospital, we needed to check her in at admitting. The woman who helped us showed no concern for our worry. My breasts by this time were engorged and hard as rocks. I was in such pain physically from my breasts, my caesarean, and my emotions that I cried at the table as she so slowly took our information. I believe it took over 30 minutes. She never asked us how we were or how she could help. We were first-time parents and had no gumption to demand the help that I needed at the time. I wish that woman would have taken the time to see that some care was needed and offered it to us, to me. That was our first impression of that hospital and it struck such a sour tone. Thankfully, the doctors, nurses, lactation expert, and staff redeemed the admitting office during our 60-day stay."

A final family story is from Jessica Spooner. Jessica shares her family's experience of being supported to participate in skin-to-skin care, which their hospital referred to as kangaroo care. Jessica and her husband not only participated in this practice, but even came up with a very inventive idea in the process!

"Our son was born at 27 weeks' gestation and spent 92 days in the NICU. From day 1, both my husband and I were encouraged to participate in skin-to-skin contact, or kangaroo care, as much as possible, and preferably on a daily basis. The recommendation was to spend at least three consecutive hours in kangaroo care, between my son's scheduled "cares" times, to provide the least amount of disruption to my son and his need for good sleep. My husband and I took that advice to heart and generally participated in 6 hours' worth of kangaroo care per day, 3 hours with each of us. It was pretty cute to see my tiny 27-weeker snuggled up in my husband's chest hair.

"My husband, however, with his love for coffee, sometimes had difficulty participating in kangaroo care for the whole 3 hours without stopping for a bathroom break. Because he wanted to comply with the 3-hour minimum recommendation, he requested a "portable loo" to urinate in so he wouldn't have to stop kangaroo care. Now that's dedication! This

(continued)

(*continued*)

wound up being quite the joke in the NICU; I'm not sure anyone else has ever made such a request in the NICU!

"When we left the NICU after 92 days, we dropped off a poem of our story, complete with stickers of my husband's head on a kangaroo. We thought it would be hilarious if my husband marketed his own Kangaroo Care Portable Potty."

> *The nurses said "It's important to kangaroo"*
> *It's good for his brain and development too*
> *But three whole hours you must do*
> *To ensure baby gets his sleep too*
> *But what, oh what, is a dad to do*
> *When nature calls halfway through?*
> *Do not worry, do not be blue*
> *The nurses can fetch you a portable loo*
> *You'll feel fine, as good as new,*
> *Once you've used Cory's Kangaroo Loo*
>
> —*Spooner Family*

RECOMMENDATIONS/SUGGESTIONS FOR BEST PRACTICE

1. Assign a family-support specialist to check in with families throughout the NICU stay.
2. Provide and encourage ongoing staff education on how to provide psychosocial support to NICU families.
3. Always provide culturally sensitive education, material, and communication.
4. Have welcoming and easy-to-understand signage.
5. Have an educational checklist for families to track what they need to learn and what "tasks" they need to master prior to discharge.
6. Fully implement family-centered developmental care practices.
7. Encourage early and frequent skin-to-skin care with all family members.
8. Honor and support the feeding choices of parents.
9. Offer family-centered multidisciplinary rounds.
10. Assist families in communicating with extended family and friends.
11. Create a comfortable and safe space for families away from the bedside.
12. Offer peer-to-peer support activities and events.
13. Provide parent educational materials.
14. Include social work, psychologists, and family support specialists as regular staff on the unit.
15. Establish telemedicine for baby–parent connections when parents are unable to physically be in the unit.

16. Include siblings and integral members of the family.

17. Establish parent self-care programs.

RECOMMENDED RESOURCES

Excellent websites and resources are available to staff who are interested in becoming more proficient and confident in providing psychosocial support to their NICU patients and families (Figure 6.2).

Each unit can create its own parent educational checklist that meets the discharge educational requirements of its institution, but here is an example of what one might look like (Figure 6.3).

When units have family-focused multidisciplinary rounds implemented, having a form that allows families to write down their thoughts prior to rounds so that they feel prepared to speak is extremely helpful. In additionally, when families cannot be present at rounds, these forms can be filled out and left for the multidisciplinary medical team to review during rounds. This way, the medical team can still receive parents' feedback and concerns and leave feedback for families (Figure 6.4).

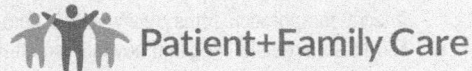

Online Education:
1. https://www.mynicunetwork.com
2. http://www.nationalperinatal.org/webinars
3. http://www.dandlelion-webinars.com

Website Recommendations:
1. http://nann.org
2. http://www.academyonline.org
3. https://www.awhonn.org
4. http://www.nationalperinatal.org
5. https://www.marchofdimes.org/baby/the-nicu-family-support-program.aspx
6. http://handtohold.org/healthcare-professionals
7. http://www.babyfirst.com/en/developmental-care/family-centered-care
8. http://coinnurses.org
9. https://www.aap.org/en-us/about-the-aap/Committees-Councils-Sections/Neonatal-Perinatal-Medicine/Neonatologist/Pages/Neonatologists.aspx
10. http://nna.org.uk
11. http://www.patientfamilycare.com
12. http://www.preemieparentalliance.org
13. http://preemieworld.com

Figure 6.2 ■ Recommended resources to improve psychosocial support for NICU families.

Books:
1. *Developmental and Therapeutic Interventions in the NICU* by Elsie Vergara
2. *Developmental Care of Newborns and Infants: A Guide for Health Professionals* by Carole Kenner and Jacqueline M. McGrath
3. *Trauma Informed Care in the NICU: Evidence Based Practice Guidelines for Neonatal Clinicians* by Mary Coughlin
4. *Transformative Nursing in the NICU: Trauma-Informed Age Appropriate Care* by Mary Coughlin
5. *Supporting Siblings and Their Families During Intensive Baby Care* by Linda Rector

Journal Article Recommendations:
1. Psychosocial program standards for NICU parents: https://www.nature.com/articles/jp2015141
2. Recommendations for involving the family in developmental care of the NICU baby: https://www.nature.com/articles/jp2015142
3. Recommendations for peer-to-peer support for NICU parents: https://www.nature.com/articles/jp2015143
4. Recommendations for mental health professionals in the NICU: https://www.nature.com/articles/jp2015144
5. Recommendations for palliative and bereavement care in the NICU: a family-centered integrated approach: https://www.nature.com/articles/jp2015145
6. NICU discharge planning and beyond: recommendations for parent psychosocial support: https://www.nature.com/articles/jp2015146
7. Recommendations for enhancing psychosocial support of NICU parents through staff education and support: https://www.nature.com/articles/jp2015147
8. The neonatal intensive parenting unit: an introduction: https://www.nature.com/articles/jp2017108?WT. feed_name=subjects_medicalresearch&foxtrotcallback=true

Figure 6.2 ■ Recommended resources to improve psychosocial support for NICU families. (*continued*)

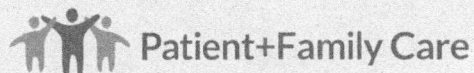 Patient+Family Care

Important points:
- ✓ This is only a guide! There may be more information the staff needs to share with that is important.
- ✓ YOUR questions and priorities are equally important; therefore, fill in the blank spaces so that we know what *you* want to hear about and learn.
- ✓ There is going to be a lot of information shared with you during this stressful time, so don't expect to remember everything. Even if it is checked off, ask staff to repeat information for you!

Baby Care Education
- ☐ Changing diapers
- ☐ Taking temperatures
- ☐ Understanding baby's temperature ranges
- ☐ Swaddling
- ☐ Understanding baby's cues
- ☐ Skin care
- ☐ How to give a bath
- ☐ How to prepare feedings
- ☐ How to pump breast milk
- ☐ How to store/thaw/prepare breast milk
- ☐ How to prepare formula
- ☐ How to feed baby
- ☐ Appropriate feeding schedule/amounts
- ☐ Number of wet/dirty diapers to expect
- ☐ How to administer medications
- ☐ Sleep/wake cycles
- ☐ How to suction nose and mouth
- ☐ Umbilical cord care
- ☐ How to trim nails
- ☐ Infant choking and CPR
- ☐ How to prevent illness in babies
- ☐ Signs and symptoms of illness
- ☐ When to call the doctor
- ☐ Importance of follow-up visits
- ☐ Signs and symptoms of illness

- ☐ How to dress baby
- ☐ How to properly position baby
- ☐ Safe sleep practices
- ☐
- ☐
- ☐
- ☐
- ☐

Discharge Preparation Checklist
- ☐ Car seat obtained and education on proper positioning
- ☐ Importance of follow-up appointments
- ☐ Pediatrician selected and follow-up appointment made
- ☐ Have adequate supplies of:
  - ○ Diapers
  - ○ Blankets
  - ○ Clothing
  - ○ Feeding supplies
- ☐ Have a safe place for baby to sleep
- ☐ Understand safe sleep practices
- ☐
- ☐

Figure 6.3 ■ Parent education checklist.

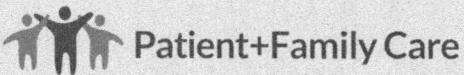

Behavioral:

Heart:

Breathing/Lungs:

Feedings:

Pee/Poop:

Current Questions:

Parent needs today/current struggles:

Upcoming family needs:

Figure 6.4 ■ Parent multidisciplinary rounds participation form (front and back).

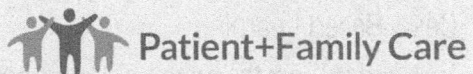

Date:_____

*In your absence today, the multidisciplinary rounds team wanted to provide you with the following updates and also address your noted concerns:

Behavioral:

Heart:

Breathing/Lungs:

Feedings:

Pee/Poop:

Current Questions:

Parent needs today/current struggles:

Upcoming family needs:

Figure 6.4 ■ Parent multidisciplinary rounds participation form (front and back). (*continued*)

Case-Based Learning

L.M. and H.L. are the parents of Henry, born at 28 weeks' gestation. Their previous child, Kayla, was born at 30 weeks and is now 5 years old with mild developmental delays after her 6-week NICU stay.

L. and H. mention that the NICU environment is much different than 5 years ago, when Kayla was born. They comment on the bed in the room for them to sleep in, the rounds that occur each morning that they participate in, and the unlimited visiting hours. You reply that the NICU has recently undergone remodeling and has adopted a new family-centered developmental care best practice. This practice is known as NIPU—Newborn Intensive Parenting Unit, and they will be experiencing family-integrated care.

QUESTIONS

1. How is this model different from family-centered care?
2. What should L. and H. expect during this hospitalization?

ANSWERS

Family-integrated care (FICare) incorporates what Hall, Hynan, et al. (2017) describe as an undervalued and underutilized natural resource to improve neonatal outcomes—the family–infant relationship. Family-centered developmental care (FCDC) enhances bonding between parents and baby, which has been shown to influence neurodevelopmental outcomes by improving physiological stability and reducing stress. This optimizes neuroprotection, brain growth, and psychosocial and cognitive development.

L. and H. will be oriented to the NIPU's physical improvements in sleeping, kitchen, and laundry space. They can expect to be full partners in Henry's caregiving all day, every day. The healthcare team will meet with them daily and as needed if Henry's condition changes. They are invited to provide input about Henry and to ask questions freely during rounds. They are encouraged to ask for clarification of unfamiliar words and to read Henry's medical record if they would like.

They will be given information about the benefits of skin-to-skin contact with Henry; they will use kangaroo care as early, often, and long as possible. They will bathe him and take his temperature, along with other care activities. They should not worry about their abilities to care for Henry, as their participation will increase as Henry stabilizes and as they are ready, with staff serving as facilitators and mentors for them. They will be shown how to recognize and respond to any signs of stress and how to console and relax Henry. They'll know his feeding cues and ways he takes his breast milk best. By the time they go home, they will feel confident about caring for Henry and will know him inside and out.

L. and H. will meet other parents who are going through similar experiences. Henry's sister will visit, as will grandmas, grandpas, and others they choose. They will

(continued)

(continued)

have access to social workers, case managers, and a psychologist if they desire. All told, Henry will be receiving the best kind of newborn care possible in today's NIPU.

REFERENCE

Hall, S. L., Hynan, M. T., Phillips, R., Lassen, S., Craig, J. W., Goyer, E., ... Cohen, H. (2017). The neonatal intensive parenting unit: An introduction. *Journal of Perinatology, 37*(12), 1259–1264. doi:10.1038/jp.2017.108

REFERENCES

Cooper, L. G., Gooding, J. S., Gallagher, J., Sternesky, L., Ledsky, R., & Berns, S. D. (2007). Impact of a family-centered care initiative on NICU care, staff and families. *Journal of Perinatology, 27*, S32–S37. doi:10.1038/sj.jp.7211840

Craig, J. W., Glick, C., Phillips, R., Hall, S. L., Smith, J., & Browne, J. (2015). Recommendations for involving the family in developmental care of the NICU baby. *Journal of Perinatology,35*. S5–S8. doi:10.1038/jp.2015.142

Discenza, D. (2018). Providing equal family-centered care in every NICU. *Neonatal Network, 37*(1), 45–49. doi:10.1891/0730-0832.37.1.45

Hall, S. L., Cross, J., Selix, N. W., Patterson, C., Segre, L., Chuffo-Siewert, R., ... Martin, M. L. (2015). Recommendations for enhancing psychosocial support of NICU parents through staff education and support. *Journal of Perinatology, 35*, S29–S36. doi:10.1038/jp.2015.147

Hall, S. L., Hynan, M. T., Phillips, R., Lassen, S., Craig, J. W., Goyer, E., ... Cohen, H. (2017). The neonatal intensive parenting unit: An introduction. *Journal of Perinatology, 37*(12), 1259–1264. doi:10.1038/jp.2017.108

Hall, S. L., Ryan, D. J., Beatty, J., & Grubbs, L. (2015). Recommendations for peer-to-peer support for NICU parents. *Journal of Perinatology, 35*, S9–S13. doi:10.1038/jp.2015.143

Hynan, M. T., Steinberg, Z., Baker, L., Cicco, R., Geller, P. A., Lassen, S., ... Stuebe, A. (2015). Recommendations for mental health professionals in the NICU. *Journal of Perinatology, 35*, S14–S18. doi:10.1038/jp.2015.144

Ionio C., Colombo C., Brazzoduro V., Mascheroni, E., Confalonieri, E., Castoldi, F., & Lista, G. (2016). Mothers and fathers in NICU: The impact of preterm birth on parental distress. *Europe's Journal of Psychology, 12*(4), 604–621. doi:10.5964/ejop.v12i4.1093.

Mosher, S. (2017). Comprehensive NICU parental education: Beyond baby basics. *Neonatal Network, 36*(1), 18–25. doi:10.1891/0730-0832.36.1.18

Rector, L. (2007). *Supporting siblings and their families during intensive baby care*. Baltimore, MD: Paul H. Brookes.

HELPING FAMILIES MAKE THE HOSPITAL A HOME

7

"Many infants admitted to a neonatal intensive care unit have complex medical conditions requiring care from multiple subspecialists and prolonged hospitalizations" (Welch, Check, & O'Shea, 2017, "Abstract" section) and can spend weeks, months, or even years in the hospitals. Families can also spend an ample amount of time at the hospital, making it feel like a second home—minus the comfort. Some NICUs remodeled after private room recommendations came out, and parents have been lucky enough to have their child's NICU room be more of a family living space, which can be quite comfortable and feel more like a home. These units are not the norm though, and it will take decades before neonatal units are all remodeled to meet these new design recommendations; as a result, staff need to find ways to make the unit feel more like a home for families.

MAKING THE NICU A NURSERY

When parents find out they are expecting, many of them start setting up and decorating a baby nursery. They pick out a theme and go crazy! Unfortunately, when their baby ends up in the NICU, they do not get to take their baby home to that cute nursery, and a hospital Isolette with pumps and monitors surrounding their bed is far from what they envisioned as their baby's first little nesting area.

NICU staff should encourage families to make the NICU space as comfortable and personal as possible. Some ideas on how to do this may include:

- Decorating crib cards
- Hanging up family photos
- Adorning the bed with personal blankets
- Dressing the baby in personal clothes
- Having stuffed animals nearby
- If there is wall space, putting up decorations

137

The primary goal is to inspire families to make the space feel like their space and to truly make it theirs. This also provides them something else they can control, and when they already feel so out of control and powerless, this helps give them an outlet to be creative and feel they are able to do something for their child that only they can do.

CELEBRATING MILESTONES

Parents, especially first-time ones, love to celebrate and capture all of a baby's "firsts." You typically will see new parents taking photos and videos of the first time baby gets a bath, the first time baby sits in a swing, the first time baby is held by every family member, the first time baby eats a solid food, the first time baby crawls. In the NICU, capturing and celebrating firsts should be no exception. Staff needs to celebrate even the smallest of milestones to encourage families and highlight the incremental achievements their baby is making, even if they may be quite small. The milestones that should be celebrated could include, but are certainly not limited to, the following:

- First time skin-to-skin with each family member
- First time off supplemental oxygen
- First time feeding at breast
- First time feeding by bottle
- First time taking a full feeding by mouth
- Every time the baby reaches a new pound in weight
- Every time baby reaches a new gestational age
- The day baby reaches its due date
- Each time baby reaches a month of age
- When baby's umbilical cord falls off
- When baby has its first tub bath
- When baby starts/completes phototherapy
- When baby is off IV fluids
- When baby makes it to an open crib
- When baby stops having apnea/bradycardia spells
- When baby first wears clothing
- When baby gets to start Back to Sleep protocol
- When baby has its car seat study/challenge
- When mom and dad get to room in

- When discharge education is in the final stages
- When baby is discharged!

There are many ways to commemorate these milestones. Using the unit's digital camera is one way and then printing off photos and putting them into cute scrapbook cards for the family is always fun. Then the cards can be placed into a scrapbook and kept as a chronological story of their journey. There are also many different "journey bead" programs available through websites or family support organizations that allow families to put together a necklace, bracelet, or keychain that commemorate each milestone. Journey beads serve as a connection among parents, their baby, and their healthcare team that celebrates the celebration of milestones, growth progression, and the parent experience.

One very dependable and respected company that offers not only a beautiful journey bead program, but also special crib notes, wrist bands, a NICU journey book, and inspirational memories, designed exclusively for NICU patients and their families, is Peekaboo ICU. Peekaboo ICU was created by a NICU nurse, who wanted to find a way to provide support to parents as they face the emotional journey of the NICU, empower them with knowledge, and offer them support and encouragement. Most recently, Peekaboo ICU launched a mobile app designed to inform, inspire, and engage parents as they navigate their way through the NICU.

Whether units purchase already developed programs from an organization such as Peekaboo ICU or develop a program of their own, the important factor is finding what works best for each unit so that all staff members feel comfortable with being consistent with the process and families know they can expect the same level of support from all care team members.

HOSPITAL HOLIDAYS

Inevitably, some families spend holidays in the hospital, which can be a very difficult time. "The spirit of holidays, celebration and most importantly the time for families to come together for perhaps the only time in the year" (Beresford, 2017, p. 245, para. 1) can be completely disrupted when parents have a child in the hospital. The hospital, unit, and each staff member need to prioritize making the holidays as stress free and cheerful as possible.

Every family will come with its own traditions on how it celebrates holidays, so staff should inquire about what it is that makes holidays special for each family and do what they can to bring those traditions into the unit. In addition, the unit should host activities and events that families can partake in that relieve stress of families during the holiday time so that they can try to enjoy the season. Here are some examples of ways that the unit can help make each annual holiday a little more special for families (Figure 7.1):

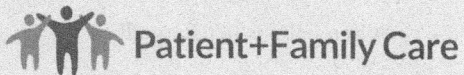

	New Year's	• Get a small party hat and take a picture of the baby wearing the hat. • Put the photo of the baby in a cute new-year picture frame. • Have the parents write down their goals and wishes for their baby's new year on the frame.
	Valentine's Day	• Have craft supplies available and allow the family to make a fun valentine for their baby. • Ask friends and family members to bring or send a valentine to place at the baby's bedside! • Decorate the room with lots of hearts! • Decorate the unit with Valentine decorations.
	Easter	• Put together a small little Easter basket for the baby's first Easter and include a little stuffed bunny, small plastic eggs, a little hardback Easter book, and a candy (or healthy carrots) that parents/family can snack on when they are visiting! • Host an Easter egg hunt for siblings.
	St. Patrick's Day	• Put four-leaf clover cutouts and decorations around the unit. • Dress babies in green outfits and make a photo frame that says, "I'm a lucky charm."
	4th of July	• Bring in colorful glow sticks that are safe and "bright" and let families have their own version of a firework show with their baby. • Adorn the bedside with fun decorations. • Have parents make a list of what their baby can do independently.
	Halloween	• Dress babies up for the occasion. • Host "trick-or-treating." • Have families come and paint a small pumpkin and have a contest.

Figure 7.1 ■ Ways to celebrate the holiday in the NICU.

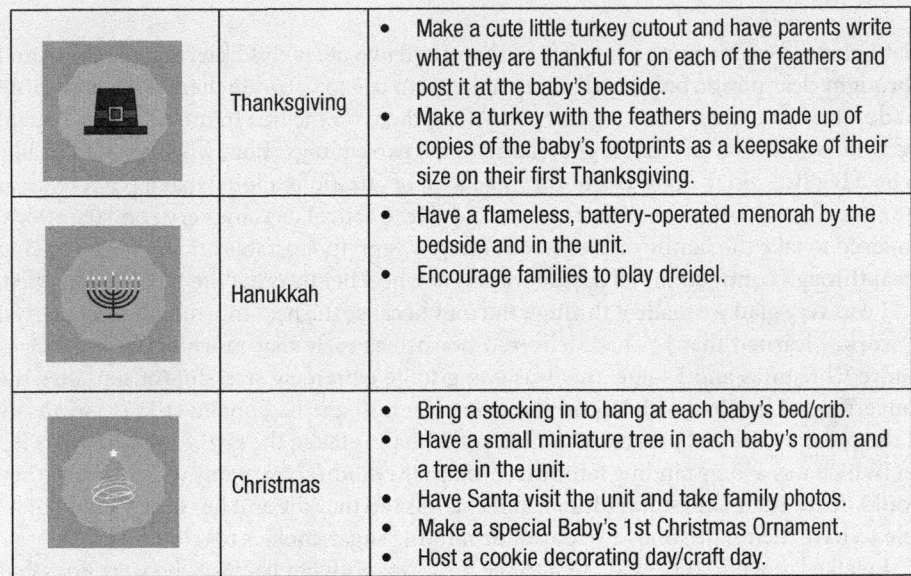

	Thanksgiving	• Make a cute little turkey cutout and have parents write what they are thankful for on each of the feathers and post it at the baby's bedside. • Make a turkey with the feathers being made up of copies of the baby's footprints as a keepsake of their size on their first Thanksgiving.
	Hanukkah	• Have a flameless, battery-operated menorah by the bedside and in the unit. • Encourage families to play dreidel.
	Christmas	• Bring a stocking in to hang at each baby's bed/crib. • Have a small miniature tree in each baby's room and a tree in the unit. • Have Santa visit the unit and take family photos. • Make a special Baby's 1st Christmas Ornament. • Host a cookie decorating day/craft day.

Figure 7.1 ■ Ways to celebrate the holiday in the NICU. (*continued*)

Author's Personal Story

I met the Y. family mid-December when J.Y. was on bed rest on our antepartum unit. J.Y. was having twins and was in preterm labor at 23 weeks' gestations, so she was receiving medication to try and stop her labor and prolong her pregnancy. When I first went to her room to introduce myself as her family-support specialist, what I was immediately struck by was how wonderfully her room was decorated for the holidays. I quickly learned that she loved Christmas, so her friends spent an afternoon decorating her room to bring the holidays to her.

She had a Christmas pillowcase and comforter on her bed; battery-operated Christmas lights around her window; a small table-top artificial tree in the corner of her room adorned with lights and ornaments; a small Bluetooth radio by her bed softly playing Christmas music on Pandora; stockings for her, her husband, her two older children, and her babies hanging off the wall; and holiday scented oil that made the room smell like fresh pine needles. I had to admit I felt like I was visiting her home, where she had made it feel like a winter holiday haven. J.Y. told me that she planned on staying in that hospital bed through the holidays to keep her babies in utero safely, so she wanted to be prepared to still enjoy her holidays.

Over the next 2 weeks, I visited J.Y. to provide information and education about what a potential NICU admission and journey would look like. I particularly loved the visit

(*continued*)

(continued)

that I planned one evening when her husband and two older children could be there, and I brought clear plastic bulbs and plenty of items to use to decorate them with, and we all made Christmas ornaments together and hung them on the tree in mom's room. I spent the time with the family that night talking to the two siblings about what it would be like to be a big sister in the NICU and they had a lot of questions about what a NICU was; at the ages of 6 and 8, they were very mature and able to articulate some very good questions. I offered to take the family on a tour, but mom was pretty unstable and had been having breakthrough contractions all day, so we had to wheel her through the NICU on her bed.

I was very glad we made it through the tour because the next morning when I arrived at work, I learned that J.Y. had delivered her babies early that morning. It was 5 days before Christmas and I knew this was going to be extremely stressful for her after the conversation I had had with her the day prior. Her husband had not had time to wrap any of the presents she had purchased online yet, he hadn't taken the girls to sit on Santa's lap yet (which was a longstanding family tradition), they didn't have plans yet as to what they would do for their Christmas dinner, and she was sad that she and her girls would not be able to have their Christmas Eve day of decorating sugar cookies together.

I walked down to the NICU first to see if J.Y. was with her babies, who were boys, but no one was in the room. I then went to her postpartum room and found her in her bed crying. I approached her bedside and asked permission to sit with her for a little while and she broke down into more tears as she said yes. J.Y. confided in me that she was overwhelmed and she really did not think that her babies' first Christmas was going to be spent in a NICU, and they were so sick and so little that she didn't even know if they were going to survive. She was fearful of her daughters having a terrible holiday, and what would they think having to spend it at the hospital? Or if they spent it at home, how would she enjoy the day without seeing the twins? I handed her a box of tissues and let her express all of her anxieties and frustrations about her twins' condition and about the holiday stresses on top of it all until she could calm down.

Once she was able to collect herself, I asked if I could return with something for her. I left to go to the NICU and came back with a slip of paper that showed her a calendar of that week's holiday event calendar. Much to her surprise, we had everything she needed; an afternoon for parents to wrap gifts while children had holiday story time, Santa family photos, a holiday craft day, a sugar cookie decorating party, a full holiday meal for all families, Christmas Mass in the chapel; if they wished, we could sneak presents under the unit tree for the kids so that they could have a Christmas morning here at the hospital too. If I remember correctly, her words to me in that moment were "It's a Christmas miracle."

Our hospital and our unit go to great lengths to make sure that holidays are special for families, because we realize that it can be overwhelming to have to spend time away from family, friends, and traditions. J.Y.'s girls had a wonderful time seeing Santa in the hospital, and when they went to see their baby brothers, the entire family was able to capture their annual family photo with Santa just like every year before, without having to leave their

(continued)

(continued)

new babies out. A year later, J.Y.'s family came back and shared with me that it actually was one of their most favorite and memorable Christmases ever. They decorated sugar cookies with other families, dad came and wrapped presents while his girls had holiday stories read to them by the local librarian volunteer, they hid gifts under the tree, and on Christmas day, they opened gifts at home and then a gift at the hospital beside their baby brothers. It was quite magical, and despite having to be away from home, the girls lit up telling their baby brothers about all the new toys they got and they had fun filling their stockings with stuffed animals, new clothes, and handmade drawings they made just for their brothers!

Family Story

Another family that had to spend the Christmas holiday in the NICU was the Phillipson family. Emilie shares her experience of having to spend her first Christmas with her son in the hospital.

"Christmas of 2016 will always stand out as both the worst and best Christmas, and surely the most memorable for our family for the rest of our lives. Truthfully, Christmas and holidays in the NICU are just that—they're in the NICU, where you don't want to be but can't stand to leave. Christmas is no exception, but with the encouragement from family, friends, and NICU staff, we made it to the other side with all of the good and bad memories in tow.

"Our son was born at 32 weeks as a result of spontaneous preterm labor. We checked into the hospital the evening of December 5th, he was born on the 7th, and we were discharged 26 days later on December 30th. Normally during this time, my husband and I would be decorating our home, picking out our perfect Christmas tree, taking strolls in the icy wonderland, spending time cooking, and eating with extended family. In the late hours of the night, we'd enjoy cups of hot cocoa by the fireplace while watching our favorite holiday films, just soaking up our last Christmas as a family of two. And then the completely unexpected, traumatic birth of our first child happened, and we were sent into the whirlwind of the NICU life with endless unknowns of beeping, cords, schedules, and missed firsts. I didn't get to hold my son when he first cried, or nurse him when he was hungry. He felt the pain of a half a dozen needles before he felt the comfort of his mother's arms. Neither of us had any idea what to expect anymore, only that what we both knew to be true was no longer. More than anything, this is what is most difficult about spending time, and holidays in particular, in the NICU: Not only is your holiday season lackluster, missing out on usual family traditions with your new little one, but it is also overflowing with missed expectations of what your first days and holidays were *supposed to be like*. A NICU parent must learn that their first experiences with their baby are not less, just different, and time is needed to process and realize these emotions. Sometimes, a great deal of time.

"There were a few nurses who really stood out to me during our stay. I really appreciated the staff who understood that my son and I were a codependent pair and who were there to support my efforts and mama emotions, as well as him medically. My son had been given a 'first Christmas' outfit after his early arrival, but getting a tiny human who is

(continued)

(*continued*)

wrapped in tubes and cords dressed into unnecessary oversized clothing is no easy feat. I appreciated the nurse who encouraged me to bring in the clothes, helped me dress him, and suggested that she take multiple photos of my son and me together in his special outfit. She did not make me feel like an inconvenience, and I was so proud to be able to show those pictures to my friends and family outside of the hospital—to experience something that was normal for a new parent. It was good for this mama's heart.

"Our NICU's family support staff had organized a Santa and Elf to visit families in their rooms (a doctor for security purposes) with the baby. One particular nurse knew that I hadn't eaten all day but that Santa was leaving soon and I would miss the opportunity if I left. She tracked down the Santa crew to come to my room ASAP so that I would not miss the event and could also take time to nourish myself. The family-support staff, a local nonprofit group, and a few churches gave gifts to our family: a pair of jammies from a former NICU family, a handmade ornament, a few blankets, quilts, and knitted baby hats. As the gifts came in, I felt a little overwhelmed, but looking back, they are cherished pieces and I look forward to sharing them with our son year after year to help tell him the story of his birth and first Christmas.

"On Christmas Eve, my husband and I were having lunch in the hospital, everything had been going well, we'd taken our required safety classes, and our son had stabilized and come off of breathing support. He was eating and gaining weight well, and we were anticipating bringing him home the next day as our little Christmas present! Unfortunately, we received a phone call from the doctor right then that he had a bradycardia episode earlier in the day and that our countdown to discharge would need to start over, a hard reality to swallow on any day in the NICU—particularly *that* day. Our nurse welcomed us back into the room and asked if we were okay and if she could help us with anything. She stopped what she was doing (of course always paying attention to her patients in the background) to listen to us vent our frustrations and offer tissues and remind us of the positive things he'd done in the last few days.

"A few of the doctors and nurses later chatted with me about what our plans were for the holiday. They suggested that we have family members come to us and bring Christmas dinner to enjoy in the waiting room/kitchen if we didn't want to leave. They conveyed that we could use doctor's orders to avoid large family get-togethers if we wanted to avoid the crowds. They encouraged us to go and be with family if that was what we wanted and that they would call us with any updates. We were welcome to play Christmas music in our room or watch movies, even bring in a few decorations. We could stay overnight as often as we needed or never, and that was okay too. Flexibility, and knowing the doctors and nurses would support us fully however we chose to make-do with our holiday, was really key to being comfortable.

"Ultimately, we chose to have family visit for a quick dinner and then spent the rest of the evening, just the three of us, snuggled up in our room, beeps, cords, schedules, and all. That was our Christmas 2016; nearly the entire month of December spent walking hospital hallways and learning to care for our extra-tiny human. No one desires to spend a holiday or any amount of time in the NICU. Christmas season that year was nothing like I ever imagined and certainly not anything I ever want to go through again, but it was our reality, and we made our own memories and created our own firsts, no matter how different I had originally imagined them to be."

RECOMMENDATIONS/SUGGESTIONS FOR BEST PRACTICE

1. Encourage and inspire families to create their NICU space to feel more like home; make the NICU a nursery.

    a. Bring in family photos.

    b. Adorn the baby's bed with personal blankets.

    c. Dress the baby in personal clothing.

    d. Put up personalized crib cards.

    e. Have cute stuffed animals nearby.

2. Celebrate and honor milestones and baby "firsts."

3. Look for consistent ways to celebrate milestones that all staff can adhere to.

4. Honor holiday traditions for families that have to spend holidays in the hospital.

5. Host holiday events/activities for families.

6. Staff should inquire about how families spend their holidays and do what they can to encourage families to adhere to traditions.

7. Have printed and posted holiday event calendars available for families.

RECOMMENDED RESOURCES

Having a holiday event calendar for families, showcasing all the supportive and peer-to-peer connection events that are available, printed and posted is very helpful. Here is an example of what one might look like during the Christmas holiday season (Figure 7.2).

Wonderful resources are available to NICU staff to help celebrate milestones for infants and families (Figure 7.3).

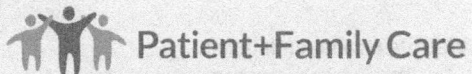

Patient+Family Care

Date	Time	Event	Location
Monday 18th	11 a.m. 5 p.m.	Ornament Making Massage Monday	Respite Lounge Respite Lounge
Tuesday 19th	9 a.m. 2 p.m.	Coffee with a Doc Trail Walk Tuesday (indoor walk due to weather)	Respite Lounge Meet at NICU Entrance
Wednesday 20th	10 a.m. and 5 p.m.	Santa Visit and Family Photos	Patient Rooms and Respite Lounge
Thursday 21th	11 a.m. and 6 p.m.	Holiday Craft Event	Respite Lounge

Figure 7.2 ■ December 18th–25th NICU events.

Date	Time	Event	Location
Friday 22nd	6:30 p.m.	Pizza and Movie Night—Polar Express Showing (RSVP for pizza at main desk)	Meeting Room H
Saturday 23rd	10 a.m.	Sibling Saturday—Holiday Reading Corner and Parent Wrapping (kids will hear stories from our library volunteers and parents will have time to sneak away and wrap presents. All wrapping paper and supplies will be provided!)	Sibling Corner and Meeting Room A&B
Sunday 24th	11 a.m. 6 and 9 p.m.	Sugar Cooking Decorating and Hot Chocolate/Treats Christmas Mass	Respite Lounge Hospital Chapel
Monday 25th	8 a.m. 9 a.m. 3 p.m.	Christmas Mass Hot Chocolate and Donuts Holiday Dinner	Hospital Chapel Lounge Respite Area

Figure 7.2 ■ December 18th–25th NICU events. (*continued*)

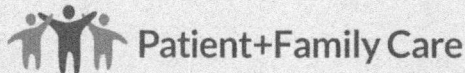
Patient+Family Care

Website recommendations:
1. http://peekabooicu.com
2. https://peekabooicu.org/220-the-caterpillar-nicu-admission-bead.html
3. https://peekabooicu.org/234-nicu-milestone-crib-cards.html
4. http://www.mykidsinspiration.com/shop/preemie-products/cat_5.html
5. https://www.everytinything.com/nicu-milestone-cards/original
6. https://www.etsy.com/market/nicu_milestone_cards
7. https://www.pinterest.com/nicuhelpinghand/documenting-your-nicu-journey/?lp=true
8. http://www.dandlelionmedical.com/products/empower-program
9. https://www.everytinything.com/nicu-journals/our-nicu-journey

Figure 7.3 ■ Recommended resources for helping celebrate milestones in the NICU.

Case-Based Learning

M.Z. and P.Z. are married parents of a term newborn undergoing neuroprotective cooling for hypoxic ischemic encephalopathy. The baby is 36 hours into the 72-hour therapy. Both parents have just arrived to the NICU for the first time because dad elected to stay with mom at the referring hospital until she was discharged. Because they are both non-English speakers, you have arranged to have a translator help with orientation to the NICU and to update the parents and answer questions about their baby's complicated condition and treatment. The translator directs the information to both parents, but only the dad replies. You ask the translator to ask the baby's mother directly to answer, but the mother does not do so.

QUESTION

1. What potential cross-cultural issues can you identify?

ANSWER

Culturally competent care is distinct from family-centered care. Both philosophies identify each newborn and its family as unique, but the global mobility adds complexity to the therapeutic relationship between family and healthcare provider. Appreciation for, and understanding of, the diverse cultural, racial, ethnic, linguistic, spiritual, and religious traditions and practices becomes ever so important during the universal crisis of NICU admission (Purdy et al., 2017). Understanding the nuances of cross-cultural competency is more than ready translation and food preferences. Other issues include communication, socioeconomic concerns, and cultural norms about decision making. In the Z. family's case, exploration yielded the information that their cultural norm is for male members of the families to discuss and determine healthcare matters.

Staff limitations due to unconscious bias need to be explored and training provided (Heitzler, 2017). Education and activities that improve self-awareness and appreciation for the range of values and cultural practices improve trust and quality of communication (Hall et al., 2015). Fragile NICU relationships can be devastated by cross-cultural difficulties. Relationship building may be derailed by a lack of intuition or an exposure to family's psychocultural needs. At minimum, it takes more time to provide information via translation, and it can be difficult to assess the full understanding of the information imparted (Hendson, Reis, & Nicholas, 2015).

However, it can be as simple as asking. Once the question is posed and answered, staff must strive to be nonjudgmental and receptive to differences in lifestyles and traditions. Hall et al. (2015) describe this as culturally effective care.

REFERENCES

Hall, S. L., Cross, J., Selix, N. W., Patterson, C., Segre, L., Chuffo-Siewert, R., ... Martin, M. L. (2015). Recommendations for enhancing psychosocial support of NICU parents through staff education and support. *Journal of Perinatology, 35*, S29–S36. doi:10.1038/jp.2015.147

(continued)

(*continued*)

Heitzler, E. T. (2017). Cultural competence of obstetric and neonatal nurses. *Journal of Obstetric, Gynecologic & Neonatal Nursing, 46*(3), 423–433. doi:10.1016/j.jogn.2016.11.015

Hendson, L., Reis, M. D., & Nicholas, D. B. (2015). Health care providers' perspectives of providing culturally competent care in the NICU. *Journal of Obstetric, Gynecologic, & Neonatal Nursing, 44*(1), 17–27. doi:10.1111/1552-6909.12524

Purdy, I. B., Melwak, M. A., Smith, J. R., Kenner, C., Chuffo-Siewert, R., Ryan, D. J., ... Hall, S. (2017). Neonatal nurses NICU quality improvement: Embracing EBP recommendations to provide parent psychosocial support. *Advances in Neonatal Care, 17*(1), 33–44. doi:10.1097/ANC.0000000000000352

REFERENCES

Beresford, D. (2017). Last thoughts. *Journal of Neonatal Nursing, 23*(6), 245. doi:10.1016/j.jnn.2017.09.006

Welch, C. D., Check, J., & O'Shea, T. M. (2017). Improving care collaboration for NICU patients to decrease length of stay and readmission rate. *BMJ Open Quality, 6*(2), e000130. doi:10.1136/bmjoq-2017-000130

HELPING FAMILIES PREPARE FOR DISCHARGE AND LIFE AFTER THE NICU

"Although going home from the hospital is highly anticipated, the event evokes fright as the families assume responsibility of their tiny infant" (Lopez, Anderson, & Feutchinger, 2013, para. 1). Parents leave a unit where their medically fragile child has had 24-hour observation by trained professionals who had all of the equipment and skill required to perform life-saving measures if necessary, and babies were connected to monitors that would alert these trained staff at the earliest sign of trouble. Not only are those safety nets being left behind, but also many parents form close bonds with the staff and see the care team and psychosocial support team as family. So when families leave the NICU at discharge they feel as though those relationships are being severed. The NICU care team is a group of people who have seen their family at their absolute worst and did not waver; they were there for them in their moment of crisis and offered hope and inspiration without judgment; they were always there to lend an ear, a hand, or a shoulder to cry on; and they were the ones that parents view as the heroes who saved their child's life. Separating from the NICU environment can, therefore, be an emotionally and mentally difficult junction for parents, not to mention the physical demands that lie ahead that come with the burdens on any new parents who find themselves at home with a newborn. Neonatal care teams have the fundamental responsibility, beginning at the moment of hospital admission, to prepare families for hospital discharge.

HOW TO TAKE OVER THE CARE OF THEIR NEWBORN

NICU staff is well coached in the concept that discharge preparation and discharge teaching begin at admission. Planning for discharge and assessing for risks related to a patient and family's status, including their home environment, their available support system, and their psychosocial stability, begin at the moment of admission and continue throughout the neonatal hospitalization. "A key feature of the discharge planning process is engaging the patient and family and the multidisciplinary team. Discharge planning should be patient centered and driven by the patient's specific needs and preferences [and] patient and family engagement is critical to successful hospital discharge planning" (Weiss et al., 2015, "Discharge Planning" section).

Family engagement, from the moment of admission, is incredibly important when it comes to preparing parents to take over the care of their newborn. As discussed in previous chapters, including parents in all care-related tasks as early as possible is important to helping them feel like important members of the care team and helps them fulfill their roles as parents in the baby's life. In the context of hospital discharge, being involved in care tasks from the moment of admission helps them build much-needed confidence prior to leaving the safety net of the hospital and their medical care team, when they assume all hands-on care for their child independently. Families that have been given the opportunity to provide hands-on care with the support and encouragement of staff nearby are much more prepared and confident that they will be successful in the autonomous care of their baby.

Every neonatal unit has its own discharge education checklist, but there are universal topics that all discharging parents should be able to feel comfortable with prior to leaving the hospital with their child. These topics include, but are not limited to, the following:

- Understanding what their child's feeding plan is and how to properly prepare/store feedings
- Dressing/undressing/swaddling their baby
- Proficiency at diaper changing, bathing their baby, and keeping the skin clean
- Understanding their infant's cues and knowing signs of distress
- Understanding what medications their child is taking and why their child is taking each of them and knowing how to properly prepare each medication and how to adequately administer each medication on schedule
- Understanding thermoregulation and knowing how to accurately take a temperature, recognize a normal temperature range for their child, correct a low or high temperature, and when to call the doctor
- Understanding safe sleep patterns and environments
- Knowing car seat safety
- Understanding the importance of immunizations, ways to prevent illness, and when their follow-up appointments are and with whom
- Having a basic knowledge of infant rescue/cardiopulmonary resuscitation (CPR)
- Understanding the severity of respiratory syncytial virus (RSV)
- Recognizing ways to prevent shaken baby syndrome

If a patient is being sent home on multiple medications, it can be helpful to provide the parents with their own version of a medication administration record (M.A.R.). Both as a nurse and as a patient, I know that I have relied on a M.A.R. so that I know when my assigned patients, or when I myself, are due for medications. Having a way to track when medications are due, and a way to sign off when they have been given, can be a real stress relief for families. Not to mention that when a new parent is sleep deprived and is at home adapting to a new baby, it can become difficult to remember when and what medication has been given.

Another way staff can help ready parents for taking over the care of their child is to prepare them to become less dependent on monitors. Staff should disconnect all equipment and allow families to "room in" near the NICU prior to going home. Some units have family sleep rooms within the unit, and others have the ability to use neighboring family birthing or postpartum rooms, but either works just fine. Families should be highly encouraged to spend a minimum of 24 hours, and ideally 48 hours, in a room with their newborn to simulate being home as the primary caretakers. This offers the opportunity for parents to take the same responsibilities they will be taking on after discharge, with the comfort of knowing the NICU staff is only a few steps away if an emergency arises. Rooming-in is a nice transition for many families because it provides a trial and allows them the opportunity to be independent with an expert backup team nearby.

Prior to discharge, families should be invited to attend a discharge preparation class in which all basic newborn care is covered. During this time, parents receive education on infant rescue and CPR, car seat safety instruction, and a list of community resources. Many hospitals provide NICU-specific discharge classes, and if the NICU is large enough to host independent courses, these classes are ideal because NICU-specific content can be presented; this class also doubles as a peer-to-peer networking opportunity. However, not all neonatal units are large enough or have a high-enough census to be able to support a discharge class in a group setting. In those situations, families should be encouraged to attend a discharge class that is available to postpartum families so that newborn care topics are covered and some level of peer-to-peer networking is accomplished. Although NICU parents and term newborn parents have vastly different discharge experiences, they share the new parent experience, and there are benefits that can be gained by that connection.

If a hospital does not offer any type of discharge class, then opportunities for discharge education, in addition to the care team's education, should be sought out as an option for families. One support example for NICU families is Your NICU Baby offered by The Wellness Network. This product is available via tablet and is all web-based, so families can browse educational topics at their own pace, take a deeper dive into topics that are applicable to their child's condition, and know that all of the information has been created by experts in the field of neonatology. The platform offers information in a variety of learning styles such as written, audio, and video messages, meeting the learning needs of almost all parents. The Wellness Network is on the forefront of the importance of psychosocial support of NICU families and even offers information and education on the importance of self-care and ways to cope with the stress of parenting a medically fragile child.

HOW TO MANAGE FOLLOW-UP APPOINTMENTS

Often, when infants leave the NICU, families think the NICU journey is over. I admit that as a NICU nurse, I naively believed this for many years. I believed that the worst was behind these families and that things would be easier for them now that they were headed home. Unfortunately, that is not always the case; in fact, families sometimes look back on the NICU as an easier time.

The NICU is a "one-stop shop" where all the doctors come to the baby, all of the equipment the child needs is there and provided without a second thought, the environment is secure, everyone is required to wash their hands over and over again (and if someone has even an inclination that they might be sick they are not allowed to enter), parents have the comfort knowing someone is watching over their child 24/7, and they are able to be home and sleep at night (although when their child is in the hospital, they are stressed and worried and hate being away from their baby and often do not sleep well, and mothers wake up every few hours to pump, so very little sleep occurs). While a baby is in the NICU, any question a parent has, they can ask and have instant answers from an entire team of multidisciplinary experts who are at their fingertips.

When families leave the hospital, they now have to load up and make multiple trips to see multiple doctors and specialists with a newborn in tow, working around nap schedules, and if there are other siblings in the families, they are transporting them as well. If the child is on medical equipment, they are having to coordinate with home suppliers to deliver oxygen or supplies before they run out, and they have to make room at home to store large tanks, not to mention having to tote that around from appointment to appointment. They walk into a medical appointment with other families who are there with sick children—imagine all of the germs that they have just exposed their child's fragile immune system to! They are constantly trying to figure out how to tell their family to wash their hands or not to touch their baby, they try to avoid large crowds but have to keep going into busy medical centers for more appointments with specialists, and now every time they have a question, they have to call a doctor's office, leave a message, and wait to get a call back, only to get that call back and find out they were the wrong doctor to call.

The struggles of the NICU do not end when families are discharged, and NICU staff needs to understand that many families continue to have struggles well beyond the hospital. Care coordination efforts prior to discharge are key, and having as much support to manage all of the follow-up care and as many needs met prior to discharge helps reduce stress and set the family up for success. In fact, "transition to home is no less important than hospital care. As is seen from the [scenario] mentioned here, caregiving and parenting a preterm infant can be very challenging and demanding, especially during the immediate weeks and months after discharge" (Boykova, 2016, "Conclusion" section). NICU staff must all do their part to prepare families for the reality of life after the NICU, and one way they can do that is by helping them understand the importance of any follow-up visit they have after discharge.

Providing families with the names, contact information, location, and understanding of the importance of each follow-up appointment is critical because "attendance at NICU follow up is crucial for parents and infants to gain access to the expertise required for reassurance and support, timely diagnosis, referral to needed services and assistance with the coordination of their care, which is sometimes complex" (Ballantyne, Stevens, Guttmann, Willan, & Rosenbaum, 2012, para. 1). Without proper follow-up care, infants may miss important milestones that, without proper intervention, could negatively impact their health or development for the rest of their lives. However, it is not sufficient enough to provide families with education about the importance of these follow-up appointments. Care coordination must go a step further and ensure that families will be able to attend follow-up appointments, and if there are any barriers that may hinder a family's ability to attend, then staff need to work with families to remove those barriers prior to discharge. Again, helping set families up for success prior to discharge should be of utmost priority in all aspects of postdischarge care and follow-up.

HELPING FAMILIES FIND CONNECTION WITH OTHERS

"Graduate NICU parents have reported feeling isolated and [experience] a diminished ability to function because of the many hours per week they have to spend providing direct care and coordinating appointments for the child after leaving the hospital" (Mosher, 2017, "Discharge Education" section). If NICU graduate parents find themselves discharged in the midst of cold and flu season, these feelings are often amplified when their providers tell them to stay indoors and away from any crowds to avoid being exposed to unnecessary germs and reduce the risks of contracting RSV, which can be extremely dangerous to premature infants. Many postdischarged families "become overwhelmed after discharge by their baby's health problems, rescheduling appointments or seeing doctors unfamiliar with their baby's history or condition" (Purdy, Craig, & Zeanah, 2015, "Introduction" section), which further lead to stress and postpartum depression rates.

As discussed numerous times in this text, one proven way to reduce stress and feelings of isolation among NICU parents is to provide connection and a peer-to-peer network, and postdischarge communities for graduate families is no exception. In fact, postdischarge communities may be just as, if not more, important than in-hospital peer-to-peer connections. When families are visiting their child in the hospital, whether they participate in peer-to-peer activities or not, they at least see other families in the unit and understand they are not alone. Once they are discharged and are confined to their homes, they truly are alone in a sense, so, finding ways for families to connect after the NICU is critically important to help provide psychosocial support.

Many organizations have been successful at developing and hosting postdischarge support groups for lactating mothers. The same structure can be followed for NICU families, so there is no need to reinvent the wheel. A volunteer peer-to-peer mentor needs to be willing to lead the group, the organization needs to dedicate space and time for the group, the group needs to be publicized, and then families show up. There can be organized topics, or the group can be parent led, meaning there is no formal topic for discussion and the group is more of a meet and greet in which NICU graduate families can come and just be with one another to discuss whatever is on their minds. These meetings are well attended when they are held on hospital property and when the NICU family-support specialist attends because the specialist can answer more complex questions, assess for concerns, suggest that families seek medical care if appropriate, and provide a more professional oversight of the meeting. Many organizations transition the graduate groups to an offsite location and have more fun activities planned when the children are a little older; often these groups are completely parent volunteer led.

If in-person groups are not an option for an organization, are not something a parent feels comfortable attending, or are not events a family can attend because of various barriers, organizations should provide other support networks to reduce the feelings of isolation for families after discharge. Other support options may include call-in groups or online communities. One organization that offers really wonderful support calls is Keep 'Em Cookin'. They are specific not to NICU families, but rather high-risk bed-resting mothers who are looking to find support from other women on bed rest. What is great about their support service is that they have a live call available every week, and it is led by an expert who can answer questions and moderate. It provides an opportunity for women to meet one another and realize they are not alone. Thankfully, we live in a world where technology is at the fingertips of almost everyone, and there are a lot of options to find support online. Organizations can offer their own online support community, and Ruzuku offers a very easy-to-use platform that allows you to create your own online community. Patient+Family Care has a support group online titled "Parenting in the NICU and Beyond" that helps provide a peer-to-peer connection with education and information and is resource rich with other recommendations to parent support networks. The benefit of online networks is that they are available 24/7 and are at the convenience of the family's schedule.

It's also important to research what parent groups are available in the community. Although NICU families have their own unique story, challenges, and experiences, joining and becoming involved in new parent groups is still going to be very beneficial in helping reduce of isolation feelings and depression.

MAKING DISCHARGE A CELEBRATION

Regardless of how long a baby has been in the NICU, being discharged from the unit is a great accomplishment and is something to be celebrated. Not only has the baby gained strength and stabilized enough to no longer require intensive care, but also the parents have been able to accomplish all of the required teaching and learning, and they too have achieved many things that need to be celebrated and recognized. I often see adorable graduation pictures of babies in the NICU, where nurses put on small graduation caps and make really wonderful graduation announcements. I often think we should see the parents wearing matching hats and graduation gowns, celebrating right next to the baby in the photographs. Think about it: Parents are the ones who have to take "Parenting a NICU Baby 101" and prove they can recite back all of the important information the staff throws at them. Where is their diploma? Where is their graduation? Where is their celebration?

Staff should make the exciting, yet overwhelming and scary, discharge a true celebration for families by finding ways to really commemorate the special event that it is. Some of the most popular ways that I have seen it celebrated are:

- Have small graduate caps for the babies
- Have little diplomas for the babies
- Provide NICU Graduate plush animals
- Give families a NICU-to-home book as a gift
- Take a family photo as they leave and it put up on the "discharge" board
- Provide families with a Congratulations Basket that includes the following donated supplies:
    - Gas voucher
    - Grocery store gift card

- House-cleaning gift certificate
- NICU-to-home book
- Coffee
- Coffee mugs
- Nuts and chocolate
- Cards of encouragement and congratulations from other parents

However one chooses, units need to make sure that the day of discharge is celebrated and spent focusing on the many accomplishments both baby and parents have made during their journey!

Author's Personal Story

W.E. delivered a girl at 34 3/7 weeks' gestation, and I was assigned as the bedside nurse on the day of birth. Baby E. had been born during the night shift, and she was nicely tucked in when I arrived and resumed care at 7 a.m. I received full report from the off-going nurse and shortly after 8 a.m., W.E. and her husband A.E. arrived with their two other children. Baby E. was born while the older children were at home with grandparents, and this was their first time meeting their new sister. Since I was well trained as a family-support specialist, I quickly grabbed our unit digital camera and captured many wonderful family first photos and made sure to include the siblings as equal members of the family. They were 8 and 12 years old, so they were quite mature and very eager to be helpful big sisters. I learned from W.E. that she and her husband had been trying for years to have a third child, but they unexpectedly struggled. They didn't think they were going to be able to have a third child, so they stopped trying and were in the process of adopting when they got this little surprise. Needless to say, their older two daughters were thrilled and couldn't wait to help take care of their baby sister.

With W.E.'s permission, I invited the siblings up to the bedside and asked if they would assist in the morning care. I went through a lot of education about premature babies and what would be a little different with their sister than what we call a *term baby*, and they listened very attentively. They were careful and cautious as they assisted in taking an auxiliary temperature, changing the diaper, and helping reposition her. I promptly told them how important those things will be to help with at home and what they will need to do to help their mom after not only after she goes home, but also when the baby does. I pulled out a discharge education checklist and gave one to each girl and told them that before this little baby could go home, each of them would need to feel comfortable with all of the tasks and information on that sheet because as big sisters they would have to help to their parents and know how to care for their little sister.

Later that afternoon, W.E. and A.E. returned to the unit without their children and were appreciative about how inclusive the unit was of their children. They shared

(continued)

(*continued*)

a story about a friend they had who had a premature baby in a different hospital the previous years, and siblings were not allowed in the unit at all if they were under the age of 14. They had a real fear that their daughters were going to be left out, and they were unsure how their family would deal with that stress. They also shared that they were very grateful to know that their daughters were hearing important information about how to care for the child from the "experts" because information that came from the parents was usually shrugged off and not taken seriously.

From that moment on, the entire family was included in every aspect of care possible, including changing diapers, taking temperatures, dressing, swaddling, preparing fortified feedings, rotating the saturation probe site, changing bedding, bathing, participating in medical rounds, and administering oral medications. When discharge was nearing, I could sense there was still some apprehension as the reality of being independent was looming. Our family birthing unit was full, so we were not able to offer rooming-in as we typically do, so I coordinated with our charge nurse on the pediatric floor, and we were able to offer rooming-in on our pediatric unit. The benefit of the staffing at that particular hospital is that the staff from NICU and pediatrics float to each respective department, so the family would also know the staff on pediatrics. We arranged two nights of rooming-in, and the family was given the opportunity to stay with their infant autonomously.

Prior to transferring the family to their new room, I sat with them and asked them to walk through the next 48 hours with me and anticipate what they may need. I wanted them to think through all cares and all events so that they could process what they might need and have to go through the troubleshooting process on their own. They were able to identify that they would need the following:

- Bottles for mixing breast milk and fortifier
- Breast milk
- Fortifier
- Breast pump
- Cleaning supplies for the pump parts
- Diapers
- Wipes
- Clothes
- Medications
- Diaper/feeding log

They did not identify the need, however, for the following, and I was able to remind them that they would need these:

(*continued*)

(*continued*)

- Thermometer
- Syringes for medication administration
- Extra blankets

Once we gathered everything they would need, I also provided them with a M.A.R. and showed them how we as nurses on the floor would record medication administration. Mom was overjoyed! She shared with me that she was going to go get blank paper and make her own record because she had seen the nurses use a record sheet and she was jealous of such a useful tool. We moved them up, and in the next 48 hours, they were able to successfully care for Baby E. with the comfort of knowing that the pediatric and neonatal staff were close by if they needed anything.

Prior to discharge, we held a little graduation celebration in which the family was given graduation diplomas and we listed all of the accomplishments they had made. Because there were siblings involved, we also presented both big sisters with their own diplomas. All care team members who could come say goodbye, did, and they all took the time to mention what they noticed most about the family over their stay and celebrated the accomplishments with them. A graduation photo was taken and, with the family's permission, was pinned up alongside one of their first family photos on a bulletin board by the NICU entrance. The side-by-side photos are used as an inspiration to show how far families can come.

Two weeks after discharge, I had the honor of speaking to W.E., and she told me that although she was exhausted and overwhelmed, she felt very well prepared for all of their appointments, she was skilled in the ability to care for her daughter, and her family was well adjusted because of all of the preparation they had prior to discharge. A.E. shared with me that for him, he initially hated having to be at the hospital so long, but now he sees it as such a gift because his family was given time and preparation to build confidence in caring for a preterm baby.

Family Story

Emily Lindblad shares her story about staff preparing her for hospital discharge from the unexpected NICU admission after delivering 29-week triplets.

"'Do you have car seats yet?' I turned and attempted to focus on the words coming out of the nurse's mouth. Surrounded by beeps and wires and babies in plastic boxes, it was hard to process English at that moment, never mind intelligently respond to seemingly ludicrous questions.

"'If you don't have car seats you'd better get some. They're not going to be in here forever!' I was roughly 36 hours from the single scariest event of my life; the

(*continued*)

(*continued*)

emergency C-section that meant my tiny triplets had made their unexpected entrance into the world at 29 weeks. I couldn't understand why someone was talking to me about bringing my babies home. I could barely see them through all of the tubes, wires, and sensors covering their little bodies, and I was scared at the thought of holding them, let alone putting them in a car seat, and waltzing out of the hospital. As overwhelming as everything was, hearing someone talk about our children with such optimism was a relief.

"We knew that there was no way to predict how the next hours, days, or weeks would unfold, but simply having someone acknowledge that our time in the NICU wouldn't last for all eternity planted a little seed of hope in my heart. The tight fist of terror lessened a bit and I felt like I could breathe for the first time in days.

"Over the course of the next 65 and 66 days, respectively, that attitude, that the NICU was merely going to be a stopover on our journey as a family, wound through every interaction we had with the NICU staff. Even on the roughest days or during the panic-inducing 3 a.m. phone calls, everyone maintained a positive outlook that although there would be bumps and temporary setbacks, graduation day would eventually come. In addition to the emotional support the NICU staff provided, they strove to give each family the practical skills they would need to transition to home. We were encouraged to be as involved in our children's care as we could be, and as they grew and became less fragile, we took over a significant portion of the nonmedical care.

"In a setting where it's all too easy to feel like an outsider instead of a parent, the NICU staff made parental involvement a priority! Our particular NICU did not have private rooms, so unfortunately, rooming-in was not an option, but we were welcome to be in the NICU at all hours. We had the opportunity to take part in rounds, ask questions, have input into decisions that were made, and advocate for our children. The staff also discussed situations that arose from something as simple as all three babies being hungry at the same time and offered suggestions on how to juggle three newborns. Toward the end of our NICU stay, when the babies were taking full feeds by breast or bottle, the nurses would check in once we arrived and then leave us to care for the babies ourselves. With the mantra of 'watch the baby, not the monitor' running through our heads, we'd do our best to ignore all the beeps and focus on the cues the babies were giving us. The last week or so, when it was obvious that discharge day was not far away, the nurses would unhook all off the sensors, leaving us with three wire-free babies. Not only was this useful practice for us, but it was also immensely reassuring that if the nurses were confident enough in our parenting abilities to walk away, then maybe that meant we really could handle triplets!

"In addition to having as much hands-on time with our children as possible, the NICU also provided a number of classes for the parents, including on CPR and on infant safety and basic newborn care. These were particularly helpful because they addressed issues specific to premature babies, which would not have necessarily been covered by an outside newborn essentials or CPR first aid class. That instruction, combined with the

(*continued*)

(*continued*)

time spent caring for our children, added to our parenting toolbox and allowed us to feel well prepared when we didn't have the support of a full NICU at our side.

"The staff also realized that as unsettling as the NICU can be, parents often struggle to find resources once they leave the NICU. At first, I didn't believe we would actively miss the NICU, but there were several times, once our children came home, that I was tempted to call and get advice from one of their nurses. The NICU staff worked with us to arrange follow-up appointments with the various specialists our children needed to see, helped find a pediatrician and early childhood development team that was experienced with preemies and multiples, and spoke with our family about ways they could provide support when the babies came home. As overwhelming as the NICU rollercoaster was, to this day I am thankful for the wonderful nurses and other staff members we encountered. Every person who worked with our children made an effort to work with our family as a whole, ensuring that this was merely a challenging chapter in our parenting journey, not the entire story."

RECOMMENDATIONS/SUGGESTIONS FOR BEST PRACTICE

1. Encourage early parent participation in all infant care activities to help improve confidence in their ability to take over the caretaking after discharge.

2. Provide families with their own handmade M.A.R. if their child is being discharged on medications.

3. As discharge nears, disconnect patients from monitors, if they will not be discharged home with equipment, to encourage parents to begin watching cues rather than screens.

4. Find a way to allow rooming-in so that parents can simulate being independent care providers, yet have the safety of the care team nearby.

5. Offer discharge classes.

6. Have adequate care coordination prior to discharge to prepare families for follow-up appointments and to have discharge medical needs met.

7. Provide a written list of follow-up appointments, providers, and contact information for families.

8. Assess for potential barriers to accessing follow-up care and provide care coordination to eliminate those barriers.

9. Provide postdischarge support groups or peer-to-peer connection opportunities.

10. Assess community new parent groups and activities and encourage parent participation.

RECOMMENDED RESOURCES

Numerous resources can assist staff and families to prepare for the discharge home from the NICU (Figure 8.1).

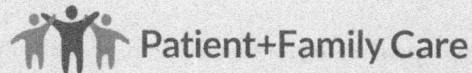

Patient+Family Care

Website Recommendations:
1. http://www.yournicubaby.com/subscription-overview
2. https://www.thewellnessnetwork.net/#nicubaby
3. http://www.keepemcookin.com/live-chat
4. https://www.ruzuku.com/
5. https://shop.plushland.com/index.php/product/nicu-mocha-sitting-bear-white-t-shirt-6
6. http://handtohold.org/resources/helpful-articles/coming-home-from-the-nicu
7. https://www.facebook.com/NICUParentingandBeyond
8. https://www.facebook.com/nicuhealing/
9. https://miracleat28.wordpress.com
10. https://www.facebook.com/NICUSurvive
11. https://www.everytinything.com/nicu-journals/our-nicu-journey

Book Recommendations:
1. *From Hope to Joy: A Memoir of a Mother's Determination and Her Micro Preemie's Struggle to Beat the Odds* by Jennifer Degl
2. *Girl in the Glass: How My Distressed Baby Defied the Odds, Shamed a CEO, and Taught Me the Essence of Love, Heartbreak and Miracles* by Deanna Fei
3. *This Lovely Life* by Vicki Forman
4. *Juniper: The Girl Who Was Born Too Soon* by Kelley and Thomas French
5. *Preemie: Love, Life and Motherhood* by Kasey Mathews

Figure 8.1 ■ Recommended resources for helping families prepare for hospital discharge.

Providing families with a home M.A.R. form to track what medications need to be given and when can be a wonderful way to help reduce stress and keep critical medications given on schedule. Hospitals should create branded M.A.R.s to distribute to families, but here is an example of how one might look (Figure 8.2).

Graduate NICU families may find that they have numerous follow-up providers and appointments to keep track of after hospital discharge. Providing families with an easy-to-read list of all of their providers, contact information, location, and importance of follow-up for each is key to provide prior to them leaving the hospital. Here is an example of what a follow-up form might look like (Figure 8.3), yet hospitals should create personalized and hospital branded forms if possible.

Celebrating graduation from the NICU is something every NICU should do for every patient and family. There are many ways to celebrate this occasion, but here are examples of how a baby and parent graduation diploma might look so that they could be given as congratulatory gifts (Figures 8.4 and 8.5).

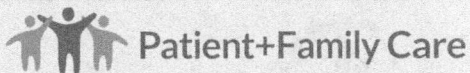

Instructions: Write down each medication when the medication is due and then schedule it for the week. Once you administer the medication, cross out that dose to indicate that it has been given.

Medication	Due	Mon.	Tues.	Wed.	Thurs.	Fri.	Sat.	Sun.
Ex: multivitamin	9 a.m. one daily	~~9 a.m.~~	~~9 a.m.~~	9 a.m.	9 a.m.	9 a.m.	9 a.m.	9 a.m.

NOTES:

Figure 8.2 ■ Medication administration record.

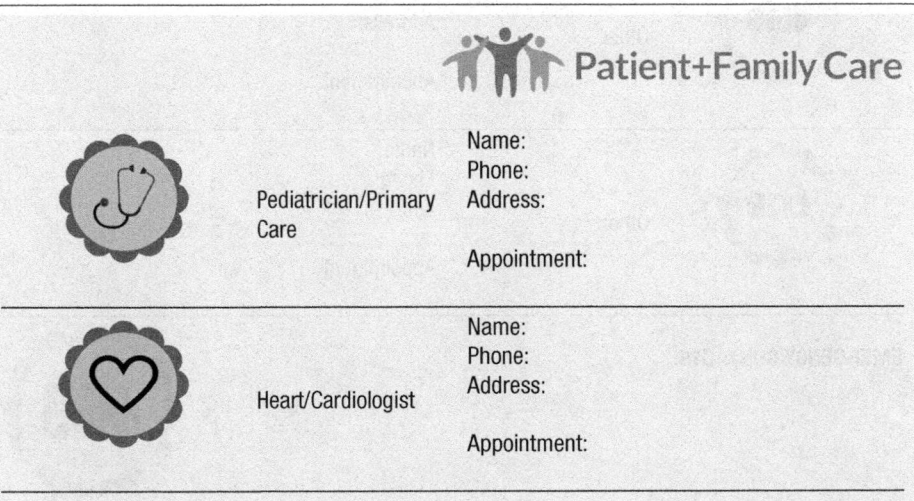

Figure 8.3 ■ Follow-up providers and appointments.

	Lung/Pulmonologist	Name: Phone: Address: Appointment:
	Eye/Optometrist	Name: Phone: Address: Appointment:
	Ear/Nose/Throat	Name: Phone: Address: Appointment:
	Stomach/Internist	Name: Phone: Address: Appointment:
	Other	Name: Phone: Address: Appointment:
	Other	Name: Phone: Address: Appointment:

EMERGENCY CONTACTS:

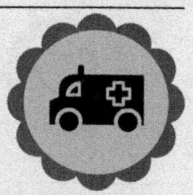

Figure 8.3 ■ Follow-up providers and appointments. (*continued*)

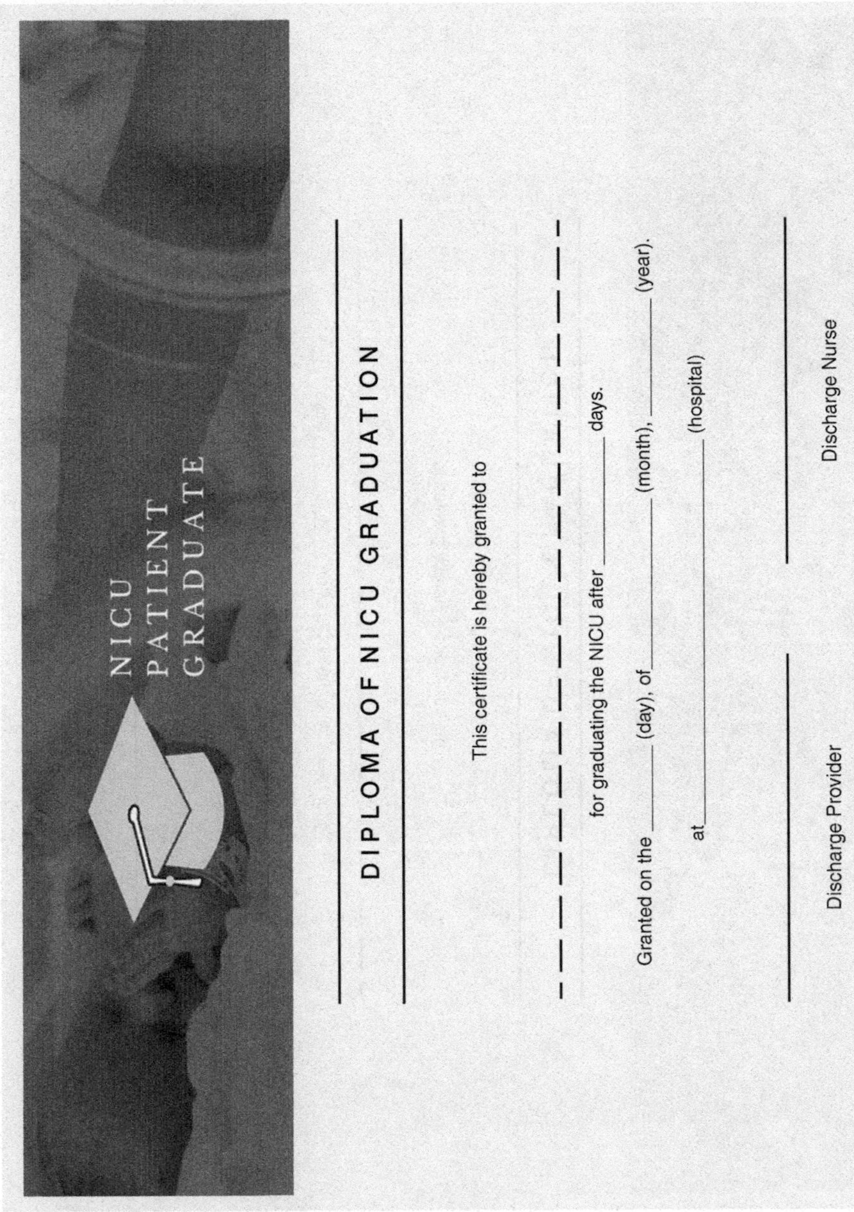
NICU
PATIENT
GRADUATE
DIPLOMA OF NICU GRADUATION
This certificate is hereby granted to
for graduating the NICU after ______ days.
Granted on the ______ (day), of ______ (month), ______ (year).
at ______ (hospital)
Discharge Provider
Discharge Nurse

Figure 8.4 ■ Sample NICU patient graduation diploma.

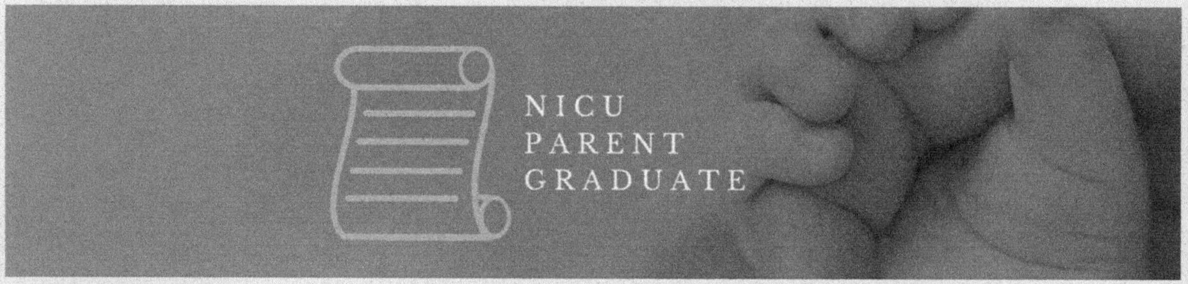

NICU PARENT GRADUATE

DIPLOMA OF NICU GRADUATION

This certificate is hereby granted to

_____

for graduating the NICU after _____ days.

Granted on the _____ (day), of _____ (month), _____ (year).

at _____ (hospital)

_____   _____
Discharge Provider   Discharge Nurse

Figure 8.5 ■ Sample NICU parent graduation diploma.

Case-Based Learning

S.Y. brings her well-appearing son, who was born at 25 weeks' gestation and had a 3-month NICU stay, for an evaluation at the neurodevelopmental follow-up clinic. She states that she has not been out of the house for a month out of fear that her baby will catch germs from being outside. She describes her daily routine of cleaning her house thoroughly. In spite of her efforts, she thinks the baby may have the flu. She bursts into tears.

QUESTIONS

1. What are the contextual features surrounding S.Y.'s emotional status?
2. What interventions might be indicated in this case?

ANSWERS

S.Y. may be suffering from vulnerable child syndrome. This condition occurs when parental perception of a child's vulnerability to illness or injury is exaggerated. It can occur with parents of preterms who see their baby as more vulnerable to illness and sometimes leads them to seek medical care when there are no physical symptoms.

In a review of the literature, Tallandini, Morsan, Gronchi, & Macagno (2015) found that length of hospitalization may be more of a trigger for this syndrome than gestational age at birth. Parenting stress and maternal anxiety about their competence to care for, feed, and interact with their baby are predictors of development of vulnerable child syndrome.

This case illustrates the importance of supporting parents in caring for their ill and/or preterm babies so that they acquire competence and therefore self-confidence. Kangaroo care is an intervention that promotes early infant–parent bonding and improves parenting confidence. Family-integrated care with open visiting, full participation, and RNs mentoring the family while they provide care is another strategy to reduce parental stress and encourage them to fully bond (Lee & O'Brien, 2018).

REFERENCES

Lee, S. K., & O'Brien, K. (2018). Family integrated care: Changing the NICU culture to improve whole-family health. *Journal of Neonatal Nursing, 24*(1), 1–3. doi:10.1016/j.jnn.2017.11.003

Tallandini, M. A., Morsan, V., Gronchi, G., & Macagno, F. (2015). Systematic and meta-analytic review: Triggering agents of parental perception of child's vulnerability in instances of preterm birth. *Journal of Pediatric Psychology, 40*(6), 545–553. doi:10.1093/jpepsy/jsv010

REFERENCES

Ballantyne, M., Stevens, B., Guttmann, A., Willan, A. R., & Rosenbaum, P. (2012). Transition to neonatal follow-up programs. *Journal of Perinatal & Neonatal Nursing, 26*(1), 90–98. doi:10.1097/JPN.0b013e31823f900b

Boykova, M. (2016). Transition from hospital to home in preterm infants and their families. *Journal of Perinatal & Neonatal Nursing, 30*(3), 270–272. doi:10.1097/JPN.0000000000000198

Lopez, G., Anderson, K., & Feutchinger, J. (2013). Transition of premature infants from hospital to home life. *Neonatal Network: NN, 31*(4), 207–214.

Mosher, S. (2017). Comprehensive NICU parental education: Beyond baby basics. *Neonatal Network, 36*(1), 18–25. doi:10.1891/0730-0832.36.1.18

Purdy, I. B., Craig, J. W., & Zeanah, P. (2015). NICU discharge planning and beyond: Recommendations for parent psychosocial support. *Journal of Perinatology, 35*, S24–S28. doi:10.1038/jp.2015.146

Weiss, M. E., Bobay, K. L., Bahr, S. J., Costa, L., Hughes, R. G., & Holland, D. E. (2015). A model for hospital discharge preparation: From case management to care transition. *Journal of Nursing Administration, 45*(12), 606–614. doi:10.1097/NNA.0000000000000273

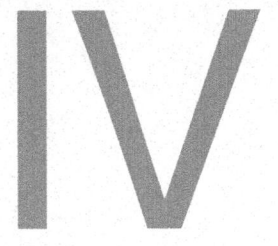

SUPPORTING PATIENTS WITH SPECIAL CHALLENGES IN THE NICU

9

HOW TO SUPPORT FAMILIES WHO ARE CHALLENGING TO CONNECT WITH

It is the goal of all clinicians, at least in my opinion, to go to work every day and be able to form a meaningful connection with every patient they care for. I cannot imagine that anyone would want to go into a caring profession and not have a desire to provide healing and build a therapeutic relationship with their patients and support systems. When caring for neonatal patients and their families, "the therapeutic relationship is an important prerequisite to effective communication between health professionals and patients in order not only to transmit information, but also to effectively address mental processes which active by it. The communication between health professionals and patients include[s] the ability to express sincere concern for the care of the patient and the patient becomes a partaker of this interest" (Moussas, Karkanias, & Papadopoulou, 2010, "Principles of Communication" section), and this becomes increasingly important when families are difficult to connect with.

Although most clinicians might idealize that therapeutic relationships would come naturally and easy with every family, unfortunately, that is not always the case. Despite best efforts, some families are more difficult to connect with for a variety of reasons. It may be difficult to connect with a family because the family itself has the following characteristics:

- Have a personality conflict with the care provider
- May be too angry about the situation to move past frustration
- May be in such shock that its members' moods and personalities have changed during a crisis and they shut out all connections with others
- Might be suffering from depression, which makes connection with others challenging
- Might have drastic cultural differences that make connection difficult
- May speak different languages, which creates a barrier to connection
- Might have sensitivity to someone of the opposite sex or of someone the opposite sex's position (For example, women in some cultures may not feel comfortable

169

speaking to men, so the male in the family is the spokesperson for the family, making connecting with the mother very challenging for any male care provider.)

- Could be coming into the NICU with a negative past experience and projecting those old feelings on to the staff
- May have low cognitive and emotional intelligence, making any connection with others difficult
- Might have low literacy levels and are ashamed of this knowledge level, so members shy away and try to hide the low understanding and avoid close relationships so that their true intelligence level will not be discovered

This list contains only a few examples, but every staff member should try to determine the root cause of why meaningful connections are not being made with families so that interventions can be attempted to remedy the limited connection. It is also important to realize that it is not always because of families that connections may be difficult. Care providers can be equally responsible for therapeutic relationships suffering within the healthcare community. Providers also contribute to the issue for various reasons, including, but not limited to, the following:

- Having a lack of education on how to provide adequate psychosocial support for families in crisis
- Being distracted by personal matters and not fully being present at work
- Not taking care of themselves and therefore not being able to fully invest in their work and the families they care for
- Experiencing compassion fatigue or burnout
- Working long hours and extra shifts, and being too overworked to be able to efficiently work to the fullest
- Expending negative cultural energy within the unit and focusing more time on gossiping, lateral violence, and attacking peers/managers
- Being more focused on personal priorities and tasks they need to accomplish in their personal lives (e.g., shopping online, working on school papers/assignments, selling items for a second job)
- Wanting to provide too much privacy to families and choosing to shut doors to private rooms when families are in with their children and then, for example, knitting or reading a novel
- Having experienced loss in the unit and disconnecting from other families as a coping mechanism to reduce the risk of being hurt again
- Having cultural barriers that are difficult to understand and not having the resources to know how to overcome them
- Having language barriers and limited resources or lacking the drive to push for the resources or adequate translation services for families

Again, the list could go on and on. As you can clearly see, there are numerous reasons why families and staff may not connect well with one another. Regardless of the reasons, units need to understand that "implementing interventions to improve communication and decision making about goals of care in the hospital required an understanding of the perspectives of patients, families, and clinicians in this clinical setting. In particular, awareness of barriers enables the development of tailored interventions that are more likely to improve professional practice compared with standard interventions" (You et al., 2015, "Introduction" section) so that optimal care and outcomes can be achieved for neonatal infants when barriers are identified and attempted to be overcome prior to discharge. All staff should attempt to find out the reasons why a connection is not occurring, attempt to remedy those reasons, and do everything possible to make some type of positive connection to positively influence the relationship not only to improve the NICU journey for the infant and family, but also to attempt to positively impact their lifelong success.

CARING FOR FAMILIES WITH VARYING LEVELS OF EDUCATION AND LEARNING DISABILITIES

Families with low educational levels and learning disabilities are some of the most challenging to connect with and to care for. Babies whose parents have some level of intellectual disability should immediately have social workers and family support specialists involved to determine all psychosocial needs and barriers that might be present because it has been shown that parents with low levels of literacy have children "with increased risk of child developmental delay, child speech and language problems, child [behavior] problems and frequent child accidents and injuries. Parental intellectual disability was also associated with increased risk of exposure to a wide range of environmental adversities such as poverty, poor housing and social isolation" (Emerson & Brigham, 2014, "Abstract" section). These data should never deter staff, however, from treating parents with the same level of respect and dignity as the most educated and sophisticated families. Parents of all ages, races, sexes, socioeconomic levels, and intellectual levels should be welcomed and treated equally as loving and capable parents in the neonatal unit.

Staff should always approach relationships with families mindfully and be open, honest, and a cognoscente of the cognitive ability of families; if there is any question at all about a family's ability to care for the child post discharge, staff should be upfront with families immediately about that concern. Initially, families may be hurt, upset, angry, and offended, but communicating that the desire of the staff is to work closely with the family to empower them to retain custody and be as fully involved in the life of their child as possible will hopefully help curb some of the tension. With proper social work support and continuous assessment by the care team, parents with lower cognitive levels or even extremely low educational levels feel supported and encouraged and are easier to connect with if they feel the staff is there to root for their success.

During the NICU journey, families are evaluated on their ability to properly care for their child in the hospital, and predictions are made about their success outside the hospital after discharge. Staff working with families should assume that all parents will be discharged home with their baby and thoroughly educate them on all discharge educational topics.

It is imperative, as it is with any family, for staff to document the parental ability to care for their child, and with these families, it is of even more importance. If there is any suspicion that a family may not be able to safely care for a child independently, either because of the inability to provide actual care for a child or because their cognitive abilities would make the living situation unsafe for the child, social work and care management teams should intensely work with the family to determine what level of social support they have and if there are close family or friends who could assist in caretaking post discharge. If there is adequate social support, the goal should always be to keep families united, but staff need to adjust their education and support to extend to all individuals who will be primary care providers in the child's life.

Providing education and sharing information with families with learning disabilities or extremely low literacy levels can be extremely challenging, so units need to have multiple ways to provide education to patients and their families so that they can meet the learning styles and literacy levels of every family. "This includes avoiding medical jargon, breaking down information or instructions into small concrete steps, limiting the focus of a visit to three key points or tasks, and assessing for comprehension. Additionally, printed information should be written at or below a fifth- to sixth-grade reading level. Visual aids, graphs, or pictures can enhance patient understanding, as can more concrete presentation of numerical information" (Hersh, Salzman, & Snyderman, 2015, para. 1).

CARING FOR FAMILIES WHO HAVE VERY LIMITED RESOURCES AND SUPPORT

Families, who have limited resources and/or limited support from their own family or community may be extremely difficult to connect with while they have a child in the NICU. When families struggle to meet their own basic needs on a daily basis, they already are living their lives fighting a daily battle. Having a baby adds an additional layer of stress, and adding the complexity of that baby being born premature or ill, with potential lifelong complications, may add such levels of stress that families may "falsely minimize or avoid [their] stressful situations, which lowers the probability of resolving their problems" (Lever, 2008, "Excerpt" section) and can drive a frustrating wedge between them and the providers that try and care for them.

As a nurse who has cared for patients in denial, I can attest that these patients and families can cause extreme frustration and annoyance; no matter how many times I would try to explain to them the severity of their child's condition or would attempt to discuss with them the reality of potential long-term health consequences so that we could problem solve and prepare for discharge, they would appear to blatantly disregard what I was telling them. I felt like everything I said went in one ear and out the other. Yet "following Freud's work in the early 20th century, denial has been understood as a psychological defense that can, under the right circumstances, be a protective and normative. In this model, denial is viewed as supporting the patient by preserving hope in the face of poor prognosis" (Williams, Olfson, & Galanter, 2015, para. 3). With this knowledge, it should be no surprise that many NICU families, even those that are not already facing extreme stress and worry in their lives, have some level of denial when on the roller coaster of the NICU journey.

Sometimes, families who are experiencing poverty, have limited resources, or struggle to cope with the stress they are under in the NICU may disconnect and have very limited visitation to the unit. If there are already financial struggles, the family may choose to focus more on work and maintaining their jobs so that they can have control over being able to bring in what financial security they can to provide basic living necessities for themselves and their child on discharge. Others may have such limited resources that they do not even have the means to get to hospital. This could include limited or no transportation, no childcare for older children, no ability to pay for meals once at that hospital, or limited clothing and access to showers, making them ashamed of their appearance. Other families may be homeless and have to spend their time searching for ways to find food to survive day to day, and that becomes their priority. When parents have so many other life events taking priority, not being physically present on the unit makes connections extremely difficult and staff has to mettle through finding ways to build meaningful relationships with these families.

Regardless of why parents may or may not be present or why they are difficult to connect with, providing full social work, case management, and family-support specialist services are of utmost importance throughout the entire NICU journey. Social work and case management teams are well educated in community resources, and together can help connect families to the available services in their community. These highly sensitive, empathetic, and resourceful professionals aim to provide "a means for improving client health, wellness and autonomy through advocacy, communication, education, identification of service resources, and service facilitation" (Sminkey & Ledoux, 2016, "Advocacy as a Foundation" section). As care team members who are acting as two of the utmost patient advocates, case managers and social workers "are required to perform a comprehensive assessment to identify the client's needs. In addition, [they] must identify options and provide choices, when available and appropriate" (Sminkey & Ledoux, 2016) to patients.

The entire NICU multidisciplinary team wants to collaborate and work together to identify these clients' needs and find options available within the system and within the community that will help meet those needs, but "the patient with special needs requires a case manager able to sensitively advocate on his/her behalf, to logically discuss pros and cons of each option, and to collaboratively reach consensus as to the most appropriate interventions as part of the patient's care plan" (Treiger & Powell, 2017, para. 6). When resources are identified, social workers and/or case managers often are the most qualified for presenting families with this information so that they can continue to provide ongoing care-coordination efforts throughout the NICU stay, into discharge planning, and beyond the hospital discharge. When families realize that individuals involved in their child's care are actively engaged in finding resources for them, that the care team is for them and not against them, they typically become more involved in care and start to be more open to the care team. That is when meaningful connections are made.

ADDRESSING THE UNIQUE NEEDS OF TEEN PARENTS

A unique subset of NICU parents that can be a challenge for today's NICU nurse is teen parents. "In 2016, there were 20.3 births for every 1,000 adolescent females ages 15–19" (Office of Adolescent Health, 2016, "Teen Births" section, para. 1), which was a slight decline from the previous year. With "the increasing age of the workforce [being] a global phenomenon" (Graham et al., 2014, "Aging Across the Globe" section), the generational gap that is present between the aging nursing force and the teen parent is a real issue and creates a barrier between staff and families that often is based on judgment, lack of understanding, shame, and varying levels of maturity. The generational gap tends to be based on different beliefs based on core values such as "work ethic, moral values, respect for others, political views, attitudes toward different races and groups and religious beliefs" (Adcox, 2017, "The Generation Gap Today" section) that can greatly hinder the ability for meaningful connections to be made.

Many teen parents have shared that they have "experienced many negative health care encounters that have contributed to disengagement and mistrust of the health care system. To engage this high-risk population in health care, practitioners are encouraged to consider their own biases when servicing this population and work toward fostering positive, nonjudgmental interactions, and supportive environments" (Harrison, Clarkin, Rohde, Worth, & Fleming, 2017, "Conclusion" section). It is important to remember that nurses are to always care for patients in a nonjudgmental way, and treat all patients equally without bias or discrimination. When working with teen parents, this ethical principle is even more significant because they may be dealing with negative societal impressions caused by the young age at which they became pregnant, they may be dealing with the disappointment of family members, there may be internal struggles with how their choices impact their religious upbringing and beliefs, they may or may not have support from others because of their life choices, and they are developmentally not fully mature and may battle with many of the new challenges they are facing.

It should be also understood that "young mothers may be more at risk for problems adjusting to the changes associated with childrearing for many reasons; developmentally, physically, emotionally, and cognitively they may not be prepared for the challenges of motherhood. Studies of teen fathers find that they want to be involved but often encounter barriers to involvement, including lack of money, lack of parenting skills, unstable relationships with the mother or her family, and increased psychosocial stress and anxiety" (Walsh & Goser, 2013, para. 1). Research also shows that "children born to teen parents are more likely to have developmental and academic delays, and often have literacy difficulties and significantly lower standardized test scores. They are 50% more likely to repeat a grade and are less likely to complete high school than children born to non-teen parents" (Ricks, 2016, "The Focus of Teen Pregnancy" section). Moreover, these teen parents will be dealing with the pressures of family, peers, social media, school, and future goals, so finding ways to connect with them and provide comprehensive psychosocial support should be of utmost importance for the entire multidisciplinary team. In addition, providing comprehensive support should be very targeted by case management and social work teams to help teen parents meet all of their physical, emotional, mental, and developmental needs.

The primary focus areas of supporting teen parents should include the following:

- Developing independence as parents
- Encouraging strong co-parenting relationships between the mother and father, if they are in a healthy and nonviolent relationship
- Finding local community resources to help meet the needs for caring for newborns
- Connecting parents with present and past teen parents to develop important peer-to-peer connections and support

- Supporting their decision making and including them as equal members of the care team

- Collaborating with their school to facilitate their meeting academic goals

- Offering and providing education materials that meet their learning-style preferences and that are at their academic level

- Assisting them in finding independent housing if they desire to live and parent autonomously

- Referring them to psychology to begin professional psychosocial support so that they have someone who can help them work through the challenges of becoming a parent during such a transitional time of their life

For units that have a high percentage of teen parents or are a large enough unit to support a teen parent support group, regularly scheduled support groups or teen parent activities should be planned so that while teen parents are in the NICU, they can connect with other young parents and find a meaningful peer-to-peer connection. Units that are unable to supply that level of support should find ways to refer patients to community groups and safe online support networks.

Author's Personal Story

I met T.S. as a family-support specialist on day 5 of her daughter's life. T.S. had delivered her little girl at 26 6/7 weeks' gestation, only 6 weeks after finding out that she was pregnant. T.S. was 16 years old, was a junior in high school, and had been dating a young man for 4 months. This young man, P.L. was also 16 years old and was a junior at a different high school. When I entered the NICU room, the two of them were sitting on opposite sides of the baby's Isolette on tall chairs, both texting furiously on their cells phones, and did not even seem to notice that I had entered the room despite the knock on the door and my greeting.

After washing my hands and quickly reviewing the dry erase board in the room, I cautiously approached the bedside as not to alarm them. I still at this point did not believe they knew I was in the room and I didn't want to startle them. I said hello once again and T.S. looked up and acknowledged me at that point. She said "Hi," offered me just enough time to introduce myself, then was back to typing swiftly on her phone. Initially, I was really put off and started to judge these two as disrespectful and rude children. I was labeling them as "typical teenagers" who were more interested in their electronics than anything else, including their child.

I caught myself in this judgmental thinking and remembered that their world was just that; it was their world and their experience. I had no knowledge at all as to what they had been through, what they were going through, and what their priorities were. I interrupted them briefly and asked when a good time would be to come and talk to them, and T.S. answered an hour later. I thanked her and decided to remember that with

(continued)

(*continued*)

developmental family-centered care, communication and psychosocial support should occur on the family's schedule, not my own.

I returned an hour later and found T.S. alone in the room still on her phone. It appeared she was taking pictures of her and her daughter and posting them or sending them to her network of connections. When I walked in, she politely put down her phone and turned her attention fully to me. I admit I was pleasantly surprised, and I felt foolish for initially thinking negatively about her behavior. I washed my hands, reintroduced myself, and pulled up a chair to sit next to her for a little while. I wanted to have a very early initial conversation about my family-support specialist role and the things that we could accomplish together during her daughter's stay. I learned in the next 20 minutes that T.S. and P.L. were together and planned to co-parent together even though P.L. was not the biological father; that they both planned to transition to the local high school offering a teen parent program so they could finish high school and also parent; that she lives with her best friend and her parents, who were kind enough to let her come live with them during her pregnancy because her family had not gotten along since they found out she was pregnant; that she was not looking to have any kind of relationship with the biological father (in fact, she hadn't told him that she was pregnant with his child); that she and P.L. were going to be moving in with her older sister, who was 24 years old and a single mom, when the baby was discharged; and that her personal life goal was to go to college and become a fashion designer while P.L. wanted to study criminal justice and become a police officer.

I was a little blown away by her clear and concise goals, and internally I was pretty apprehensive about how successful she would be because I had some red flags that stood out to me quite immediately:

1. She did not have support from her parents, and she did not mention others who would be involved to offer support.

2. She was living with a best friend and her family who agreed to let her live with them during her pregnancy, but were they going to let her stay there longer? Now that she had delivered the baby, would she have a place to live if she was not welcomed back or chose not to return home to her parents?

3. She planned to change schools and join a teen parent program, unaware that the local program was full and had a long wait list.

4. She planned to move in with her sister who was a single mom, and I wondered what type of relationship she had with her sister, and what type of supportive relationship her sister would be if she was busy being a parent herself.

5. She had not told the biological father that she was pregnant and had his baby.

6. She did not mention that she or P.L. had a job, so how were they going to support themselves and this child?

(*continued*)

(continued)

This list was just my initial thoughts after 20 minutes, so it didn't surprise me that after the next 2 months of caring for T.S. and P.L. that my list of concerns grew exponentially. During their daughter's stay, which was filled with days when the clinical team was worried about her medical stability, T.S. would come into the unit with an entourage of friends, at all hours of the weekdays, and spend their time at the bedside taking photos of themselves with the baby, who was still extremely fragile, and then gossip about school rather than focus time and energy on the many educational tasks and learning that was piling up. Weekends were quieter, and visits were limited to T.S. and P.L. coming in alone or coming in accompanied by P.L.'s parents. I noticed that during the week, when T.S. and P.L. were surrounded by friends, their personalities were lively and happy, but on the weekends, they were more solemn and quiet.

After several weeks of this habitual behavior, I scheduled a meeting with the two of them to share my observations, and I reviewed with them that multiple staff members, including the neonatologists, nurses, social workers, case managers, and myself, had all attempted to meet with them to provide really important updates and information but felt as though those pieces of information were not being received. Both T.S. and P.L. looked puzzled and confused and admitted that they did not recognize that any of this had occurred, and I re-emphasized that the NICU is a place where staff and parents work together to care for babies, and that we wanted to help them gain confidence in their roles as parents and caretakers. To do that, we needed them to start providing us some of their attention and maybe limiting some of their social visits with friends that were occurring in the unit.

T.S. broke down into tears. She confessed that she was struggling on so many fronts that she didn't even know what to do or where to go for help. She was desperately trying to act brave and put together, but in reality, she was falling apart. She didn't have her family around to lean on; her friend's family had asked her to leave, so she was staying with random friends who were getting their parents to agree to let her stay for a night or two at a time; she came to the unit with friends because that was the only time they wanted to be around her anymore; she was too afraid to stay long in the unit and learn about her baby because she didn't know how to bond with her daughter and was too scared to get attached because what if she failed and her baby got taken away; and she was so far behind in school, she was afraid she was going to have to repeat her junior year. She felt disconnected, lost, and defeated. My heart just hurt for her, and frankly, it also hurt for our entire team!

All along, the entire staff and I did everything we could to try and connect with her and provide her with psychosocial support to avoid this very outcome. Yet despite our best efforts, here she was. She was sad and felt alone, and I felt like we had failed her in every way possible. It was time to press the restart button and try again. The reality was, she and P.L. were still coming to the unit frequently and they had great support from his parents. Not all was lost!

From that moment, the social worker and I had regularly scheduled meetings with this young couple. We used the first meeting to set realistic and agreed-on goals together not

(continued)

(*continued*)

only for their daughter (who was the patient), but also for the two of them as parents and as individuals. Our incredible social worker helped connect them to a local teen parent program that housed teen mothers and offered teen parenting programs. Since T.S. was still not comfortable reaching out to her parents, she agreed to try a group home setting where young pregnant and new mothers lived together and supported one another with the oversight of women who volunteered their time to mentor these young ladies. P.L. was allowed to visit during day hours but could not stay the night, which allowed them time to be apart and focus on catching up with schoolwork. Our social worker also found a tutor who was willing to donate time to help the two of them get caught up and talk with the administration at the school. With the support of the tutor and with the completion of one summer class, T.S. would be able to remain on track to move on to her senior year as scheduled. Our social worker and I also helped with the following tasks:

- Re-enlisted the support of the NICU psychologist to provide professional mental health support and adequate postpartum depression screening
- Enrolled T.S. and P.L. in a new parenting course that was offered through the county health department and offered at no cost to families who qualified
- Enrolled T.S. and P.L. in a job-resource program in which young parents are supported in finding work so that they can have flexible schedules to focus on their family, yet also have financial means to support their family
- Found donations from various community resources to obtain diapers, clothing, a car seat, blankets, and a crib to meet some of their newborn basic needs
- Ensured that, between myself and bedside nursing staff, T.S. and P.L. were learning to care for their child and feeling confident in the required discharge education so that there would be ample time to review everything multiple times to reinforce confidence
- Assisted in identifying a pediatrician and other specialty providers so that all follow-up care and appointments could be made prior to discharge
- Walked through scenarios of how they would get to follow-up appointments and helped remove identified barriers prior to discharge
- Provided all education in various methods and at their educational level
- Found community programs and events for new parents that T.S. and P.L. might enjoy
- Held an educational hour for T.S. and P.L.'s friends to explain premature birth, the lifelong risks and potential complications of prematurity, ways to help reduce the risk of infection and illness after discharge, and ways to support new parents (which they *loved*)

(*continued*)

(*continued*)

Although all of these interventions supported this young couple in the remaining weeks of their NICU journey and ultimately led to them leaving the NICU, when their daughter was 39 weeks and 4 days old, with confidence and a realistic postdischarge plan, these interventions also led to our staff learning so much from them. We learned that despite our best efforts, we can't easily connect with every family every time. We also learned that you cannot give up! You have to support families from the moment they arrive in the NICU to the moment they leave, because you never know when you will make a connection that will leave a positive impact on their life or in their story.

Family Story

Patricia Heyward shares her story of being a teen mom who gave birth to a 28-week infant who spent 81 days in the NICU.

"On September 26, 2017, I went in for a regular OB check when I was referred to a high-risk doctor because my daughter's growth at 28 weeks was measuring only 24 weeks. After getting my ultrasound, the doctor insisted on having me admitted to the hospital and being closely monitored. I was diagnosed with sIUGR, and my daughter's placenta was very thin and not giving her enough blood or nutrients. My first night in the hospital, my daughter dropped her heart rate three different times, each when I was either napping or on my way into a deep sleep.

"On the second day at 4:30 in the morning, a nurse ran into the room waking me to put an oxygen mask on me and made me lie on my side. It took 5 minutes to get my daughter's heart rate to go back up to where they wanted it, and I cried and insisted on having a doctor come take my daughter out of me before something bad happened. That morning I got another ultrasound, and my daughter failed her biophysical profile; also, she was not practicing breathing. With that, and also with her heart rate dropping, I was told that my baby was in distress and I was going to have an emergency C-section in the next couple of hours.

"The neonatologist came to talk to me at that point and explained that with my daughter being the size of a 24-week baby and weighing only 520 grams, she might struggle quite a bit, but the resuscitation team was going to do everything in their might to save her. I was prepared for my C-section 10 minutes later, and before I knew it, we were welcoming my princess into the world. She was very tiny, only 1 lb 2.3 oz. The first couple of days were scary because you never know what to expect with babies being so small. After a week, I finally got to hold my daughter, hooked up to IVs, oxygen, and also a PICC line. I remember the nurses being very nice, helpful, and also encouraging at that time. Before this NICU experience, I had a 32-week son born due to preeclampsia, and he ended up passing away after only 2½ months being on this earth. I felt like I rushed my son out of the hospital, and I feel like if I would have just let him stay until

(*continued*)

(*continued*)

his due date, we would have discovered he had reflux and could have tried to treat it. But being a young mom and not knowing things about the medical field made things even more difficult. Not having the right pediatrician and being only 16 with a child with really no support or guidance was the worst. When it came to my daughter I was very humble and patient, and I prayed for her and every baby in the NICU every single day. My daughter beat all odds being only 1 lb at birth. She had no brain bleeds, no PDA, and needed only support breathing. During our NICU stay, my daughter stopped breathing multiple times and it was so hard for me to try and bond with her because of what happened to my son. I didn't want to get attached to another baby and then have the same thing happen to me all over again.

"I insisted my daughter stay hospitalized until her due date and until she was 4 lb and could fit into her car seat. Not every nurse was helpful or encouraging though. I had multiple nurses think that just because I was underage, they could tell me what they felt like I 'needed' to do with my daughter or how I needed to move back with my mom from my own home because I would need adult supervision. As a young mother, you will always be looked at as someone who does not know anything or does not know what is best for your child. In our NICU, I felt like an outcast. I felt like I was the youngest one there. There were no support groups or any teen parent groups. Even at the NICU lunch-ins I would sit all alone because I knew no one wanted to talk to the 'teen mom.'

"Looking back, what would have been helpful being a teen mom in the NICU is having other mom's my age to converse with and not have to feel so alone on the journey. Feeling like you are the only teenager going through that experience and the only young mom who has a baby in the NICU was really hard. I wish the nurses would be able to gather all the teen moms so we could mingle and feel less alone, support one another, and become a network of individuals who could help one another get through that tough time.

"Overall, after 81 long, fighting days, we made it out alive at 4 lb 2.3 oz. We were released from the NICU on ⅛ L of oxygen, and after being home for only a month, my daughter is now 6 lb 2.3 oz, and completely off of oxygen."

RECOMMENDATIONS/SUGGESTIONS FOR BEST PRACTICE

1. Assume that all families, even those with extremely low cognitive function or low literacy levels, will be discharged home with their babies and educate them throughout the NICU journey accordingly.

2. Have all educational material available in multiple formats and in varying educational levels to meet the needs and learning styles of all families in the NICU.

3. Keep printed educational material at or below a fifth-grade reading level.

4. Have a robust case management and social work department within the NICU multidisciplinary team to support families who need internal and external resource connections.

5. Provide education to all staff on how to provide psychosocial support to all NICU families in a nonjudgmental fashion.

6. Offer teen-specific support groups and peer-to-peer activities on a regular basis.

7. Provide comprehensive psychosocial support to all families from the moment they are admitted to the unit to the moment they are discharged.

RECOMMENDED RESOURCES

Multiple resources are available to staff to further knowledge and education about how to best support families who are challenging to connect with in the NICU (Figure 9.1).

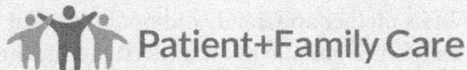 Patient+Family Care

Website Recommendations:
1. https://www.acf.hhs.gov/sites/default/files/assets/pregnant-parenting-teens-tips.pdf
2. https://www.childwelfare.gov/topics/preventing/promoting/parenting/pregnant-teens
3. http://pregnancy.lovetoknow.com/wiki/Resources_for_Pregnant_Teens
4. https://www.plannedparenthood.org
5. http://stayteen.org
6. https://www.livestrong.com/article/262052-resources-for-teen-mothers
7. https://insightstpp.org
8. http://www.healthyteennetwork.org/blog/helping-pregnant-parenting-teens-find-housing
9. https://www.teenoutreachaz.org/teen-service/teenage-pregnancy-parenting-support-groups
10. https://www.heartbeatinternational.org/6-effective-ways-to-mentor-teen-parents

Journal Recommendations:
1. Angley, M., Divney, A., Magriples, U., & Kershaw, T. (2014). Social support, family functioning and parenting competence in adolescent parents. *Maternal and Child Health Journal, 19*(1), 67–73.
2. Sherman, L. E., & Greenfield, P. M. (2013). Forging friendship, soliciting support: A mixed-method examination of message boards for pregnant teens and teen mothers. *Computers in Human Behavior, 29*(1), 75–85.
3. Akella, D., & Jordan, M. (2014). Impact of social and cultural factors on teenage pregnancy. *Journal of Health Disparities Research and Practice, 8*(1), 41–62.

Figure 9.1 ■ Recommended resources for staff who care for families that are difficult to connect with in the NICU.

Case-Based Learning

T.G. is a term 2-day-old who is 1-day postoperative repair of a tracheoesophageal fistula (TEF). During rounds, her mother is very distraught and crying. She demands that you call the surgeon because a mistake has been made because there is a tube coming out of her baby's chest when the baby's problem was in her throat.

QUESTIONS

1. What is the likely cause of this mother's distress?
2. How could this unnecessarily stressful event have been avoided?

ANSWERS

T.G.'s mother apparently did not know that a thoracotomy was needed to repair her baby's TEF and did know understand the function of a chest tube. She may have been too stressed by the situation to retain the information shared with her preoperatively or did not understand the explanation given to her by the surgical team. She may have been embarrassed that she did not understand the description of the surgery and refrained from asking for clarification. This misunderstanding could have been avoided if an assessment of her understanding was done and if a clearer description, drawing, or other teaching method such as teach back was used.

Before providing education to a family, assessment of their learning style and capacity to absorb the information being shared is critical. Healthcare providers need health literacy skills to understand how best to provide needed knowledge and teach parents most effectively about their infant. Comprehension and retention of medical terms is difficult, especially under stressful conditions. Discussions about, and consent for, procedures need to be geared toward the learning style and level of the parents. In general, patient education materials should be written in plain language, which is suggested to be at a fifth-grade reading level (Centers for Disease Control and Prevention [CDC], 2016).

Health literacy can affect neonatal outcomes in the short and long term. It is important to keep parents informed about the progress of their baby, to include them in their baby's care, and to teach them what they need to know to provide for their baby's health needs when the baby is no longer hospitalized. It is critical that we teach parents and families in ways that ensure their success.

Many NICU graduates go home taking medications; therefore, instructing caregivers in the administration of medications is a common part of discharge teaching. If not done well, without good grasp by the parents, untoward events can happen. Drug administration errors by parents, such as incorrect dose, route, or formulation, account for 70% of preventable medication adverse events (Yin, 2017). Unintentional therapeutic errors account for almost 90% of Poison Control Center calls in infants under 6 months of age (Kang & Brooks, 2016).

It is incumbent on NICU staff to ensure parental understanding of discharge care and follow-up for their infant. Not following directions because of lack of comprehension

(continued)

(*continued*)

and/or not being unaware of the importance of follow-up care can impact long-term outcomes. Lack of health literacy is linked to increased emergency room use in NICU graduates and has been shown to contribute to poor neurodevelopmental outcomes (Patra & Greene, 2017).

REFERENCES

Centers for Disease Control and Prevention. (2016). Health literacy. Retrieved from https://www.cdc.gov/healthliteracy/learn/index.html

Kang A. M., & Brooks D. E. (2016). US Poison Control Center calls for infants 6 months of age and younger. *Pediatrics, 137*(2):e20151865. doi:10.1542/peds.2015-1865

Patra, K., & Greene, M. M. (2017). Health care utilization after NICU discharge and neurodevelopmental outcome in the first 2 years of life in preterm infants. *American Journal of Perinatology*. doi:10.1055/s-0037-1608678

Yin, H. S. (2017). Health literacy and child health outcomes: Parental health literacy and medication errors. In R. Connelly & T. Turner (Eds.), *Health literacy and child health outcomes* (pp. 19–38). Cham, Switzerland: Springer International.

REFERENCES

Adcox, S. (2017, October 23). Looking at the generation gap. Retrieved from https://www.thespruce.com/looking-at-the-generation-gap-1695859

Emerson, E., & Brigham, P. (2014). The developmental health of children of parents with intellectual disabilities: Cross sectional study. *Research in Developmental Disabilities, 35*(4), 917–921. doi:10.1016/j.ridd.2014.01.006

Graham, E., Donoghue, J., Duffield, C., Griffiths, R., Bichel-Findlay, J., & Dimitrelis, S. (2014). Why do older RNs keep working? *Journal of Nursing Administration, 44*(11), 591–597. doi:10.1097/nna.0000000000000131

Harrison, M. E., Clarkin, C., Rohde, K., Worth, K., & Fleming, N. (2017). Treat me but don't judge me: A qualitative examination of health care experiences of pregnant and parenting youth. *Journal of Pediatric and Adolescent Gynecology, 30*(2), 209–214. doi:10.1016/j.jpag.2016.10.001

Hersh, L., Salzman, B., & Snyderman, D. (2015). Health literacy in primary care practice. *American Family Physician, 92*(2), 118–124.

Lever, J. P. (2008). Poverty, stressful life events, and coping strategies. *Spanish Journal of Psychology, 11*(1), 228–249. doi:10.1017/S1138741600004273

Moussas, G. I., Karkanias, A. P., & Papadopoulou, A. G. (2010). Psychological dimension of cancer genetics: Doctor-patient communication. *Psychiatriki, 21*, 148–157.

Office of Adolescent Health. (2016, June 02). Trends in teen pregnancy and childbearing. Retrieved from https://www.hhs.gov/ash/oah/adolescent-development/reproductive-health-and-teen-pregnancy/teen-pregnancy-and-childbearing/trends/index.html

Ricks, N. (2016). The strengths perspective: Providing opportunities for teen parents and their families to succeed. *Journal of Family Strengths, 15*(1), Article 11.

Sminkey, P. V., & Ledoux, J. (2016). Case management ethics: High professional standards for health care's interconnected worlds. *Professional Case Management, 21*(4), 193–198. doi:10.1097/NCM.0000000000000166

Treiger, T. M., & Powell, S. K. (2017). It may be simple, but it's not easy: Conscious case management. *Professional Case Management, 22*(3), 99–100. doi:10.1097/NCM.0000000000000218

Walsh, J., & Goser, L. (2013). Development of an innovative NICU teen parent support program: One unit's experience. *Journal of Perinatal & Neonatal Nursing, 27*(2), 176–183. doi:10.1097/JPN.0b013e31828eafd1

Williams, A. R., Olfson, M., & Galanter, M. (2015). Assessing and improving clinical insight among patients "in denial." *JAMA Psychiatry, 72*(4), 303–304. doi:10.1001/jamapsychiatry.2014.2684

You, J. J., Downar, J., Fowler, R. A., Lamontagne, F., Ma, I. W., Jayaraman, D., ... Heyland, D. K. (2015). Barriers to goals of care discussions with seriously ill hospitalized patients and their families. *JAMA Internal Medicine, 175*(4), 549–556. doi:10.1001/jamainternmed.2014.7732

10

HELPING FAMILIES BALANCE NICU LIFE AND HOME LIFE

Balancing hospital life and home life can be a challenge, and when families find themselves having to learn to juggle those two lives for weeks or months when their baby is in the NICU, the balancing act can become a tremendous task. While part of the family's life has stood still and their entire world revolves around their hospitalized child, they still have to somehow keep up with the responsibilities in their home life. They may have jobs to perform, bills to pay, laundry to do, housework and yard work to do, pets to take care of, other children to care for, vehicles to maintain, groceries to purchase, meals to make, events to attend, among other things. Let's not forget they need to find time to take care of themselves too.

In a perfect world, families who have a baby in the hospital would be surrounded by family and friends who would help them take care of all of life's responsibilities so that they would have no additional worries and could focus solely on parenting their ill or premature child. Someone would take a lead role and figure out who would pick up older children and get them to school, help them with homework, shuttle them to after-school activities, make dinner, pack lunches, do the grocery shopping, do the laundry, clean the house, care for pets, and pay the bills. How nice would it be to have an entire community of support that would help care for families so that parents could care for themselves and their baby? I can't even imagine what the immediate and long-term emotional and physical outcomes would be for infants and families if that were the case.

Sadly, not all parents of NICU babies have great support teams. Some NICU families have very little to no outside support at all and face the grueling NICU journey alone. For example, these families may be estranged from their families, may live far away from family, may be new to the area, may have been on vacation when they unexpectedly delivered early and away from their support network, might have been transported to a different city if their child required care at a higher-level facility, or may be recently separated from a spouse or significant other.

The one thing that all families have in common is they will need help from NICU staff to survive the NICU journey; they will need help psychosocially, and they will need help learning how to ask for help. So many individuals, fathers, and mothers want to appear strong and independent and feel it would be a sign of weakness if they relied on others for help. Staff need to highlight to families the importance of leaning on others during times of crisis and point out ways the unit and others can help make the juggling act a little less cumbersome. With any luck, so many balls won't have to be in the air all at once.

BALANCING OLDER SIBLINGS

Some families experience the NICU with their very first child. Other families have other children and find themselves trying to balance time at the hospital and time at home. These "parents often struggle to manage their older children in addition to coping with their newborn, making this challenging time harder for the whole family" (Wainwright, 2017, "Abstract" section). These families struggle with guilt over where they spend their time; if they are at the hospital spending time with their new baby who needs them there for bonding, feeding, and growing, they feel guilty that the other children are at home alone or are being shuttled between other family and friends. If they are at home with older children, they feel guilty that their new baby is alone in a hospital. The reality is, they can't be in two places at once, so NICU staff need to help them learn how to not only manage the guilt, but also spend time equally with each sibling, making time with both equally important. Staff caring for families who have other children need to pay particular attention to helping families include the siblings as important members of the family and should assist families in determining schedules to help create meaningful time and connections with all of their children.

In Chapter 6 of this text, we looked at supporting families in the NICU and discussed the importance of including siblings as equal and important members of the family. To elaborate on that message, encouraging sibling attendance and involvement in the unit allows families to be together and decreases the stress of separation. With encouraging sibling visitation and participation, parents are more able to be in the unit without the pressures of being separated; "the presence of parents in NICUs and their involvement caring [for] their babies, in a family centered care philosophy, is vital to improve the outcome of their infants and the relationships within each family" (Guimarães, 2015, "Abstract" section).

It is not realistic to expect that siblings can be in the unit around the clock; however, infection-control concerns need to always be kept in mind, as do the safety and health of neonates in the NICU. Although siblings of all ages should be allowed to visit at all times and studies have shown that "sibling visitations to the NICU [do] not result in an increase in the nosocomial viral infection rate" (Horikoshi et al., 2018, "Background" section), education and strict adherence to handwashing and limited visitation to those showing signs of illness should be followed. These strict guidelines also need to be enforced with siblings, and depending on the age and maturity level of siblings, visits may need to be limited to short periods so that they do not become disruptive to the healing environment.

Ideas to discuss with families for times when siblings cannot be in the unit or for supporting them in finding ways to balance time at home and at the hospital may include the following:

- If older children are in school, spend time at the hospital when they are in class and then spend evenings at home. This allows parents to spend quality time at the hospital while the other children are busy and already occupied, and then they can be available at home in the evening for dinner and homework help, keeping home routines as normal as possible.

- If children are not yet in school, find local family or friends who will watch them or take them to do fun things when parents visit the hospital without them. If they do not have family or friends in the area, assist them in finding respite nurseries or local resources that can provide low-cost childcare.

- If families live quite a distance from the hospital, assist in arranging a stay at a local Ronald McDonald House; encourage them to take advantage of the wonderful sibling activities sponsored by the House so that there is some time for family and fun outside of the hospital. If families are traveling to and from home to the hospital but live a distance, encourage an alternate schedule in which one parent stays longer at the hospital one day while the other parent is home with the siblings and then trade off the next day.

- If siblings are in school, encourage families to take time to visit the school for lunch or attend a school play, concert, or sporting event with them. As important as it is to be at the hospital with their baby, it is also important for them to remain active in their other children's life for events that are special to them.

- Facilitate activities for the families to do together that create a bond between siblings and the new baby. These may include participating in sibling support groups, asking big brothers and sisters to draw pictures to hang up at the baby's bedside, encouraging the family to bring in photos to hang up, and sending photos of the baby to the older siblings.

The important point is that even if they develop a schedule or routine that feels right for their family, they will never feel perfect! Parent guilt will be present no matter what. Staff should continually reassure them that everything will be okay and inspire them to have grace with themselves. Congratulate them on doing a great job and provide constant encouragement and positive reinforcement. They may have to change their plans several times to adapt to changing situations during the NICU journey, but with staff support, they will be able to better adapt and adjust.

BALANCING PARENTING AND RELATIONSHIPS

Mothers of preterm infants [tend] to report more health related difficulties, more depression, higher social isolation and role restriction, and less support from their spouses, than reported by fathers. Moreover, as time [goes] on, parents with preterm infants [continue] to experience greater parenting stress than those with full-term infants. (Howe, Shey, Wang, & Hsu, 2014, "Abstract" section)

NICU care providers must understand these experiences and help design programs and interventions to help improve the parenting experience for families who have infants that start out life in the NICU. In the past, studies have reported that parents who have a child with a lifelong medical condition have a divorce rate of over 70%; that is just from statistics of married couples. Imagine if the data included the numbers of relationships that are not marriages that have also ended. At a time when a parent needs a support person (whether that be a spouse, boyfriend, or girlfriend) the most, these relationships historically have been falling apart. Talk about adding even more stress to an already stressful life event!

Facing the challenge of an unpredictable event and stressful start to an infant's life can have a devastating impact on a parent's life and a huge impact on the relationship with their parenting partner. "Men and women report different reactions to stress, both physically and mentally. They attempt to manage stress in very different ways and also perceive their ability to do so—and the things that stand in their way—in markedly different ways" (American Psychological Association, n.d.). Both mothers and fathers report experiences of trauma related to the hospitalization of their child so it's not surprising that with such opposite coping mechanisms, they find themselves driving one another away and creating a distance between them that is sometimes difficult to navigate back from.

NICU staff are not marital or relationship counselors and should not claim to be. Nor should staff take on the responsibility of trying to fix relationships between parents. However, when looking at providing psychosocial support to families, if parents are struggling in their relationship with each other, that stress is certainly going to impact their stress level and, ultimately, their ability to bond with their baby and cope with the NICU journey. It is important for NICU staff to recognize signs of troubled relationships, know how to refer couples to support resources, and reassure families that stress on relationships during this tremendously stressful time of their life is normal. Staff should encourage couples to talk to each other, participate in peer-to-peer support activities, and recognize that professional support may be something they might want to consider.

Many couples do not want to admit that they may need professional support, but with the added stress of a NICU journey and potentially a life ahead of long-term health consequences due to their child's prematurity, professional support may be the best thing to help them cope through the NICU journey and beyond. Kara Wahlin, a licensed marriage and family therapist, offers a list of really great questions that couples can ask themselves to determine whether professional support is the best choice for them. If a couple can relate to the following questions, seeking help may be a ticket to better communication, improved understanding, and better relationship with each other that may save their relationship and ultimately provide a stable and healthy environment for their child and family (Figure 10.1).

Kara Wahlin is not only a marriage and family therapist, but also a NICU graduate mother of twin boys of 26 and 6/7 weeks' gestation. One boy survived and one passed away from complications of prematurity a week after birth. Kara knows firsthand what stressor parents face in the NICU and how difficult it can be to try to balance life at the

Kara Wahlin, NICU Healing

Have you and your partner experienced:

- Alienation from each other in trying to find your different parenting "roles" in this new and unpredictable experience?
- Difficulty communicating with each other after the baby is born?
- An avoidance of talking about the birth of the baby to protect your or your partner's feelings?
- Concern about your partner's level of depression and the ways that it may affect your relationship or their relationship with the baby?
- Physical distance in distinct contrast with what your physical relationship looked like before?
- Substance abuse and/or avoidance behaviors in one or the other partner in trying to "numb" memories of the experience?
- Very different ways of coping with the premature birth of your baby?
- Anxiety that is so extreme that it affects either the partnership relationship or one or the other's attachment with the baby?
- Alienation from friends and family and an inability to feel motivated to do things together anymore?
- Feelings that you live a very distinct and separate life from your partner, and that you no longer "connect" in the ways you once did?

Figure 10.1 ■ Partnership in the face of trauma.

hospital, parenthood, and a relationship. Kara has taken this experience and started an amazing organization called NICU Healing, a therapeutic program dedicated to the healing, education, and empowerment of parents and families facing the hospitalization of a premature or medically complex baby. Kara strives, with every client, to provide clinical resources that they can use to cope with the traumatic stress of the NICU environment and the parental stressors of having a premature or ill child; she also uncovers the hidden strengths of the families faced with incredible challenges. NICU Healing truly wants to help families find reprieve from the traumatic experiences they've had and to transform their trauma into powerful attachment with their child and solidarity as a family.

Parenting relationships are not the only relationships that NICU parents find themselves needing help balancing, however. All relationships are at risk of being compromised and take a toll when parents are stressed and spend time in the hospital with their child. Relationships with parents, grandparents, adult siblings, friends, coworkers, and others in their lives all are impacted. When individuals find themselves in episodes of stress or crisis, it can be very difficult to maintain relationships, which can be an additional cause of stress for parents. NICU staff can reassure families that this too is normal and recommend that communicating to family and friends through a letter or email may be beneficial, explaining what the family is going through and how their family and friends can help them through this difficult time (Figures 10.2 and 10.3).

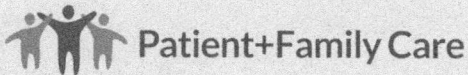 Patient+Family Care

Dear Family and Friends,
As you know, we have welcomed a new addition to our family! However, to get stronger and healthier, our baby needs a little extra help from the NICU. We have seen our child have great days and then some fairly rough days. Premature and sick infants apparently like a rush because they operate on this roller coaster, so we never know if it will be a good day or a rough day!

And what we are noticing is that we tend to have the same type of routine these days. Some mornings we can get up, feel like we can carry on a normal day, and get through all we have to do with little stress and worry. Unfortunately, other days we struggle to even get enough energy to just get out of bed and complete simple tasks. The emotions of being new parents, balancing the hospital with all of the other life responsibilities we have and trying to make sense of everything that is going on, can be a lot to deal with.

We want you to know that we will seem to go up and down, depending on the day. Please be patient with us! We need the love and support from our family and friends now more than ever, but we may also need space and time too. Do not take this personally. If you don't hear from us for a while, it's not because we are not thinking of you and not wanting to stay connected. It's just that we have other competing priorities right now too.

Thank you so much for your understanding! We are just trying to figure this all out and we are so thankful for you to be by our side during this incredible journey!

With Love,

	PHONE	FAX	WEB
2660 NE Hwy 20 Suite 610 #338 Bend, OR 97701	541-410-1921	541-382-2145	www.patientfamilycare.com

Figure 10.2 ■ Sample letter to family and friends from NICU parent.

RETURNING TO WORK

Many parents face the unfortunate reality of having to return to work prior to their baby being discharged from the hospital. Depending on what maternal and/or paternal leave parents have and contingent on how long their baby will be in the hospital, many parents face the grueling decision of whether or not to take their leave after birth or after hospital discharge. Some families take partial leaves after birth and the remainder after discharge, some have one parent take leave after birth and the other take leave after discharge, others both take leave after discharge but not after birth, and others do not even have leave and must return to work shortly after delivery. Regardless of their situation, if a parent has to return to work while their child is in the hospital, the transition back to work is stress provoking for the family, and staff should be prepared to support them through this time.

When your friends or family members welcome a baby who requires time in a NICU, they experience great days and, unfortunately, difficult days. Babies can spend anywhere from hours, to days, to *months* in the hospital, so your patience and support for them will be greatly appreciated. Also, while many parents won't ask others for help, we know that even the smallest things that others can help with will make a huge difference! Here are some ideas on how *you* can help:

- Prepare meals for them.
- Set up a meal train so that others can prepare meals too.
  - Visit https://www.mealtrain.com to set up a meal calendar and send it to other family and friends.
- If they have other children:
  - Find time to watch them and take them do something fun and special.
  - Help pick them up from school or daycare.
  - Help with homework and school projects.
  - Take them to their after-school or summer sports/activities.
- Help watch and take of their pets so that they can spend more time at the hospital.
- Spend an afternoon doing yard work for them.
- Ask if you can help wash and fold laundry for them.
- Offer to clear their house or help hire a housekeeper to come in and help.
- Create travel packs for taking to the hospital.
  - Include healthy snacks.
  - Include bottled water and/or juice boxes.
- Purchase books about premature babies and give them a gift.
  - Find countless books that are either medically focused and provide information about the development of premature and sick infants or books that have been written by other NICU parents that focus on the emotional aspects of caring for a fragile infant.
- Try to take them out to dinner or to sneak them away for lunch or even coffee (time with friends and family will be good for them).
- Offer to drive them to and from the hospital.
- Purchase gas gift cards to help lessen the cost of traveling back and forth.
- Go to the grocery store and get them basic things to make sure they have things at home:
  - Milk
  - Bread
  - Sandwich meat
  - Protein bars
  - Peanuts (if they are not allergic)
- Ask what would be helpful to them and have them create their own list of ways to help.

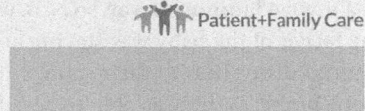
Patient+Family Care

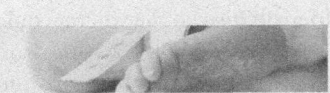

Figure 10.3 ■ Ways that family and friends can help NICU parents.

Some important things to consider, and help prepare families for when returning to work, may be the following:

- If families have other children, time at the hospital and at home is even more challenging to split and balance because now their day is spent at work. Their free time is now much more limited and is divided between hospital, home, and other life responsibilities.

- If breastfeeding/pumping, mom needs to have a breast pump and the ability to pump while at work. Coordination with her employer ensures that she has a private space to pump several times a day, that there is a safe place to properly store the expressed milk, that she has a way to adequately transport the expressed milk from work to home or the hospital, and that her employer supports her breaks to pump.

- If both parents are working, they might visit the hospital together or take turns. Often, fathers visit the hospital on their way to work in the morning, and mothers visit on their way home in the evening, or vice versa.

- Depending on where their place of employment is located in relation to the hospital, traffic patterns or traffic times may impact their ability to visit the hospital or their visitation plans.

- When they are at work, the medical team needs to know the best way to reach them if there were an emergency and for daily updates.

The most important way that staff can support any parent having to return to work is finding techniques to help them feel connected to their baby, finding ways that they can stay involved in the care planning and decision making, performing care on the parents' schedule, and being flexible to meet their needs.

Author's Personal Story

I met N.B. after a bedside nurse put in a referral for her to have a family-support specialist consult. Before our first meeting, I read her son's NICU chart and learned that he was a 32 week and 4-day-old infant at birth and was now 2½ weeks old. Medically speaking, he was stable and was what we considered a feeder/grower and was doing well. N.B. was 39 years old and this was her fourth child. The other three children were 8 and 5 years old, respectively, with the 5-year-olds being a set of identical twin girls. The family lived in a town 45 minutes away, so N.B. was staying at the local Ronald McDonald House, and the father of the baby was staying at home with the older siblings so that there would be limited disruption to their school and extracurricular activities. N.B.'s husband worked from home, so he was able to see the children off to school and pick them up, and he would travel up to the hospital with the entire family on the weekends, when they would stay together at the Ronald McDonald House.

(continued)

(*continued*)

I entered N.B.'s room and I found her tearful and facing away from her child, even though she was cradling him in her arms. I grabbed some tissue and asked if she would be okay if I came in and sat down with her for a little while. She agreed and I sat with her in silence after I introduced myself and allowed her the space to be with her emotions. After she collected herself and was able to stop crying, she apologized; I immediately told her that she should not apologize for being emotional, that being a new mother was stressful, exhausting, and emotional, and adding the NICU component on top of it all amplified all of those experiences. Her reaction was normal, and she was allowed to feel and be any way she needed to be.

I asked N.B. if there was anything in particular that was upsetting her or if she felt it was the hormonal and expected emotional reactions to motherhood. She opened up and shared the following things with me:

- She missed her older children terribly! Every time she held her son, she felt overwhelming guilt that she wasn't at home with her other children. Her husband would come up on the weekends with the girls, but by the time they arrived on Saturday morning, visited at the hospital, went back to the Ronald McDonald House to spend time together as a family, she felt the weekend was already over and they were heading back again on Sunday.

- She hated missing everything at her children's school. She was a dedicated volunteer and routinely spent every Tuesday and Thursday mornings in their classrooms and felt that she was letting not only the teacher, but also her girls, down. She had several big classroom projects that she had signed up to take on, and she was now falling behind on her work and she felt like she was failing.

- She felt like she and her husband were drifting apart. She was lonely and scared, and desperately wanted to talk to him. However, she felt like when they talked on the phone. he was short with her; when they saw each other on the weekend, he was distant; and they argued more now than they ever had before.

- She was missing her friends and didn't know how to reach out to them. When she talked to them, she tried to tell them how she was feeling and what the NICU experience was like, but none of them seemed to understand, so she felt she almost scared them all off because they weren't calling her, weren't visiting, and weren't including her in their weekly coffee book club meeting invites anymore.

N.B. was clearly struggling with many issues and there was no way we were going to be able to work through all of them in one sitting. I assured her that together we could work through all of her concerns and that she was not going to have to face any of her anxieties alone, but we would have to tackle them one at a time. It was almost time for her son's care, so I tasked her with writing out all of her worries that night and then to prioritize them. We could then meet again the next morning and together create a plan. I also tasked her with

(*continued*)

going back to the Ronald McDonald House early that evening to eat a warm, nutritious dinner and to get to bed at a decent hour. I educated her on the importance of sleep, and with her pumping around the clock, sleep was very important.

I met with N.B. the next morning and she looked like a different person. She looked rested and she had a big smile on her face. She came up to me with a journal and was proud to show me she took her assignment from the night before seriously. She wrote down all of her concerns in detail, ate a great dinner that had been prepared by a local Rotary Club, and after taking a nice hot shower, got to bed early and slept well between her scheduled pumping. Just journaling and writing down everything relieved her of a lot of her stress.

We sat down to go through her priorities and were able to easily work through almost all of her issues that one day at some level. When it came to her children, I asked her if their school district had early-release hours on Wednesday. She said they did, so I asked what she thought about being in the NICU Wednesday morning for her son and then heading home to pick up her girls when they got out of school at 2 p.m. She could then spend the afternoon with them and her husband, have a family evening, go to their school on Thursday morning to volunteer, and then come back to the hospital for Thursday afternoon care. That would give her another afternoon and night with her family, a night a week back at her own home, an additional night a week with her husband, and a day back in the classroom. She lit up and immediately crossed three things off her list at once. I told N.B. that while that idea sounded good at the time, that didn't mean it was a foolproof solution for all of those concerns. I recommend that she should trial it to see how it worked for her and her family and make adjustments as needed.

N.B.'s friendships was the next priority on her list and we spent time talking about how most people have no idea what it is like to be in the NICU. I asked her that before entering the NICU with her son, if she knew what it was like for a parent to be in the NICU with their child? She admitted she did not and seemed to instantly have a newfound sensitivity for what her friends were going through. I asked if she would leave the NICU to attend the book club if her friends invited her, and she said no. I asked her to consider that maybe her friends were respecting her time at the hospital and that is why they weren't inviting her. I encouraged her to consider talking to them or sending them a letter if she didn't feel like talking to them in person to let them know how she felt; I provided a sample letter of what other parents had provided to family and friends.

Last, we talked about her relationship with her husband. I disclosed to her that I was not at all skilled or trained to give her any advice at all, that staff in the NICU were there to provide support to her and her husband, but we were not trained counselors. I offered to provide her with resources within our community and online that might be beneficial. I encouraged N.B. to also continue meeting with our unit social worker and psychologist, with whom she had already been meeting and had established a trusting relationship. Before we wrapped up our conversation that day, she took me up on my offer of receiving

(*continued*)

(*continued*)

a list of resources; I informed her that I would check in on how things were going for her in a few days in regard to her relationships.

I realized with N.B. that sometimes parents are so overwhelmed with all they are dealing with that they just need someone to sit down with them, encourage them to really think about what it is that is bothering them, and help troubleshoot ways to work through those issues. NICU staff have the luxury of seeing interventions that work or don't work for hundreds of families throughout their careers and can share those ideas with other families who have never been in that situation and just needed some creativity and inspiration. Thankfully for N.B., I was able to share some of those previous success tactics that seemed to work really well for her.

Family Story

Alex Ortega, a mom experienced at what it was like having premature deliveries, shares her courageous story about being admitted on antepartum bed rest and having to be separated from her husband and two older children while all she could do to maintain her pregnancy as long as possible to give her unborn son the best possible chance at survival. At first, she didn't realize that the struggle of balancing home life and hospital life would continue once she went home from the hospital and ended up realizing that, in fact, the balancing act became more difficult when she returned home.

"When they admitted us to the hospital for severe preeclampsia, I remember looking at the nurse with tears in my eyes, ... but what about my family? Everything as we knew was going to change.

"Forget the fact that I was resigning from my full-time job immediately, or the fact that I was so sick. What about my family? How were they going to manage without me? What we didn't realize was that Mom being stuck in the hospital, for what we naively thought was going to be 15 weeks, was soon to become the least of our problems.

"Our son, our third beautiful preemie baby, Theodore Ronin Alexander, would enter the world a few short weeks later, at just 28 weeks' gestation, changing our lives and our family dynamic forever.

"After having delivered our son prematurely and having had been admitted to the birth center for so long, I think that I was not only in shock from the recent events, but also so very homesick. I incredibly underestimated my readiness and my ability to manage my home life while attempting to be a parent to the NICU's latest micropreemie admit.

"This naive, almost blissful, fog dissipated quickly once we were home. Once I returned home after being in the hospital for a month, the reality and the weight of the situation came to a head. I sat on my bed; my older kids climbing on me and loving me (they had missed me SO much), my husband pulling them off of me and turning on their new movie *Moana*. I sat there desperately trying to figure out how to get my breast pump to work, still sore and

(*continued*)

(*continued*)

bleeding from the emergency delivery of Theo just 2 days prior. My womb and my heart aching to just have my child with me, as one, once again, and it hit me; How was I going to do this? How does *anyone* manage taking care of older children, a house, and a husband while they have a brand-new baby in critical condition in the hospital? That takes a supermom, and I felt far from it. I couldn't even figure out my breast pump, for crying out loud.

"Thus began my struggle with not only being a new preemie parent, but also a mom to my big kiddos and a wife to my husband. I had to learn how to balance everyone, and I had to learn fast. It felt like there was no right answer at all. I thought finding that sought-after balance would never happen. It felt like the balance of home–husband–NICU was most certainly unattainable after all. I thought I would never be able to get caught up on the laundry that I knew was piling up, nor the dishes that laid in my sink. I thought for sure my older kids were going to forget who I was, and if they didn't, they would resent me for missing so much of this precious time with them, time I could never get back. I was afraid that I wasn't spending enough time with my newborn baby in the hospital and we wouldn't be able to create that special bond that mothers and their children had, and don't you dare forget the fear: the constant fear that something was going to happen to him while I wasn't there and I wouldn't be able to get to him on time, I wouldn't be there when he really needed me. The fear that I would, yet again, fail as his mother. I was convinced that if I did make it through this painful journey, my marriage most certainly wouldn't. I was afraid that this would all change me and not for the better. The constant anxiety I had that I would become someone who was a stranger to my family and my husband was crippling. What if he can't love me after this? What if I'm too broken? I had read all of the scary stories of marriages failing during or after a long-term NICU admission, and I had seen the less-than-pleasing statistics. I felt like it was inevitable that we were on our way to being one of those numbers or one of those sad stories. My heart was telling me that this wouldn't be the case for us, that we would beat the odds, but my mind was telling me something entirely different.

"This one particular night, I ended up just collapsing in the doorway of my extremely disheveled house, in absolute sorrow and hopelessness. Tears flowed from my eyes, but they were straight from my soul. (I had just returned home from seeing Theodore and received some rather saddening news. He was extremely sick and quickly worsening, so I'm sure that added to my distressed state of mind.) I sat on the floor in a mess of my kids' coats and shoes (that hadn't been put away in Lord knows how long), and through the sobs and tears, I told my husband I couldn't do it, that there simply wasn't enough of me to go around. I remember telling him over and over again that I couldn't do it. That God had made a mistake when he chose me to be Theodore's mom; I wasn't strong enough. I was failing everyone. He just walked over to me and just sat on the floor of our entryway and held me as I bawled, not saying a word, but allowing my heart to get out what I needed to. I told him I was exhausted. I was so completely and absolutely drained to my core. I was emotionally and mentally depleted. We had two kids at home, my step-son on the weekends, and our poor 28-week preemie was fighting for his life in the hospital just down the street. He was so close, but he felt like he was half a world away. I was functioning in my daily life as a shell of my former self. I

(*continued*)

(*continued*)

was so empty and felt so lost. I felt sad and guilty when I wasn't with him but felt the same sadness and guilt when I was, because I was away from my family and my other children. In my mind, I was failing them too. I don't know if I took it especially hard because of the type of person I am (I'm the type of person who feels like my true purpose in this world is to be a mother, it's my everything, and my family is my entire world), but the pain I was feeling not being able to be there for ALL of my kids and my husband was crushing to my soul. I felt like I was dying from the inside out, and I knew then, I had to make a change.

"We had to make this work; we had no choice. The world didn't stop just because we had our baby extremely premature. Our older children's worlds didn't stop just because they had a really sick baby brother. We had to learn how to function as a family again, in a world that never slowed down, that never missed a beat. I had to learn. I had to learn that the guilt I was feeling was okay and that the sadness and heartbreak was okay. I had to learn to allow myself to feel my emotions. Acting tough and keeping a smile on my face obviously wasn't working anymore. I had to come to terms with the fact that I did miss out on enjoying the last half of my pregnancy and even grieve, it if need be. I had to allow myself to heal and quit pushing myself too far and remind myself that this situation was only temporary and that one day, when I left those secured double doors, I would no longer be empty handed and my heart wouldn't ache. I would be leaving with my son in my arms; we just had to get there. I forced myself to understand that my kids weren't going to hate me, that my husband was still going to love me, and once we made it through this battle, we would be okay. Everything was going to be okay!

"I was now a mom of a micropreemie fighter, and a mom of two amazing preschoolers (one being special needs) and one awesome bonus kid from my husband, and I was a wife. It was time to step up . . . and be the warrior I needed to be and the warrior I knew deep down I could be, because this was our life for now. We didn't know if it would ever go back to what we knew as 'normal' or what that normal would even look like once Theodore came home; however, I did know one thing, I was going to do it. I was going to make it work, and we would learn to adapt to our new world, as would my family, and in the end, my baby boy would come home.

"I just had to remember: It's not forever, it's just for right now."

RECOMMENDATIONS/SUGGESTIONS FOR BEST PRACTICE

1. Assist families in finding ways to ask for help from others and provide resources in the community that can help meet any needs they may have.

2. Encourage and welcome sibling involvement in the NICU.

3. Assess the relationship status of parents and recommend professional support if relationships are struggling.

4. Provide support for parents in learning how to communicate with friends and family to help ease the stress of balancing relationships.

5. Provide families with journals and encourage them to write about their feelings throughout their NICU journey to help alleviate stress and decrease anxiety.

RECOMMENDED RESOURCES

Multiple resources are available to staff and families to help them learn to balance home and hospital life (Figure 10.4).

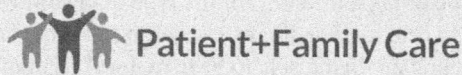 Patient+Family Care

Website Recommendations:
1. http://www.patientfamilycare.com
2. http://www.nicuhealing.com
3. http://www.foryourmarriage.org/married-life/
4. https://guidedoc.com/help-your-relationship-with-free-marriage-counseling
5. https://www.mealtrain.com
6. https://www.mindfulreturn.com/nicu
7. https://www.thecut.com/2016/09/how-to-handle-work-when-your-babys-in-the-nicu.html
8. https://monbaby.com/safesleep/support-for-nicu-families-technology-advances-in-the-nicu
9. http://handtohold.org/resources/helpful-articles/resources-every-nicu-family-should-know
10. http://handtohold.org/support/sibling-support
11. http://www.preemiebabies101.com/nicu-sibling-support
12. http://www.prematurity.org/baby/siblings-baby-nicu.html
13. https://www.today.com/parents/family-paved-way-siblings-visit-preemies-nicu-t117326
14. https://www.healthcaretoolbox.org/latest-news/23-f-remember-the-family/377
    -helpingsiblings-cope-in-the-nicu.html
15. http://micropreemie.net/blog/connect-siblings-nicu-babies
16. https://www.thebump.com/a/breastfeeding-and-work
17. http://www.breastmilkcounts.com/working-moms/pumping-at-work
18. http://www.workandpump.com
19. https://www.hygeiahealth.com/blog/pumped-pumping-moms-tips-returning-work
20. http://www.parenting.com/article/tips-pumping-breast-milk-work

Figure 10.4 ■ Recommended resources for helping families balance home life and hospital life.

Case-Based Learning

F.Y. is a 38-year-old mother of 6-day-old twins born at 29 weeks' gestation. The twins were conceived with assisted reproductive technology after she experienced several pregnancy losses after the birth of her first child 10 years ago. She is hesitant to bring her 10-year-old to the hospital to see his siblings because of behavior that worries her. His soccer coach told her that he intentionally kicked a teammate and was unrepentant. In addition, he has been uncooperative at home and more aggressive with their dog than previously.

(continued)

(*continued*)

QUESTIONS

1. What are the contextual elements that may be at play for the 10-year-old sibling?

2. What actions might you take to help support this family?

ANSWERS

The sibling may be feeling unattended to but cannot verbalize his emotions. He may be jealous of the attention that his tiny siblings are receiving. His mother is no longer home every afternoon to pick him up from school and take him to soccer practice. She is tired when she comes home from the hospital and may be spending less time with him due to stress and exhaustion.

Sibling rivalry is alive and well and lives in the NICU! However, many NICUs have programs to improve family dynamics. Childcare, family areas, and playrooms are wonderful additions to NICU design. Child life therapists offer activities such as drawing pictures and writing songs for the new baby. Role playing, diaper changing, and baby care with dolls empower the older sibling and allow them to practice until the time comes for them to participate in newborn care (Maree & Downes, 2016).

Sibling visitation in NICUs down to the age of 2 is not uncommon. However, tending to a curious, busy toddler while attending to a critically ill newborn is a parenting challenge unlike any other. Integrating the family does not stop at the parents; siblings and grandparents are also mentored by NICU RNs using this model of care. Older siblings can participate in supervised kangaroo care. They may bond and learn important lessons about their tiny siblings when they help diaper or help feed them. This can help them feel important, instead of left out (Kory & Fredian, 2017).

Sometimes, sibling visitation must be limited because of infectious diseases. Peluso, Harnish, Miller, Cooper, and Fujii (2015) concluded that the number of infants with respiratory syncytial virus (RSV) in the NICU can be reduced by excluding sibling visitors under 13 years of age during the RSV season. In these circumstances, school-age children may understand a clear explanation of the reasoning and benefit from praise for not giving germs to their sibling or other fragile babies. Booklets of photographs of their tiny sibling to share at school may be a way for them to feel special, too. Handwashing before touching the baby is a good thing to teach everyone who visits while in the hospital and at home.

REFERENCES

Kory, N., & Fredian, G. (2017). Incorporating family centered care in the NICU: An integrative literature review. Retrieved from http://via.library.depaul.edu/cgi/viewcontent .cgi?article=1154&context=nursing-colloquium

Maree, C., & Downes, F. (2016). Trends in family-centered care in neonatal intensive care. *Journal of Perinatal and Neonatal Nursing, 30*(3), 265–269. doi:10.1097/JPN.0000000000000202

Peluso, A. M., Harnish, B. A., Miller, N. S., Cooper, E. R., & Fujii, A. M. (2015). Effect of young sibling visitation on respiratory syncytial virus activity in a NICU. *Journal of Perinatology, 35*(8), 627–630. doi:10.1038/jp.2015.27

REFERENCES

American Psychological Association. (n.d.). Gender and stress. Retrieved from http://www.apa.org/news/press/releases/stress/2010/gender-stress.aspx

Guimarães, H. (2015). The importance of parents in the neonatal intensive care units. *Journal of Pediatric and Neonatal Individualized Medicine, 4*(2), e040244. doi:10.7363/040244

Horikoshi, Y., Okazaki, K., Miyokawa, S., Kinoshita, K., Higuchi, H., Suwa, J., . . . Fukuoka, K. (2018). Sibling visits and viral infections in the neonatal intensive care unit. *Pediatrics International, 60*(2), 153–156. doi:10.1111/ped.13470

Howe, T., Sheu, C., Wang, T., & Hsu, Y. (2014). Parenting stress in families with very low birth weight preterm infants in early infancy. *Research in Developmental Disabilities, 35*(7), 1748–1756. doi:10.1016/j.ridd.2014.02.015

Wainwright, L. (2017). Children with newborn siblings in a neonatal unit: Learning from support programmes in the USA. *Journal of Health Visiting, 5*(1), 26–31. doi:10.12968/johv.2017.5.1.26

11

SUPPORTING FAMILIES FACED WITH NEONATAL TRANSPORT

It is critical to provide psychosocial support to families in the NICU and to help families feel connected when parents and infants cannot be together around the clock. When newborns and their families are separated due to neonatal transport, the sensitivity and need to provide psychosocial support magnifies exponentially to ensure that the emotional and physical well-being of both infant and parents are met. Medical providers and care teams at both the sending and receiving facilities, along with the transport team, play equally significant roles when it comes to providing education, information, and emotional support to families that face separation from their newborn. Family-centered care in transport scenarios is more than a multidisciplinary team approach; it is a multiunit, multiteam, and multisystem approach.

Transport teams, who skillfully transport critically ill patients, should also be trained to skillfully and empathetically support families prior to the physical transport of their infant. The transport team interacts with a family for only a short time, typically only during the stabilization and loading of the patient. Although the team needs to be proficient at providing medically complex care while communicating compassionately with families, it is the care team at the hospital where mom delivers and recovers who needs to take on the primary support role of the family. Staff at the hospital where the infant is being transferred takes on a more long-term support role, as they will be at the facility where the family will eventually transfer and will need psychosocial support to cope with the NICU journey ahead.

CARING FOR FAMILIES WHOSE INFANT IS TRANSPORTED OUT OF A FACILITY

As soon as the need for neonatal transport is determined, staff should begin preparing the family for what to expect and how to prepare for the transport. Information should include the following:

- Why the baby needs to be transported to another facility
- What type of transport their child will have (helicopter, fixed wing, or ground)

- What safety risks are associated with the type of transportation their child will have
- Who will show up from the transport team to support the stabilization of the infant
- What the team will do to stabilize the infant
- What paperwork will be required and what paperwork can be done prior to the team arriving, which should be started immediately
- How the family can be involved in the stabilization process and where they can be while the team is working with their baby
- What equipment to expect to see
- If anyone can accompany the baby on the transport, what will need to be done to prepare to depart
- Where the baby is being transported
- What the receiving hospital is like (e.g., where the hospital is, what the unit is like, who works there, who the care team is)

During this transition, parents are often very overwhelmed and scared and "experience a wide range of emotions that will soon be magnified by distance, by strange surroundings, by lack of normal support and by extended lines of communication. Therefore, these specific family fears should be validated and not taken lightly" (Mosher, 2013, "Supporting Families Prior to Transport" section). A family-support specialist assigned to a family from the moment transport is decided can accompany them through the whirlwind that is ahead of them. If no family-support specialist is on staff, a dedicated staff member who can focus solely on the emotional support of the family should be a goal for the supervisor in charge of staffing the unit so that someone can dedicate uninterrupted time to meet the emotional needs of the family during the transport period.

A family-support specialist, or other support staff, can provide several interventions to help prior to the family–infant separation. These interventions may include, but are certainly not limited to, the following:

- Using photography: A digital camera should be on the unit for many reasons, but in this case, it can be used to capture photos of the baby and the family. Photos of the baby can be printed and given to the family so that they have a way to "see" their child after the separation, and photos of the parents and/or family can be printed and sent with the transport team so that the baby can "see" the family during the separation. Many times, the transport team tapes the photographs inside the Isolette, giving families a sense of security that their child will feel like a part of them and allow them to feel that they will be with the child during transport.
- Trading scented blankets: If possible, a blanket the baby was wrapped in after birth, and prior to transport, should be left with the mother and family so that the scent of the newborn can be left with them. This scent may help the mother with bonding and attachment, and it may, in fact, assist her to have something

that smells like her child when she is pumping breast milk. More important, if at all possible, something that has the mother's scent should be sent with the newborn. It has been proved that "smells that are familiar to the baby, such as the smell of the mother, have soothing effects on infants" (Badiee, Asghari, & Mohammadizadeh, 2013, "Introduction" section).

- Provide mom with a plush toy: The mother and infant bonding process has tremendous implications for both mother and child, and when a mother and infant are separated, it leaves an emptiness that is impossible to fill until the dyad are reunited. It is hoped that, with a neonatal transport, mom stabilizes after the delivery and can be reunited with her child within 24 to 72 hours. However, that may not always be the case, and even if it is, those 24 to 72 hours can seem endless. Providing mom with a plush animal or toy as a gift "from the baby" at the time of transport can serve as a comfort for her to hold and squeeze when her arms feel empty without her child.

- Initiate hand milk expression: If a neonatal transport occurs quickly after birth because of the critical nature of a child's condition, a mother's milk supply will not be in, so attempting to pump milk will produce only a small amount; it may frustrate the mother more if she thinks she is failing to provide for her baby. The healthcare staff can help mom hand-express colostrum into a medicine cup, which can then be collected and sent on ice in a syringe, properly labeled, with the transport team. In the event feedings are started prior to mom and baby being reunited, then the initial colostrum can be with the baby for the first feeding. This also affords mom the feeling of accomplishing something only she can do for her child prior to their separation.

BUILDING RELATIONSHIPS BETWEEN TRANSFERRING UNITS

If there are hospitals where babies are frequently transferred, then a strong relationship should be formed between the sending and receiving hospitals. Building a robust relationship helps build trust between the two organizations and creates a seamless transition between one care team to the next for families. "When care is transferred across birth settings, confusion and conflict among providers with respect to roles and responsibilities can adversely affect both outcomes and the experience of care for women and newborns" (Vedam et al., 2014, "Abstract" section), so being proactive to avoid such conflict will benefit both staff and patients alike.

Learning about one another's facility so that staff can educate families about the other hospital is of utmost significance. Families' nerves can be put to ease when a sending facility can tell them about the location of the receiving facility, the NICU's location within the facility, the appearance of the unit, the unit's culture, the staff, the providers, the amenities, and the support services available. It also helps to be able to answer questions that the family may have about policies and procedures. To learn this much about the other hospital, staff should be encouraged to visit and even spend part of a shift shadowing staff to really get a feel for the other hospital's philosophy and environment. In addition, a welcome kit for the receiving facility should be given to the family at the time of transport; it should contain information about the facility so that they have tangible information that they can read through when they feel ready and when they want to review all the information at a later time. Having this information in their hands is also beneficial so that they can share it with other family and friends; this way, their support network is also aware of the important information.

Welcome kits should include, at minimum, the following:

- A map with directions on how to travel from the sending hospital to the receiving hospital
- A map of parking lots and where the best place to park on campus is to be nearest the NICU entrance
- Parking pass (if receiving hospital requires patients to pay for parking)
- Where the NICU is located at the receiving hospital on a campus map
- Contact information so that the family can call the unit and receive updates about their child at any time
- A list of local area hotels and motels and other services such as laundry mats, gas stations, and grocery stores
- Ronald McDonald House information, if a local house is an option
- Hospital amenities
- NICU welcome letter
- NICU-specific visitation policies
- NICU educational material
- NICU tour video DVD (should also be featured on hospital website)
- Sheet with frequently asked questions
- Deli/cafeteria voucher

Staff also need to be mindful about "talking up" the receiving facility staff. Even if they don't know them well, they need to speak highly of them to help build up parental confidence in where their child is going. The last thing parents need to hear are nurses speaking negatively about other nurses, not to mention that "intimidating and disruptive behaviors can foster medical errors, contribute to poor patient satisfaction and to preventable adverse outcomes, increase the cost of care, and cause qualified clinicians, administrators and managers to seek new positions in professional environments" (Lachman, 2014, para. 1).

The sending facility staff needs to call and provide a thorough report to the receiving facility that includes not only the medical aspects of the patient coming their way, but also details about the psychosocial aspects of the family's situation, including, but not limited to, the following:

- Who the parents are
- Who the parents identify as their family and support network

- Where the family live and what their living situation is

- What is known about their current working situation/leave plans

- What emotional state is

- What support has been given until that point

- What learning style preference the family has reported they have

- What education had been provided to the family until that point and how it was received

- How the family can be contacted

- If there are any known needs/concerns

- If there is a mental health history

- If the family has any known coping strategies

Once the baby is transported, staff need to prioritize continuing to care medically for the mother, providing psychosocial support to the family during the separation until the mother is stable enough for discharge, making the mother as comfortable as possible, and assisting the family in connecting with the receiving hospital as frequently as they would like. It is also incredibly important to support the mother in pumping every 3 hours and properly labeling and storing her breast milk so that the milk can be transported with the family when they go see their baby for the first time. Assisting the mother with pumping can truly help a mother in feeling as though she is doing something for her child while they are apart.

When a family is medically stable to be discharged, the staff should send them off to the receiving facility comfortably and equipped with things they need. For example, providing mothers with extra nursing pads, feminine pads, pumping supplies, and a full water bottle would be a great way to send her off. That way, if the family goes right to the hospital to see their child, the mother will have some basic necessity items and they will not have to stop at a store to pick up those items. Sending fathers or support persons with a full bottle of water as well would be a nice gesture and would encourage them to stay hydrated and take care of themselves.

CARING FOR FAMILIES WHOSE INFANTS ARE TRANSPORTED INTO A FACILITY

Staff at a receiving facility needs to start providing support to families well before they arrive at their hospital. As soon as a patient is accepted for transport, staff should begin learning about the family and begin preparing to provide comprehensive psychosocial support. A phone call to the family should be made as soon as possible, after a report is received, for staff to introduce themselves as the care team who will be caring for their child once the transport team arrives. As the receiving care team, information can be shared with the parents as to what room or bed space the baby will be admitted to, who all will be working on the admitting team, what the initial care goals will be, and how the family can directly contact them if they want to call back to the unit and speak to the admitting team. The admitting nurse should assure the family that another phone call will occur once the admission is completed and then follow through and call the family with an update as soon as the patient's admission is complete and the patient is stable.

Units should have technology available which allow families to "see" one another when separation is inevitable. This type of technology is wonderful when families are faced with neonatal transports, but also comes in handy when families have to stay out of the unit because of illness, when a family member has to travel, when a parent is incarcerated, when a parent is deployed overseas, or for any other reason a parent or sibling cannot be physically in the unit for a time. Technology should be brought in and connected with the family so that the parents can see that their child is stable and tucked in to the new bed. Having the ability to see their child calms so many of the parent's nerves, and having this type of technology also allows staff to introduce themselves to parents "face-to-face," which helps begin to build a trusting relationship. While the face-to-face connection is established, staff can show the family the unit so that when they arrive for the first time, it won't seem so foreign.

If a parent accompanies a child on transport and arrives in the unit with the baby, then the parent should be welcomed and included in the admission just as any new parent should be. See Part III Chapter 5 of this book to review how to include families in the admission process and assure that the accompanying parent or family members feels connected to their child as much as possible.

Until the mother and entire family can be reunited with the baby, the receiving facility should frequently provide updates, use technology to provide connection, record events in a NICU journal, and take lots of photographs for the family. Not only will these simple gestures mean a lot to the family, they will help provide keepsakes to will help fill the gaps of the time lost between the parents and the baby caused by the separation.

Author's Personal Story

I was a member of the critical care air transport team for 2 years and was activated to attend the impending delivery of an infant at 26 2/7 weeks' gestation at a hospital 1 hour away from our level-three NICU. Thankfully by helicopter, our team was able to arrive in 13 minutes after we took off and reached altitude. Our transport team consisted of myself (a neonatal nurse), a respiratory therapist, and a critical care adult nurse, and the pilot, of course. We arrived at the critical access hospital and were welcomed by the delivery team that was composed of a family practice doctor and two labor and delivery nurses. I had been to this hospital before for deliveries and had taught these particular nurses neonatal resuscitation, since I was a regional neonatal resuscitation program instructor. Because of my previous visits and educational engagements, it was a familiar environment and a familiar team of staff. They were welcoming, highly skilled, and well prepared for the pending high-risk premature delivery.

(continued)

(*continued*)

Our team walked quietly into the patient room where the mother was in active labor and waited patiently by the door until she was through a contraction before we went all the way into the room to introduce ourselves. After we told her and her mother who we were, we explained to her what we would plan to do at the moment of delivery, what she could expect with the stabilization process, and what the transport process typically looked like at that hospital. We told her that we would be over in the corner quietly setting up everything we would need to perform life-saving interventions for her child, and if we set it all up, we hopefully wouldn't need any of it. But we would have it all out and ready to go just in case we did.

The mom continued to labor, we set up our resuscitation table, the labor and delivery nurses were incredible at helping us, and after 20 minutes a 1-lb 3-oz baby girl was delivered and quickly placed on the warmer for us to begin resuscitation. As the leader of the resuscitation, my primary role and responsibility was to run the resuscitation and perform the main tasks such as intubation, umbilical lines, and chest tubes. Being in that role leaves very little time to focus on the family, which was a difficult reality for me as someone who also functioned as a family-support specialist the other half of the time. Yet because I had established such a great relationship with the team at this hospital, they knew the importance of family support and they knew how important frequent communication was, and they would step right in and take over that role.

As the transport team and I actively resuscitated and worked to stabilize the premature patient, I spoke out loud so that the entire team and the labor and delivery staff could hear everything we were doing. The labor and delivery team could then relay all of the information to the family in terms that they could understand and were there to answer questions. If there was anything that we said that even they didn't understand, they could recognize when it was an appropriate time to approach the team to ask clarifying questions and then would go back to the family and offer additional information. As much as I could, I would turn around and address the family in person and always tried to point out really positive things to the mother and grandmother. In this situation, I remember specifically telling them that her daughter had beautiful long fingers and fingernails already, and the grandma smiled and said her mother had really long nails when she was born too.

Fast forward to us being done with the stabilization and getting ready to head out and me driving the adult team a bit crazy. They eventually got used to it, but at first they would get so inpatient with me because before we could leave I would always take the transport Isolette over to the mom's bedside, if the baby was stable enough to tolerate the additional time, and allow mom to see the baby and hold its hand through the port holes for a few minutes. I really felt it was important for them to have a little skin-to-skin time, even if it was just hand-to-hand, and spend some time explaining to the mom and family about the transport Isolette, the equipment, the medications and IV fluid, the respiratory support, the plan for transport, the care we would be giving in flight (or during ground transport), and the admissions process when we got to the hospital. I suppose I always put myself in the mother's position and would not want to hear that a stranger was taking

(*continued*)

(*continued*)

my baby away before I could see or touch the child. So we went to the mom's bedside and I spent enough time to go over all of that information with mom and had her sign the consent form to transport. I then presented mom with a transport welcome bag from the receiving hospital that included the following:

- A welcome letter with congratulations on the birth of the child and contact information to the unit
- A stuffed animal for mom
- A DVD that contained a video tour of the unit where her baby was transferring
- A map with directions from her hospital to the hospital where her baby was transferring
- A campus map of the hospital where her baby was transferring with the NICU highlighted on the map and the recommended parking area highlighted
- A meal voucher for the cafeteria
- A NICU book that included frequently asked questions and a glossary of NICU terms
- A business card of the NICU manager stapled to the bag
- A flier to the local Ronald McDonald House and an application to stay, with the NICU social worker's business card attached
- A flier with local area hotels that provide discounts for hospitalized families

I very briefly informed the mother of what was in the bag and told her that the hospital staff would be going through the information with her in more detail. The staff at the hospital were well prepared to go over all of the information with the family. They even knew how to contact our hospital social workers to help initiate the process of getting families on the wait list to stay at the Ronald McDonald House and to assist with transportation support, if that was a barrier for the family.

Being a family-support specialist as the second part of my job, I had convinced the transport team to get a digital camera, and we took it with us on all transports. I took a picture of mom and baby together before we left and then I took pictures throughout the entire transport: the loading-up process, care of the baby during flight, the flight view, the unloading process at the hospital, the crew entering the hospital with the baby, the receiving team admitting the baby, and the baby all tucked in nicely after report and handoff was complete. The transport team then would burn all the photos onto a CD and print copies off as well and present them to the family so that the family would have images of the entire transport and could see what they missed. It was a way to give them a small keepsake and eliminate the question "What was the transport like?" that so many parents have.

(*continued*)

(continued)

As soon as the baby was stabilized and handed off to the receiving hospital staff, I called mom and told her that the transport went smoothly and that her daughter tolerated the flight really well and that she was now tucked in nicely in her new bed. I answered all of her questions and then handed the phone over to the nurse who was going to be caring for her for the rest of the shift. It was a nice way to perform handoff and to give a warm handoff to the mom as well.

Family Story

This first story comes from Kelly and Scout Cloud, who are the parents to twins, McKenna and Bryson. They experienced a unique experience, and an extremely stressful experience, of having to be separated when one of their twins was transported to a hospital 3½ hours away and one was not.

Kelly: "Two weeks into our stay at the NICU, we got the news that our son Bryson would need to be transported to a hospital almost 4 hours away. In the days leading up to that news, Bryson was not doing well. His color had changed, his stats were off, and he wasn't breathing well. I will never forget walking into his room to see the nurses working on him to bring him back to breathing on his own when he had hit his low point. We got the news that Bryson would be leaving our home town so this other hospital could monitor the pulmonary saddle embolism that had developed inside him. The amazing doctor who refused to stop investigating Bryson's condition until we had an answer was the one to break the news to us. To this day, I believe we wouldn't have Bryson here on Earth without this doctor's dedication to our son.

"After we got the news, things quickly grew busy, and decisions had to be made quickly. Bryson would have to fly in an airplane versus the helicopter because of air pressure concerns. This meant we wouldn't be able to go with him. My son would be flying and I couldn't be with him. My son would be settling into a new bed in a new hospital and I couldn't be with him. My son would be in the care of people I had never met and I couldn't be with him. These overwhelming feelings of sadness, worry, and anger were lessened, though, when one of the nurses we had grown to love came to me and told me she would be able to fly with Bryson and stay with him until he got settled, since she was the one who was going to be on his transport team. Knowing that she would be with him calmed my fears."

Scott: "The primary feeling that we both had was fear. We had no way of knowing what was going to happen, and I think it's human nature to immediately jump to the worst-case scenario, which both my wife and I did. We decided that Kelly needed to stay with McKenna in Bend, and I would go out of town to be with Bryson. Because the plane needed an extra flight nurse, I had to drive over, which added even more stress to a situation that already felt very out of control. One thing that the staff and transport

(continued)

(*continued*)

team did before Bryson and I left, which we are grateful for now but kind of resented at the time, was take a 'family portrait' with Bryson in his flight Isolate and Kelly and I standing around him. At the time it felt like this was going to be the last picture of us together, and if it had been, I would have been happy to have that one last picture of us all together. Thankfully it didn't come to that end! The other thing that was stressful and could have gone better was when I got to OHSU, I wasn't exactly sure where to go and I had to wander around quite a bit to find the right place to get hooked up with McDonald house. Maybe having a single sheet with contact info or at least basic info on the things that all NICU parents will need once they hit the new city would have been very helpful."

Kelly: "Looking back on the situation, I think it also would have been helpful to prepare parents for the differences between the two hospitals. Scott loved the deep medical explanations that the teaching hospital provided. He made it a point to be there when the doctors and students made their rounds and listen to the in-depth discussion. I, on the other hand, did not enjoy that part as the details were just too much to handle at that time in my life with everything going on. There really is a significant difference in the experience; not that one is better than the other, but the transition could be difficult. In addition, the unit we started at, and where McKenna was, was a single-room unit and Bryson was transferred to a unit where there were pods. That environmental difference was a big change as well. The staff warned us about that, but it would have been helpful to know more about what those differences were and what they meant."

Scott: "The care our twins got at both hospitals really was top notch, and we couldn't have asked for better nurses and doctors. Bryson and McKenna are thriving 5-year-olds and have no developmental concerns."

This second story comes from Rachel Evans, who wound up unexpectedly delivering prematurely on vacation far from home and far from her support network. During her child's NICU stay, he experienced not one, not two, but three different transports and experienced stays at three different NICUs.

"I found out I was pregnant only 2 months following delivery of my first son. I was surprised nonetheless and overjoyed. My pregnancy was unremarkable and I felt great. My OB cleared me to fly across country to California for a quick Memorial Day get-away. While in California, my husband attended a sporting event, and I toured the area where we were staying. I spent a full day with my 8-month-old, enjoying the Aquarium of the Pacific in Long Beach and walking through the local shops. When I was ready to return to the hotel, I called and the Holiday Inn Shuttle arrived to drive me back. The driver opened the doors and went to bring a foot-stool for me to step up into the van. However, impulsively, I hiked my right foot up onto the running board, held my 20+ pound son on my left hip, and pulled myself into the van. I felt something 'pop.' My first contraction occurred at 4:30 a.m. I didn't realize I was in labor. Throughout the next day, I felt contractions, but thought I was feeling Braxton-Hicks–type contractions. For goodness sake, I was only 26 weeks pregnant, what else could it be? My husband, who is a RN, returned to the sporting event,

(*continued*)

(*continued*)

not knowing what I was experiencing. It didn't cross my mind that I was in a dangerous situation. Later that evening, when he returned, I continued to feel contractions. By 7:30 p.m., they were coming more frequently and felt too real to be fake. My husband, the nurse, examined me. With a look on his face that I'd never seen before and a sound to his voice that I had never heard before, he said, 'We need to go to the hospital—now.' Thankfully, a hospital was literally just blocks away.

"When we arrived at the emergency department, I began to hemorrhage. I was immediately registered and whisked away to the Labor and Delivery floor. Forgive me, there are chunks of time in this experience that I do not recall. Most of the experience, however, I remember in great detail. During my career as a medical speech pathologist, I've heard my patients describe this loss of memory to me, and now, I fully understand what they mean. I fully recall the name of the nurse who sat with me for what seemed like hours while I experienced contractions, gushes of blood, and efforts to stop the baby from coming. At one point, she locked eyes with me and said in the most soothing voice, 'You're having this baby tonight.' In a voice filled with fright and panic, I said, 'I know.' I will never forget her name, her voice, and something she said to me. She said, 'I'll see you tomorrow.' Such a casual phrase, one I've said many times as I've left patient's rooms. In a hospital, schedules are simply outlines. They change rapidly, and healthcare professionals, flexibly and seamlessly, adjust to the needs of their day. They prioritize patients based on acuity and a host of other variables. There were many times over the years that I said the same phrase, 'I'll see you tomorrow,' well-intended and meaning it at the time, but because of needs of the next day, I didn't get to go back to see that patient. Nurse Barbara said it, meant it, and the next day—*a day she was not scheduled to work*—she arrived at my room to see how I was. That meant the world to me. And, that changed my own healthcare practice. Never, since that experience, have I ever told a patient 'I'll see you tomorrow' without arriving at their hospital room to do just that: see them tomorrow. No matter if it meant I left a few minutes later or meant I skipped a meal, I've always seen them tomorrow.

"The next person I met was Cindy, a wildly curly haired, NICU nurse. She entered my room sometime the next morning, sat gently on my bed, and updated me on the condition of Sage, my fragile 2-lb, 14-inch baby. Sage was taken emergently from me at 11:36 p.m. the previous evening. My husband, George, could not be with me as he was in the waiting room with our 8-month old. Immediately after Sage's birth, the staff allowed George to see me and Sage, who wasn't breathing. Emergency efforts to breathe life into Sage occurred, and we were left with wonder about his condition. Would he survive? Would these efforts to give him life leave him with a life of hardship and incapacity? Not knowing if these thoughts will span just a moment or a life span, I also clutched on to hope. We were 3,000 miles from home, no familiar faces, a hotel room, and a cold hospital where my second child was just born 3½ months prematurely. What else could I have but *hope*? As Cindy sat on my bed and explained Sage's fragile medical status, she explained that he was breathing with the assistance of a ventilator, his eyes were shielded from the bright lights of the Isolette, and his breathing, heart rate, and oxygen levels were being monitored. He had multiple IVs and an oxygen saturation probe. She described

(*continued*)

(continued)

the next 72 hours as crucial. In my field, I've been in the ICUs almost daily. I understood all these monitors. But it was never personal. She allowed me time to ask questions; however, my mind seemed blank. I heard the words and tried processing all that she explained, but I'm not sure how much I understood. Then she told me it was time to get up, walk to the NICU, and meet my son. I was terrified to see him. I felt physical pain from my surgery and emotional pain from delivering Sage too early. Cindy took hold of me and guided me to the NICU. She explained the hand-scrubbing process, gowning up to protect the babies, and the sterile procedures of the NICU. She walked me through the NICU, where other babies were sharing similar experiences to Sage's. Nurses, physicians, respiratory therapists, phlebotomists, and radiology technologists walked through the unit, in what seemed like, choreography.

"The sounds of the monitors seemed deafening. Cindy stayed with me and re-explained everything, now that I was there and seeing Sage. He was so tiny with his belly rising and falling so quickly, purple bruises on the right knee, and on the brink of life. I couldn't think of him as cute and I felt skeptical to bond with him. I couldn't hold him, and I didn't want to attach myself to him if I thought he was going to leave me. It was as if Cindy could read my mind and my emotions. She just hugged me. That was the first of many hugs throughout our time in the NICU. We met many more nurses, all who seemed honest and sincere in the way they provided daily updates. The NICU had an open-records policy and we could read the medical record whenever we wanted. The nurses and staff understood our unique situation. In fact, they went beyond any expectations to help us. They offered to help George obtain his RN licensure in their state so he could work, temporarily, to offset our expenses. They searched classified ads for housing, understanding that we were staying in a Holiday Inn for the duration of our time. One RN even offered to arrange a play-date for our other son and hers. They were spectacular and most appreciated. They assured me that they would call me with any updates on Sage's status, test results, physician consults, etc. And they did. I never felt guilty for not being at NICU 24/7. In fact, they encouraged us to take breaks away from the NICU. I felt confident in their care.

"During an experience such as this, the mind races and thinks crazy thoughts. Three specific ones kept popping up. I envisioned Sponge Bob soaking up the excess fluid that flooded Sage's brain. I equated us with the cast of Gilligan's Island. They embarked on a '3-hour tour' that lasted several seasons. We went to California for 3 days and were expecting to be there for months. And, I embraced the story of Peter Pan. Remember how Tinker Bell falls ill and Peter requests that all the children around the world clap their hands? If they do, Peter pleas, Tinker Bell will get well. At the end of the story, Tink *always* gets well. We received prayers and positive energy from around the country and throughout the globe. While we were in California, I received many beautiful letters from friends and colleagues (this was pre-Facebook, and texting wasn't like what it is now). Every day, when I sat by Sage's Isolette, I read every card and letter to him. One was just a bit more powerful than the others. It was sent to me by a social worker with whom I worked. She experienced the NICU 2 years earlier when she delivered twins at 24 weeks. Madeleine truly understood what I was experiencing and her words were powerful. She

(continued)

(*continued*)

advised me not to look for progress every day. Some days would be great and filled with gains. Other days would feel like regression with loss of progress. Instead, she advised, examine a chunk of time, maybe 2 weeks, and then see all the progress made. Words are power and I grasped onto that advice. Those words equaled more hope. I share those words with my patients when they are enduring their own recovery.

"The NICU is a roller coaster, full of ups and downs. I don't like roller coasters. Sage sustained a grade III intraventricular hemorrhage, developed hydrocephalus, spent his first 10 days on the ventilator, endured four lumbar punctures, and received 23 blood transfusions. Then after 30 days in the NICU, Sage developed necrotizing enterocolitis (NEC), a common and serious intestinal disease among preemies. Sage became very sick, and this appeared to be life-threatening. We were told that he needed a medical consultation and the physician specialist did not have privileges at the hospital. Consequently, Sage needed to be transferred two miles down the road to a children's hospital. Not only did that mean moving Sage to another NICU, it meant establishing new relationships and trust with new staff. This hospital was our home for those 30 days and my emotional roots were grounded there. Sage looked gray and dusky, and he was placed back on the ventilator. I read the cards and letters to him with a bit more earnest now than I previously did. I placed my seemingly huge index finger in the Isolette and held his tiny one. I told him that I loved him and I would never forget him, that I would think about him every day. But, if it was too much for him to fight this infection, it was OK for him to be at peace. I said good-bye, not expecting him to survive the night. It was at that moment that I learned Sage's personality. He demonstrated his will, persistence, strength, tenacity, and fight for life.

"We transferred and settled in to the new NICU. I remember a sea of babies in the NICU and a staff that seemed overwhelmed. I don't recall anyone's name. I remember large looming signs that advocated breastfeeding, 'Breast is Best.' I couldn't breastfeed my preemie. I carried enough guilt as it was, and now, I continuously read a sign reminding me that I couldn't even feed my baby in the 'best' way. I knew we had to be there for Sage, and the care he received was exceptional. But there was no emotional connection between the staff and our family. Sage received treatment for his serious infection, and surgery was a possibility if he did not respond favorably to his cocktail of heavy-duty antibiotics. Sage responded quickly and the NEC was reversed. All of a sudden, we learned we would be returning to our original NICU. He no longer needed the medical care at the children's hospital. We transferred back to our NICU family and were welcomed with hugs, kind words, and encouraging praise. Sage thrived over the next few days.

"The next person I met was the social worker. We learned that *discharge* plans were pending!! It was decided that Sage had improved so much and so quickly that he should be transported home. Initially, we were told to expect a length of stay of 3 months. Sage was now 2 months old and planning for transport. Social workers are the unsung heroes of any hospital. They coordinate an inordinate number of details. We were told about the pending discharge on a Thursday, and by Monday, the social worker arranged for a Learjet flight from California to Miami followed by ground transportation from Miami

(*continued*)

(*continued*)

International Airport to Miami Children's Hospital. She secured an accepting neonatologist and received all necessary approvals from the insurance company. We would be leaving California after 2 months and heading home. We left the hospital amid hugs, tears, and well-wishes. I never forget the outpouring of sincere kindness and medical expertise that our family received throughout Sage's stay there.

"On the tarmac, I met the team involved in our 7-hour air ambulance flight of my critically ill preemie. I was greeted by the pilot, co-pilot, EMT-paramedic (EMT-P), and a nurse. They ensured Sage was prepared for the flight, establishing his medical stability and securing all the necessary equipment. Sage, my now 10-month-old son, and I departed. The flight went well, and the RN stayed with Sage while the EMT-P remained at the back of the jet with me. He helped entertain the other baby. After some time passed, I learned that we would be landing in Texas to re-fuel. However, other arrangements were in progress as well. Apparently, Sage's feeding pump malfunctioned. The skilled and resourceful RN engineered a temporary way of fixing the pump, but a new one would be needed for the remainder of the flight. As we landed, an ambulance met us and the new and old pumps were exchanged. Seamless coordination. We were back in the air before I knew it. We landed in Miami, and Sage was whisked off to his third NICU.

"The children's hospital he was being admitted to is world-renowned for excellence in pediatric medicine. We felt fortunate to have this hospital at our back door. The NICU is vast, and it is a learning institution. Physicians and residents changed frequently with gaps in communication among themselves. Thankfully, Sage was quite healthy at this point of his life, and he just needed to eat and grow. I never felt comfortable at that NICU. I returned to work at this point and went to the hospital every day afterward for a few hours. I felt like I was chastised for doing so and for not being at the side of the Isolette throughout the day. I needed to work to maintain healthcare benefits. We were scolded for having too many visitors on a particular weekend afternoon, placing all the babies at risk for infection. Then the staff realized they were scolding the wrong family. A physician, who began briefing us one day on Sage's progress, got called away, and stated she'd return to continue speaking with us. She never came back. I was concerned about Sage's physical, cognitive, and feeding/swallowing development and requested physical/occupational and speech pathology consultations. Following the initial reluctance of the medical staff, I was obliged. However, the OT and SLP never evaluated Sage. PT saw him inconsistently. In spite of the setting, Sage thrived. He consumed greater amounts with improved tolerance. He gained weight. IVs were discontinued. Brain scans showed resolution of the accumulated ventricular fluid, and everything looked great. I arrived to his Isolette one afternoon to find an appointment card indicating a date for a follow-up appointment with the pediatric ophthalmologist. This was how I found out Sage was being prepared for discharge. I inquired with the RN caring for him that day, and she nonchalantly said 'I guess so' when I asked if that meant Sage was coming home soon. She didn't know any more than I did. Sage passed another milestone, his 'car seat test.' *He was coming home!!*

(*continued*)

(*continued*)

"These 3 long months of ups and downs were coming to a close, and he'd be home. We could move forward as a family under one roof. My hopes were high. I arrived at the hospital after work, knowing that the next day, I would arrive at MCH one last time. Then, I was told that the discharge was canceled. Apparently, a . . . RN . . . who cared for Sage no more than a few times expressed that she doubted my ability to effectively feed my baby. With that, the discharge was canceled. In a flash, my feelings of hope, expectation, anticipation, and excitement transformed to sadness, anger, and disappointment. Words are powerful and the words of this RN destroyed the moment we longed for. Arrangements were made for me to stay 24 hours in the NICU and provide total care for Sage. I fed him, changed him, bathed him, administered medications, and monitored his vital signs—all while under the watchful eyes of the medical team. Early Saturday morning, the neonatologist expressed that I passed the test and could go home. Once again, Sage was deemed appropriate for discharge. Sunday afternoon we arrived at the NICU. I waited with our, now, 11-month-old son while George went to see Sage. The next thing I knew, George was walking out with Sage in his infant carrier, apnea monitor in tow, and discharge papers in hand. *Sage was officially released 3 days before his due date.*

"The next year included frequent follow-up visits to the pediatrician, medical specialists, and twice-weekly sessions with physical therapy. Sage grew and met each and every established milestone. He overcame any obstacle and outgrew any signs of prematurity. Today, Sage is an honor student and an exceptional athlete. Sage is my *hero*.

"The experience changed me. Perhaps, it softened me. I found golden moments amid dark days. I grasped on to *hope*, which empowered me and allowed me to find strength and resiliency. I strive to bring hope and empathy with me to the bedside when I meet my own patients. As a healthcare provider myself, I aspire to establish a sincere connection and express myself effectively, honestly, and hopefully with my patients and their families. I truly understand the impact that has on those who are at their most vulnerable state, wearing their emotions on the inside out. I understand that words have power."

RECOMMENDATIONS/SUGGESTIONS FOR BEST PRACTICE

1. Prepare families as early as possible for what to expect with a neonatal transport.

2. Use photography to capture photos for families prior to neonatal transport.

3. Print photos so that the family has photographs of their child after the separation, and send printed photos of the baby's parents with the baby.

4. Trade scented blankets (or scented hearts) with mom and baby prior to transport so that they have a way to recognize one another's scent during the separation.

5. Provide mom with a plush animal after the baby leaves the unit with the transport team so that she has something soft to hold and cuddle.

6. Initiate hand milk expression prior to transport and send expressed colostrum with the transport team so that mom's milk can be given to the baby as soon as feedings are offered.

7. Initiate breast pumping as soon as possible.

8. Develop relationships between teams at the sending and receiving facilities.

9. Have transport care kits for families if transport teams do not supply them to families.

10. Have receiving care teams call families prior to admitting patients to introduce themselves and establish a connection as early as possible.

11. Have receiving care teams call families as soon as admission is complete to provide an updated report.

12. Have technology available to allow families to "see" one another when separation is inevitable.

13. Have receiving facility staff provide frequent updates to the family until the entire family is united.

14. Have receiving facility staff take photos for the family and record daily events/updates in a NICU journal until families are reunited.

RECOMMENDED RESOURCES

Multiple resources are available to help families cope with the reality of being separated because of neonatal transport (Figure 11.1).

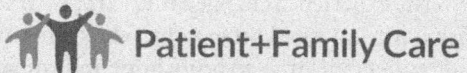 Patient+Family Care

Website Recommendations:
1. https://www.caringbridge.org
2. http://handtohold.org
3. http://holdingtinyhands.com
4. http://www.parentresourcenetwork.org
5. http://peekabooicu.com
6. http://preemiecare.org
7. http://www.preemieparentalliance.org
8. http://preemiestoday.com/default.jx
9. http://preemieworld.com
10. http://share.marchofdimes.org

Journal Articles:
1. Mosher, S. L. (2013). The Art of Supporting Families Faced with Neonatal Transport. *Nursing for Women's Health, 17*(3), 198-209. doi:10.1111/1751-486x.12033.
2. Duritza, K. (2009). Neonatal Transport: A Family Support Module. *Newborn and Infant Nursing Reviews, 9*(4), 212-218. doi:10.1053/j.nainr.2009.09.006.

Figure 11.1 ■ Recommended resources for helping families separated by neonatal transport.

Case-Based Learning

You are caring for a term baby delivered by scheduled repeat C-section at a community hospital 185 miles away. The baby was transferred to the NICU after failing to transition normally because of a ductal-dependent cardiac lesion. The closest NICU is not a surgical center, hence the long transport. Mom and dad are remaining in their community, as they intend to drive together with their 3-year old when mom recovers from surgery. Your NICU has a webcam system that enables the family to see their baby and talk to the NICU team members.

QUESTIONS

1. What are the contextual features of this family's situation?
2. How can technology help support this family during this crisis?

ANSWERS

A NICU experience is highly stressful and causes disruptions in bonding and risk for issues with attachment. The stress is increased by distance: travel time and expense, separation from a support system and normal everyday life, and a stay in a foreign environment, all the while worrying about the baby's survival. Distance may also add stress because of worries of communication with the infant's care providers (Epstein et al., 2017).

Technology may support communication, which may reduce stress. Visualization of their baby, however, can go either way stress-wise. In their study assessing stress due to the infant's appearance, Globus et al. (2016) found that some parents' stress may increase with webcam use because they couldn't touch their babies to comfort them or change their position.

Overall, although technological interventions can't replace in-person communication and interaction, they show promise in supporting communication with the healthcare team, relieving parental stress, and promoting attachment. Further studies and additional kinds of technology are on the horizon (Rhoads, Green, Gauss, Mitchell, Pate, 2015).

REFERENCES

Epstein, E. G., Arechiga, J., Dancy, M., Simon, J., Wilson, D., & Alhusen, J. L. (2017). Integrative review of technology to support communication with parents of infants in the NICU. *Journal of Obstetric, Gynecologic & Neonatal Nursing, 46(3)*, 357–366. doi:10.1016/j.jogn.2016.11.019

Globus, O., Leibovitch, L., Maayan-Metzger, A., Schushan-Eisen, I., Morag, I., Mazkereth, R., ... Strauss, T. (2016). The use of short message services (SMS) to provide medical updating to parents in the NICU. *Journal of Perinatology, 36*, 739–743. doi:10.1038/jp.2016.83

Rhoads, S. J., Green, A., Gauss, C. H., Mitchell, A., & Pate, B. (2015). Web camera use of mothers and fathers when viewing their hospitalized neonate. *Advances in Neonatal Care, 15(6)*, 440–446. doi:10.1097/ANC.0000000000000235

REFERENCES

Badiee, Z., Asghari, M., & Mohammadizadeh, M. (2013). The calming effect of maternal breast milk odor on premature infants. *Pediatrics & Neonatology, 54*(5), 322–325. doi:10.1016/j.pedneo.2013.04.004

Lachman, V. D. (2014). Ethical issues in the disruptive behaviors of incivility, bullying, and horizontal/lateral violence. *Medsurg Nursing, 23*(1), 56–58. Retrieved from https://pdfs.semanticscholar.org/09a6/b719c1d6384ed47d1f79cbf69dbf9cb3fe6f.pdf

Mosher, S. L. (2013). The art of supporting families faced with neonatal transport. *Nursing for Women's Health, 17*(3), 198–209. doi:10.1111/1751-486X.12033

Vedam, S., Leeman, L., Cheyney, M., Fisher, T. J., Myers, S., Low, L. K., & Ruhl, C. (2014). Transfer from planned home birth to hospital: Improving interprofessional collaboration. *Journal of Midwifery & Women's Health, 59*(6), 624–634. doi:10.1111/jmwh.12251

SUPPORTING FAMILIES WHO EXPERIENCE A POSTPARTUM MOOD DISORDER

12

Research has shown that "20 to 30% or higher of NICU parents experience a diagnosable mental disorder during the first postpartum year. An additional proportion of NICU parents will experience subclinical levels of symptoms" (Hynan et al., 2015, "Background" section). Postpartum mood disorders are an extremely serious issue for women after delivery, and the stresses of the NICU can amplify symptoms and the severity of a woman's mental health complications. NICU staff are by no means trained or certified to treat a postpartum mood disorder but should absolutely learn how to assess and identify symptoms of a mood disorder so that they can recognize when a mother is experiencing an illness that warrants a referral to treatment and/or professional support.

Why should staff worry about a mother who has a postpartum mood disorder? If NICU staff has the best interest of the NICU baby and family in mind, they need to understand that "maternal distress early in a child's life has long-term effects on child behavior. Generally children of depressed mothers do not fare well" (Purdy, Craig, & Zeanah, 2015, "Emotional Distress" section), and maternal depression can lead to "later impairments in growth and development of their baby and child" (Hynan et al., 2015, "Background" section). Fathers too experience depression and mood disorders while their children are in the neonatal period, but research is not nearly as robust to show the impact their mood state has on the developing child. NICU caregivers need to continuously assess the family's emotional state and mitigate any adverse effects of parental distress to provide optimal outcomes for the infant in the initial neonatal period and for long-term outcomes.

The critically important task of screening for postpartum depression and perinatal mood disorders falls on the responsibility of NICU providers because the American Academy of Pediatrics (Earls, 2010) recommends that postpartum depression screening should occur at 1-, 2-, 4-, and 6-month visits, using the Edinburgh Postnatal Depression Scale. When infants are in the NICU, those routine well-child visits are disrupted, and the parents are seeing NICU providers at those pivotal postpartum times instead of pediatricians.

ASSESSING FAMILIES FOR POSTPARTUM MOOD DISORDERS

"There is a great need for PPD screening in the NICU and this has been consistently supported in the literature" (Cherry et al., 2016, "Relevance" section), yet very few bedside clinicians receive adequate training to learn what these reliable predictors are. All bedside caregivers should be educated on what historical predictors increase a family's risk for having postpartum depression and screen all families in the NICU for these predictors. Although bedside caregivers are not able to necessarily do all the treatment with positive results, they should be screening and documenting the findings and placing appropriate referrals so that families in jeopardy can receive appropriate help in a timely manner. Initial "screening should be done within the first week [with] both mothers and fathers [as] screening for emotional distress is best done early to evaluate parents whose babies are in the NICU for only a few days" (Hynan et al., 2015, "Recommendations for Screening" section). This initial assessment provides both a baseline for future assessments and insight as to what initial interventions a family may need.

The initial screening should include assessing families for potential present predictors for postpartum depression that may also place them at higher risk for other perinatal mood disorders. These predictors include the following (Beck, 2003):

- History of depression
- History of low self-esteem
- History of prenatal anxiety
- Major life stressors
- Limited social support
- Difficult infant temperament
- Single marital status
- Unplanned/unwanted pregnancy
- Low socioeconomic status

The benefit of screening for these predictors universally can help open the conversation with families about the high percentage of NICU families who experience a postpartum disorder in an attempt to normalize the reality of the problem because "[f]requently, mothers try to hide what they are feeling due to stigma associated with mental illness following childbirth" (Cherry et al., 2016, "Introduction" section). When staff inform parents that all families are screened because such a high rate of NICU families experience postpartum mood disorders after delivery, it tells parents that they are not alone in feeling overwhelmed and depressed, which increases the likelihood of them opening up about the severity of their own symptoms. Initial screening, when performed by bedside caregivers, also provides families with the comfort of questions being asked by someone they already have an established relationship with, rather than a new caregiver coming in and asking them questions blindly. Some units have family-support specialists perform initial screenings, especially if those specialists have established a relationship with a family prior to delivery, to take advantage of an even more established trusting relationship in the hopes that families open up even more fully about any mental health issues they might be struggling with.

There are many initial screening tools available, and a screening tool should be developed that is customized to meet the needs of each hospital based on the support services available. The basic predictive questions, as well as a welcome letter to the family explaining that the unit provides a layered level of support to assist them in coping with their perinatal mental health needs, should be included (Figures 12.1 and 12.2).

Patient+Family Care

Person Completing the Form:	☐ Mother	☐ Father	☐ Sibling	☐ Other (specify)

Highest Education Completed:	☐ Less than high school	☐ Some college	☐ Come graduate school
	☐ High school/GED	☐ Graduated college	☐ Graduated graduate school

Are you a part of a spiritual community?	☐ Yes	☐ No	Which one?_____

Please tell us who lives in your home (include the patient, yourself, and others):

	Relationship to pt.	First and last name	Age
1.	Your baby		
2.	Yourself		
3.			
4.			
5.			
6.			

Patient's Parents/Guardians Relationship Status:	☐ Single	☐ Partnered/ married	☐ Separated/ divorced	☐ Other

Figure 12.1 ■ Psychosocial assessment tool: NICU.

Tell us who you can count on to provide the following: (check all that apply)							
	Spouse/ Partner	Baby's Grandparents	Extended Family	Friends	Work Associates	Other (describe)	No One
A. Parenting							
B. Childcare							
C. Emotional Support							
D. Financial Support							
E. Information							
F. Everyday tasks (e.g., meals, errands, rides)							

Do you see having trouble with any of the following during your NICU stay? (check all that apply?)				
	No	Unknown	Yes	If yes, please comment:
A. Transportation				
B. Housing				
C. Food				
D. Money/income/paying bills				
E. School/work responsibilities				
F. Meeting basic needs				
G. Finding resources				
H. Maintaining relationships				
I. Getting medications				
J. Medical expenses				
K. Emotional/mental health				
L. Balancing life responsibilities				

Figure 12.1 ■ Psychosocial assessment tool: NICU. (*continued*)

Thinking of the adults in the home (including yourself) Please check one box for each answer:	YES	NO
1. Has anyone experienced periods of high anxiety fear or worry?		
2. Has substance abuse ever been an issue for someone in the family?		
3. Has anyone experienced long periods of depression or sadness?		
4. Does anyone have difficulty concentrating, focusing, or have been diagnosed with attention deficit disorder?		
5. Have there been relationship difficulties, conflict, or discussion of separation recently?		
6. Has anyone been (or is currently) in jail?		
7. Does anyone have a serious or chronic medical illness or condition? Explain:		
8. Does anyone have a mental health condition? Explain:		
9. Have you experienced a major life stressor within the past year? How many? Explain (examples include change in employment, loss of job, death of a family member/friend, divorce):		
10. Other family life stressors:		

Since your baby was born (check a response for each of the following questions below):	Not at all	Sometimes	Often	Very much
1. Have you had bad dreams or nightmares about your baby?				
2. Have you become jumpy since your baby has come to the hospital?				
3. When you think about your baby being in the hospital, do you tremble, does your heart beat fast, or do you begin to sweat?				
4. Have you been crying more frequently than normal lately?				
5. Are you having difficulty sleeping when your baby is sleeping?				
6. Is it hard to make yourself come to the hospital and visit your baby?				
7. Have you lost interest in things you used to like to do?				
8. Are you staying hydrated, eating well, and staying connected with family and friends like you did before you had your baby?				

Thank you for completing this form!

Figure 12.1 ■ Psychosocial assessment tool: NICU. (*continued*)

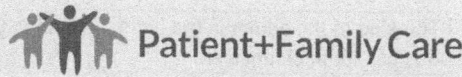

Dear NICU Parents,

Congratulations on the birth of your child/ren. We would like to welcome you to the NICU. We recognize that this time may not be the joyous time you imagined it would be because having a newborn in the hospital is such an emotionally trying experience. Yet we want you to know that your NICU team is here to support you and you will not be going through this experience alone.

Our unit offers several layers of support that all families have access to, and we hope that you will find them helpful during your time with us.

1. Trained Staff: All of our employees are trained in providing the best care possible to patients and their families. They know how to provide comprehensive psychosocial support to NICU families and screen all families for postpartum perinatal mood disorders, understand the importance of family in the life of the child, include siblings as integral members of the family unit, and provide milestone recognition and celebration for families along the care continuum.

2. Peer-to-Peer Organization Support: Our unit partners with peer-to-peer organizations in which support is focused on connecting current NICU families with graduate NICU families. Research shows that there can be reductions in stress and anxiety, as well as perinatal mood disorders, if NICU families can connect with others who have been in the situation before them to share stories and ask questions. Peer-to-peer mentors can bring hope, inspiration, and encouragement to your journey, and we encourage you to participate in our many parent activities and parent support groups. Look for the posted activity calendars around the unit for events that are coming up soon.

3. Mental Health Professionals: We have skilled and licensed trained professionals on staff who can offer clinical support for families that need mental health support. A high rate of NICU families experience perinatal mood disorders, including postpartum depression, and our team of professionals are ready to help treat and refer families on to further treatment if appropriate. Our team includes licensed clinical social workers and clinical psychologists and is ready to provide you all the support you need.

If there is anything you need during your stay, that you feel could help make your journey less stressful or more supportive, please let us know. As a unit we want to help make this experience as stress free as possible for you and your family.

Again, congratulations on the new addition to your family! We are happy to be a part of your journey and look forward helping your family grow and thrive!

Sincerely,
NICU Manager

Figure 12.2 ■ Sample letter to NICU parents from NICU manager.

Families should be continuously monitored for signs and symptoms of perinatal mood disorders and then referred to treatment and therapy as appropriate. Although postpartum depression is most often what individuals think of when they think of perinatal mood disorders, a spectrum of disorders can affect mothers; caregivers should be cognizant of and know how to recognize the signs and symptoms of them (Figure 12.3).

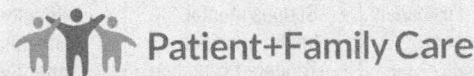
Patient+Family Care

Perinatal Mood Disorder	Definition	Signs/Symptoms	Treatment
Baby blues	• Temporary and short term • Normal response to changing hormone levels and exhaustion • Typically starts 48–72 hours after birth and lasts up to 2 weeks postdelivery • Affects 70%–80% of women and 25% of men	• Mood swings and irritability • Sadness/bursting into tears • Feeling overly sensitive • Physical and mental exhaustion • Anxiety and worry • Feeling empty and lonely • Feeling stressed and overwhelmed • Difficulty coping • Difficulty sleeping	• Talking about feelings • Performing self-relaxation techniques • Getting plenty of rest • Staying well hydrated • Eating well • Exercising daily
Postpartum depression	• Serious mood disorder • Develops anytime after birth but typically within the first few weeks and lasts up to 6 months to 1 year after birth, and can first appear in men up to 1 year after birth • Affects 20% of women and 25%–50% of their men partners • Creates feelings of sadness, anxiety, depression, and exhaustion that can inhibit mother's ability to care for newborn	• Mood swings with irritability and anger • Fatigue • Excessive crying • Withdrawal from family and friends • Inability to bond with baby • Loss of appetite • Feelings of loneliness • Feelings of guilt and being trapped • Lack of motivation • Lack of concentration	• Talking about feelings • Performing self-relaxation techniques • Getting plenty of rest • Staying well hydrated • Eating well • Exercising daily • Participating in counseling • Taking antidepressant medication

Figure 12.3 ■ Perinatal mood disorders: signs and symptoms and treatment.

Postpartum panic disorder	• Serious mental health condition • Triggered condition that results in excessive worry, fear, and anxiety that can cripple new mother • Affects 4%–10% of new mothers, but may be an underreported statistic	• Difficulty concentrating and remembering things • Trouble completing tasks • Easy distraction • Indecisiveness • Inability to relax • Insomnia and fatigue • Loss of appetite • Excessive worry, anxiety, and fear • Agitation and irritability • Agoraphobia • Suicidal thoughts or attempts • Panic attacks	• Talking about feelings • Performing self-relaxation techniques • Getting plenty of rest • Staying well hydrated • Eating well • Exercising daily • Participating in counseling • Taking antidepressant medication • Taking antianxiety medication
Postpartum obsessive-compulsive disorder	• Severe clinical diagnosis that needs diagnosis as soon as possible • Characterized by new mother's constant and repetitive thoughts and behaviors that can be in response to perceived danger toward baby • Affects 3%–5% of new mothers and some fathers • Develops 2–3 weeks after birth	• Unwanted images of hurting baby • Concerns about accidentally causing baby harm • Intrusive thoughts about suffocating or stabbing baby • Fear baby will develop serious disease or illness • Fear that they will unintentionally sexually molest baby • Obsessively checking baby while sleeping	• Talking about feelings • Performing self-relaxation techniques • Getting plenty of rest • Staying well hydrated • Eating well • Exercising daily • Participating in counseling • Participating in CBT • Taking antidepressant medication • Taking antianxiety medication

Figure 12.3 ■ Perinatal mood disorders: signs and symptoms and treatment. (*continued*)

| PPTSD | • Occurs after real or perceived trauma before, during, or after childbirth
• Like other forms of PTSD, women experience forms of flashbacks
• Up to 30% of women experience some form of PPTSD after childbirth, but 3%–7% experience full-blown PPTSD | • Repetitively experiencing traumatic event in intrusive way
• Actively avoiding triggers
• Hypervigilance
• Feelings of detachment from reality or people
• Suffering from anxiety for no apparent reason
• Difficulty sleeping, concentrating, and remembering
• Constant state of distress | • Talking about feelings
• Performing self-relaxation techniques
• Getting plenty of rest
• Staying well hydrated
• Eating well
• Exercising daily
• Participating in counseling
• Participating in CBT
• Participating in EMDR
• Taking antidepressant medication
• Taking antianxiety medication |
| Postpartum psychosis | • Serious and devastating mental health condition that causes severe hallucinations, paranoia, and delusions, and mothers completely detach from reality
• Appears weeks to months after birth
• Affects 1–2 of 1,000 women who give birth
• 10% of women who suffer from postpartum psychosis carry out suicide or infanticide | • Initial symptoms: increased restlessness, insomnia, and irritability
• Sudden onset of other symptoms then occurs and includes delusions and hallucinations
• Serious agitation and anxiousness
• Full insomnia
• Hyperactivity
• Irrational behavior
• Confusion
• Trouble concentrating
• Sudden angry outbursts
• Severe mood swings
• Aggression toward others
• Suicide or infanticide thoughts/attempts | • IMMEDIATE
• Undergoing hospitalization and intensive psychiatric therapy
• Taking antipsychotic medications
• Taking sedatives
• Participating in psychotherapy
• Participating in electroconvulsive therapy |

CBT, cognitive behavioral therapy; EMDR, eye movement desensitization and reprocessing; PPTSD, postpartum posttraumatic stress disorder.

Figure 12.3 ■ Perinatal mood disorders: signs and symptoms and treatment. (*continued*)

PROVIDING LAYERED LEVELS OF EMOTIONAL SUPPORT TO FAMILIES

Layered levels of emotional support should be available to all families in the NICU throughout their entire NICU stay; it can come from bedside caregivers, peer-to-peer support mentors, social workers, family support specialists, case managers, pastoral care, and embedded psychologists in the unit. "NICUs should also have referral mechanisms in place for psychological and psychiatric treatment outside the NICU for those parents whose symptoms require clinical levels of care beyond the capabilities of the NICU" (Hynan et al., 2015, "Recommendations for Layered Levels" section).

The first layer of support, which all families in the unit should receive, is comprehensive support from bedside caregivers. As discussed earlier in this text, NICU caregivers should all be educated and adequately trained on how to provide psychosocial support to NICU families. This includes the following:

- Staff "[interacting] with them in ways that will enhance their coping both during their NICU stay and post discharge" (Hall et al., 2015, "Rationale" section)
- Staff receiving adequate education and training to be able to provide psychosocial support to NICU families
- Units providing consistent family-centered developmental care
- Family-support specialists being on staff to provide antenatal consults and establishing pre-NICU relationships if possible
- Provision of family access to the infant 24/7
- Sibling participation being equally important members of the family
- Family participation in multidisciplinary rounds
- Bedside shift reports in which families participate and are included
- Use of technology to facilitate connection between infants and family when family cannot physically be in the unit with the child

The second layer of support should include an "active peer-to-peer support organizations, ideally with a position for a paid parent support coordinator embedded in the NICU staff" (Hynan et al., 2015, "Recommendations for Layered Levels" section). These trained mentors can help coordinate and facilitate peer-to-peer mentor activities, family support groups, sibling events, and other peer-to-peer connection opportunities that have been proved to reduce stress and anxiety among NICU families. All families should be encouraged to participate in unit events and activities, which should be offered at a minimum of once a week and more often if possible. A published and posted calendar of these events should be posted in several prominent places around the unit where not only families can see them independently, but also staff can see them and easily be reminded to share them with families to encourage participation.

The third level of support involves additional paid staff members who are responsible for further supporting the physical and emotional needs of families. These staff members are integral in the care-coordination efforts of each NICU journey and include licensed clinical social workers, case managers, and mental health professionals. "All NICUs with

20 or more beds [should] have at least one full-time masters' level social worker and one full-time or part-time doctoral level psychologist embedded in the NICU staff" (Hynan et al., 2015, "Recommendations for NICU Mental Health" section). These caregivers are vital in helping care for families whose mental health needs are more demanding and need more attention. The recommendations are for units of this size because they typically care for more critical babies, so inherently, the stress level of parents is higher, the more unstable their children are. "Larger NICUs should have proportionally more NICU mental health professionals on staff" (Hynan et al., 2015, "Recommendations for NICU Mental Health" section) to meet the needs and demands of the patient population.

Having professional mental health providers on staff has many benefits. Hynan et al. (2015, "Recommendations for NICU Mental Health" section) provide a list of the many benefits that include the following:

- Being able to conduct research in the following areas:
  - The use of assessment devices, test interpretation, and outcome evaluation
  - The risks for the development of psychological disorders in the NICU parents
  - The parent–infant attachment therapy
  - The effects of parental emotional distress on the child–parent relationships and the parental couple
  - The long-term outcomes of the child, both physical and emotional
- Being able to provide clinical services for families:
  - Assessments, interpretation of tests, and outcome evaluations
  - A variety of treatment approaches
  - Differential diagnoses of perinatal mood disorders and psychiatric disorders, as well as identification of subclinical symptoms
- Being able to provide education to NICU staff about the centrality of the parent dyad–infant relationship in all interactions and communication with families who are:
  - Guilt- and shame-ridden
  - Distressed and angry
  - Possibly struggling with substance abuse
  - Bereaved
  - Coping with prior traumas and perinatal losses (including multiple trials of assisted reproductive technology and miscarriages)
- Having the ability to support staff through education and debriefings. "Because debriefing sessions can elicit strong and sometimes opposing emotions and views, it is important to have a qualified professional leading the discussion" (Hall et al., 2015, "Methods of Staff Support" section)

In addition, and very important, embedded psychologists on the team are able to perform more complex mental health screenings with families. Bedside caregivers can perform initial screenings and refer high-risk patients to social workers and psychologists, but patients who are at high risk for suffering from severe perinatal mood disorders greatly benefit from being screened by a licensed psychologist who can properly screen, treat, and refer to further clinical services as appropriate.

ENCOURAGING INTENTIONAL PARENTAL SELF-CARE PRACTICES

"Stress emanating from the birth of a premature of sick neonate has received considerable attention and is associated with concurrent parental anxiety and depression" (Busse, Stromgren, Thorngate, & Thomas, 2013, "Introduction" section). As a universal layer of support, all families should be educated by NICU staff who "focusing on self-care during the time of NICU crisis will be critical in establishing healthy behaviors and self-care practices that will improve the overall physical and emotional health of parents, which in turn will aid in providing a healthy environment in which their child can thrive and flourish" (Mosher, 2017, "NICU Admission" section). When staff provide this education to families, they are fostering an environment that reduces stress and anxiety and hopefully subsequently reduces the incidence of perinatal mood disorders.

As discussed multiple times in the text, a parental self-care program should be standard of care in the unit, and the N.U.R.S.E. Self Care Program is one that is easy to use, easy to follow, and adaptable while families are in the unit and at home postdischarge. In looking at the model, some examples of N.U.R.S.E. goals families might make during the NICU journey might include the following:

- N (nourishment): Eat a minimum of three balanced meals a day, pack high-protein snacks when visiting the NICU, stay hydrated.

- U (understanding): Seek information on the new diagnosis they just received on their baby's heart condition.

- R (rest/relaxation): Practice deep breathing twice a day for 5 minutes, step outside for 5 minutes twice a day to get fresh air, get a minimum of 4 hours of uninterrupted sleep.

- S (spirituality-not religious): Spend 10 minutes a day journaling about their experiencing, which can lead to increased understanding.

- S (spirituality-religious): Spend 10 minutes a day reading scripture or spending time in prayer.

- E (exercise): Take a walk all the way around the hospital campus once a day.

Parents can also be encouraged to participate in other self-care relaxation techniques and should be supported in trying multiple practices until they find one that feels like a good fit for them. Self-relaxation techniques can include, but certainly are not limited to, deep breathing, yoga, meditation, guided imagery, hot baths, reading, journaling, exercise, sleep, reduction of caffeine intake, avoidance of alcohol consumption, laughing, spending of time with family or friends, and relaxing music.

Author's Personal Story

M.S. was the father of a 31-week-old boy who had been transferred to our unit several weeks earlier at 28 weeks, just after birth, when his wife went into spontaneous preterm labor at one of our community hospitals. I was the family-support specialist working with this family, had met them shortly after their admission, and had been checking on them routinely every few days. M.S. and his wife, R.S., were first-time parents and had struggled with infertility for 6 years. After multiple miscarriages, they turned to infertility specialists and attempted intrauterine insemination several times without success. Finally, this couple sustained this pregnancy to 28 weeks with in vitro fertilization (IVF). The week leading up to R.S. delivering, she had been working long days and getting very little sleep and she blamed herself for the premature delivery. She was convinced the stress she was under at work was what caused her body to reject the baby inside her. Despite multiple providers trying to explain to her otherwise, she believed she had gone into preterm labor because of something she did; she was feeling guilty and shameful, like she had let down her baby, her husband, and all of their dreams of having a perfect family.

M.S. was sitting quietly by his son's bedside when I walked in to check in on their family that particular day and I was surprised to see him alone. Typically, both he and his wife were at every visit together. For the past 3 weeks, they arrived together at 9 a.m. for the morning care, they would stay all day so they could participate in all care throughout the day, they would be present for multidisciplinary rounds at 2 p.m., R.S. would pump every 3 hours at the bedside, they would go eat in the hospital café together for lunch, and then they would leave to go home for the night after 9 p.m. care after meeting the nurse assigned to their son for the night shift. I heard that R.S. called to check in at midnight when she would wake up to pump, and M.S. would call to check in at 6:30 a.m. as they were getting up so that he could hear how the rest of the night went before the night shift would leave and report off to day shift. They had a very prescriptive routine that had not waivered for 3 weeks, so I was taken aback to see M.S. alone.

As I approached M.S., he looked more tired than usual, and I could sense that something was going on. I looked around the room quickly and did not see R.S.'s purse, jacket, or pumping bag, so I asked if he was okay if I pulled up a chair and sat with him for a few minutes. He only nodded, and at that moment, a single tear trickled down his face. I also grabbed a box of tissues from the counter and placed them in my lap so that if he was going to need them I would have them handy as I sat with him. I pulled my chair up next to him and started out our meeting just as I started every other one, looking at his son and checking in on him and asking how things were going. This apparently was a good distraction because M.S. immediately perked up and said that his son was weaned down to room air the night before and was maintaining great oxygen saturation rates thus far. I congratulated him and his son and told that little guy to keep up the great work! I looked up at the dry erase board and one of the nurses had taken a great photograph of the baby and made a little card saying "I am on room air" with the date and time and posted it for

(continued)

(*continued*)

the family. It made me smile, and I made a point of recognizing the cute keepsake and recognizing the huge accomplishment.

I sat back down and asked M.S. how everything else was going. His persona turned more somber again, and initially, he just sat silently and shook his head. He finally blurted out "I don't know what to do. My wife is really struggling, and I don't know how to help her. She was so upset today she couldn't even make it out of bed to come visit." I knew right then and there that things were not good for R.S. and our team likely had been missing signs of distress for the past few weeks.

I thanked M.S. for sharing with me the reality of what was going on because I knew that took courage, and that I hoped he would excuse me for just a moment. I quickly returned with the initial perinatal mood disorder screening that had been completed shortly after admission. Based on the screening tool, neither him nor his wife scored alarmingly high for being at risk for any level of postpartum mood disorder, and although the stress of their infertility and the fact that R.S. felt she was the cause of the premature birth were certainly huge stressors, there were no other large predictors that alerted us that she would be at risk for developing postpartum depression or other postpartum disorders. I reviewed with him other signs and symptoms of perinatal mood disorders and told him that from what I had observed, and what the other staff had documented as observing, she didn't seem to exhibit any signs of struggling. I questioned him if today's behavior was something sudden? He verbalized to me that no, these symptoms were not sudden at all. She, in fact, had been exhibiting many of the symptoms I listed but was hiding them from staff really well because as a lawyer, she always had to be so put together and professional. She didn't want to let anyone see her be anything but that. M.S. shared with me that his wife had been extremely irritable and insecure, had been crying a lot, had many fears, wasn't sleeping well in between any of her nighttime pump sessions, wasn't eating well, had to be reminded to take a shower, and felt very distant. I truly was blown away because each time I had an encounter with this family, she seems so put together, so happy, so attentive to her husband and baby, always looked well groomed and put together, and had a very robust milk supply (which led me to believe she was sleeping well, eating right, staying hydrated, and managing her stress). How could the vision of how we thought she was doing be so drastically different from the reality of how she was doing?

I instantly flashed back to my own postpartum experience after my second child. I suffered pretty severe postpartum depression and not a single person noticed until I showed up for my 6-week postpartum obstetrical appointment. My obstetrician picked up on it right away, and I was blown away that at the end of my visit, he started talking to me about postpartum depression support groups and how important it was for me to consider attending one. I tried to continue the charade and play it off that I appreciated the recommendation but was doing great, just had a slight case of baby blues, and was exhausted from not getting much sleep; raising a toddler and having an infant didn't foster a relaxing home environment. I remember he looked me in the eyes and told me that I didn't have to pretend to be strong in front of him because there was nothing to prove to

(*continued*)

him. He told me I was an incredible mother, raising two amazing healthy boys. But for them to stay that way, they needed a healthy mom, both physically and emotionally. I ended up breaking down right there in the office and once the floodgates opened, it was downhill from there.

I was a nurse. I was a NICU nurse for that matter. I knew how to take care of babies, sick babies even, so I should be able to take care of this baby without a problem. Yet I couldn't establish breastfeeding and for some reason I could not for the life of me figure out how to manage caring for this baby and a just barely 2-year old. The one time I tried to take a shower, I had the baby in a bouncy chair and the 2-year old came running in and tried climbing in the bouncy seat with the newborn. I went running out of the shower, soaking wet, to save the infant from being smothered, and when I turned around, the toddler was drinking out of a Sippy cup that I hadn't seen in a while and he had the strangest look on his face. It turned out it was a cup that had been in our bathroom for quite some time and had spoiled milk in it that actually made me gag and almost throw up when I twisted the cap off and got one whiff of the smell. After that, I wouldn't shower until my husband got home from work and I knew both boys would be monitored at all times by a capable parent.

While I was home during the day I wanted nothing more than to be the perfect wife and mother by getting all the laundry done, having the house clean, having dinner ready when my husband came home from work, getting the boys' naps in during the day, getting my workout in so that I could soon be back to my prepregnancy body, making time to go have lunch with my friends, and attending fun mommy and me reading events at the local library. The reality was I was in pajamas all day long, and just before my husband came home, I would quickly put clothing on so that he would think I had been dressed all day. I barely got the boys' naps in and would just be thankful on days the toddler would sleep at all. We were lucky if we made it to one story time every 2 weeks. For dinner, I either heated up frozen meals for dinner and put them in our own casserole dishes to try and make it look like I prepared the meal or would rely on meals friends would bring us. I wouldn't answer calls from friends, and when they asked why I never answered their calls, I would just tell them I was too busy to talk. Our laundry would sit in piles for days before I would finally do a single load. I was a mess. But I couldn't admit that to anyone. Before then, I always could manage caring for myself and always was known for doing so much for so many people that I was mortified to admit I couldn't handle this. I was irritable, cried excessively, felt lonely, felt detached from my son, felt extremely anxious, felt like a failure, had a loss of interests, didn't sleep well, had difficulty concentrating, couldn't make decisions, and was experiencing periodic minor panic attacks.

Being a nurse, I should have known better. I should have known that seeking help was not a sign of weakness but was a way to seek help to a relatively common phenomenon that happens to many women after childbirth. Yet I still was ashamed to seek help and allow my peers to see me in that state. I was ashamed to let my husband see me in that state, and I didn't want my family to think of me as a failure. As the oldest of all my siblings

(*continued*)

(continued)

(3) and cousins (18), I was the one who always was the example of how to do things right; I didn't want to let anyone down. So I immediately knew how R.S. had hidden her symptoms from us all. We were strangers to her, so she was able to hide her true emotions and feelings from us while she was at the hospital. When she went home, her husband saw her real emotions, and privately they were trying to manage and cope. R.S. was a highly respected professional in our community and she didn't want to be seen like she was weak and less than the strong woman that she was. I fully understood where she was at, and my heart ached for her struggle and was ready to help M.S. and R.S. get through this period of their journey.

I started by assuring M.S. that he was not going to need to help R.S. on his own and that there were many layers of support that would be available to not only her, but to him as well. I informed him that they were in this together and as he supported her through this, he too was going to need support. That together they would get through this stronger and healthier. I shared with him some basic information about the spectrum of perinatal mood disorders and the various ways that women can be treated. Together, we discussed which he felt would be the best way to approach R.S. about seeking support because the last thing we wanted to do is to make her feel attacked or as if he came running to the unit sharing information about his wife she would not have felt comfortable with him sharing.

We came to the agreement that he would go home and try some self-relaxation techniques for him and her to see if anything helped, but we both acknowledged that she likely would need more clinical support than self-relaxation and deep-breathing exercises to help her through her depression. I told M.S. that I would talk to the unit's psychologist that afternoon and request that the scheduled 1-month postpartum depression screening be moved up a little early based on the symptoms he had shared with me; by having the psychologist involved in what would appear as a universal and routine screening, it would allow an open opportunity for discussion and the revelation of these symptoms.

Two days later R.S. returned to the unit with her husband and looked a little less put together, a little more tired, and a little more withdrawn. She still tried to be upbeat in her interactions, was engaging with her husband and child, and was still dressed very nicely. But things were definitely different. Yet to this day I don't know if it was because I knew the truth and so therefore I could see through the façade, or if it was because she finally could not keep up the charades anymore. I entered the room and as usual I said hello, said hello to their son, asked for an update, and then asked an open-ended question about how things were going for the two of them. Almost before I could finish my question R.S. answered "Great." M.S. just shrugged his shoulders and I just went with it. Unfortunately, our psychologist was busy that day with a different family who was in crisis, so during my visit that day with this couple, we didn't do much other than celebrate that their son was still on room air and doing really well.

When R.S. left the room to use the restroom, M.S. snuck out to find me and told me that his wife was not doing any better and he was more worried about her now than he had been. I assured him that I had talked to the psychologist and she would be checking

(continued)

(*continued*)

in with them as soon as possible. I asked if he would like to see the social worker in the meantime, and he thought that would be a good idea. Before R.S. returned from the restroom, M.S. made it back to the room, and I left the unit to find our social worker and updated her on the conversations I had been having with M.S. Our social worker then went and had a nice check-in conversation with them. Her conversation was taken from the stance that she was visiting them as a routine check-in to see if they had any needs or new issues that had come up that she could assist with. Before she could really finish her question, R.S. said "No" and asked to excuse herself because she needed to pump. M.S. actually was brave enough to speak up and say that he did have a few new needs that he was needing support with. He proceeded to say that he was having symptoms of irritability, insomnia, sadness, loss of appetite, and loss of motivation. He was explaining his wife's symptoms but claiming them as his own to see what type of help was available, and later, I found out he was saying these things in hopes that it would encourage his wife to also speak up.

This discussion led our social worker to provide him with a list of wonderful unit-based and community-wide resources for postpartum depression that affects not only mothers, but also fathers, of NICU babies. She sat with them for quite some time and really went into detail about how common these symptoms were and how helpful these resources really are for parents. She shared with the family that not everyone was comfortable in group settings, so there were telephone options and online options that allowed patients to remain anonymous but still get the support and care that they needed. After the visit, many pamphlets and fliers were left in the room with the family and I noticed R.S. looking through them in detail. I was relieved and felt this was a great first step.

The next day, again when R.S. left the room to use the restroom, M.S. came and found me in the unit and shared with me that his wife spend a good portion of the night on line chatting with other mothers on a support group the social worker had told them about. He was thrilled! She also had called a postpartum depression hotline and talked to someone when she woke up for her midnight pumping. What surprised him the most was after that pump session, she fell right asleep and slept through the 3 a.m. alarm. He felt as though she was so relieved and already felt so much better after being able to talk to someone about everything, that she finally was able to get some sleep. What was even timelier was that our unit psychologist was available and planning to meet with both M.S. and R.S. that afternoon, and he was very excited to see how that visit went.

I checked in with M.S. and R.S. the next week, as I had a few days off after our last check in, and I was pretty shocked when I walked in their room. R.S. had a big smile on her face, which seemed genuine but tired. She also was wearing sweats, a sweatshirt, her hair in a ponytail, and glasses. I almost did a double take to see if I was in the right room! R.S. always wore outfits that looked as though she had walked off of the courtroom floor, had her hair done, had matching accessories, and wore contacts. Our visit took a very different turn this time as before I could even ask her how her son and they were doing, she opened the conversation by telling me how SHE was doing. She told me that

(*continued*)

(*continued*)

she had met with the unit psychologist three times since I had seen her last and that she had found out that her husband and I had talked about her emotional state the week prior. She glanced over at her husband, and he sheepishly smiled back at her. She looked back and me and smiled and just said "Thanks." She continued to share with me that she didn't realize how much she was struggling and how depressed she really was. She was so used to being so on top of everything, and everything about this experience came crumbling down. She was the reason they couldn't conceive and then she was the reason she couldn't keep a pregnancy to term. At least that is what she had allowed herself to believe. She was so thankful that her husband cared enough about her to seek help and speak up as though it was him that was suffering to get her the help she needed. And now, she wanted to just focus on getting her and her son healthy and strong so they all would be a happy and healthy family. She said she was going to open and honest about her emotions, she wasn't going to prioritize being put together every day, and if that meant some days she made it out of the house in sweats, well then, at least she made it out of the house to be with her son.

For the remainder of their NICU stay, M.S. and R.S. routinely participated in peer-to-peer mentor activities, they enrolled in a community yoga class, R.S. went to weekly counseling sessions, and was started on antidepressant medications to see her through the acute phase of her depression. By the time NICU discharge came, their family was emotionally ready to go home and parent their son independently. They even showed me their N.U.R.S.E. care plan for home and what goals they had for themselves for the first month at home. I was extremely proud of how well M.S. and R.S. faced their challenges together and pulled through her perinatal mood disorder with proper treatment and support.

Family Story

Julie Yarbrough, a mother who delivered extremely premature triplets just before Christmas and after spending time on hospital bed rest, shares her experience of struggling with postpartum depression after delivery.

"I was pregnant with triplets at the age of 46 in 2005. I had miscarried twice before, so this was my first real chance of having babies. I was diagnosed with anticardiolipin antibodies, which put me at high risk of a recurrent miscarriage and of late-term fetal loss. I had undergone IVF, and this was my last chance at having children. I was receiving intravenous immunoglobulin every 6 weeks during my pregnancy. I was also receiving 33 shots a week during the pregancy to protect the babies from several other problems. These injections consisted of hormones and heparin. I was also diagnosed with hyperemesis gravidarum, which lasted for the first 5 months of my pregnancy, and I was basically in bed most of that time.

(*continued*)

(*continued*)

"When I finally started feeling better, at about 20 weeks, my obstetrician placed me on strict bed rest for the remainder of the pregnancy to increase my chances of avoiding preterm labor. I was diagnosed with preeclampsia at 27 weeks and admitted to the hospital. I eventually delivered my babies at 29 weeks and 2 days via C-section. By that time, I had developed severe preeclampsia, and one of my babies was severely ill with severe intrauterine fetal growth restriction. I was scared but excited to finally be a mom. I knew that the babies were very early and would have problems. I was a labor and delivery nurse and knew more information about what could happen to these babies than most moms. They were all put on ventilators but holding their own.

"They weighed 1 lb 10 oz, 2 lb 4 oz, and 3 lb and 1 oz. I had one girl and two boys. I did pretty well for about 4 days. My husband and I couldn't touch the babies for 2 weeks, but we visited the NICU frequently. On the day I was to go home, I started having chest pressure and shortness of breath. The doctor ordered an ECG and when I got the results, they said I'd had a heart attack. I couldn't believe it. I didn't act like I had had one, so 2 hours later, another ECG was done, and it was normal. Needless to say, this was very stressful to my husband and me. I eventually went home that day with a diagnosis of anxiety. It was hard to leave the hospital without the babies.

"With each passing day, I seemed to get more depressed and anxious. I couldn't sleep, I couldn't eat, and I started to have panic attacks. I had never had panic attacks before, but I knew what they were. I had been on numerous amounts of hormones during my pregnancy, and they were stopped on the day of delivery. I steadily went downhill and finally had to call my doctor. She had me come in, and she put me on an antidepressant and an antianxiety medication. I thought I was going crazy. Here I wanted to have a child for so long and now I didn't even want to see my babies. I wanted to just stay in bed in the fetal position and not talk to anyone. My mom and my husband tried to help, but I just thought I was going crazy and that this was my new normal. All I kept thinking was how was I going to feed the babies, how was I ever going to sleep, and I was never going to have a normal life ever again.

"We would get phone calls every day from the neonatologist telling us the babies were fine or the babies were not doing well. We visited our babies every day. It was a nonstop roller coaster ride every day. I didn't want to hurt the babies or myself. I just wanted to run away. The antidepressants didn't work immediately, so I eventually started seeing a therapist. I also would see my obstetrician twice a week. She was very worried about me, and so was my husband, who also was a retired obstetrician and gynecologist. They both hadn't seen such a severe case of postpartum depression personally before.

"I forced myself every day to go visit the babies. I put my make-up on, dressed nicely, and pretended that everything was okay so no one would think badly of me. I was having a hard time pumping my breasts because I did not make much milk for these three babies. I was told to relax and quit stressing out because that would help. Eventually, I tried all kinds of remedies and medications to help bring in more milk, which didn't help. I felt like a failure. I was producing about 10 to 20 mL every time I pumped which to me was

(*continued*)

(*continued*)

nothing. I would have panic attacks every time I pumped. It was horrible. When I would go see the babies, which was two or three times a day, I would fake that I was OK. In my crazy state, I thought that the nurses and doctors would report me to CPS because I didn't care about the babies. I really didn't even want to hold them.

"At 8 days after my babies were born, both my boys got hospital-acquired pneumonia. They were very ill. One of my sons had to be flown to Portland, which was 3 hours away, because he was turning blue and needed heart surgery. There wasn't a pediatric heart surgeon where we lived. Now my husband was leaving for who knows for how long, and I was left behind to take care of the other two babies. Thank goodness for my mom. She kept me going mentally and physically and forced me to eat. My husband and our boy were gone for 5 days and were eventually flown back to our NICU.

"I felt like no one really knew how I felt and how bad I was except for my mom, my husband, and my obstetrician. Every day was a struggle for my babies and me. My other son eventually had two surgeries, one for a bilateral inguinal hernia repair and the other for an umbilical hernia repair. His intestines twisted, and he needed emergency surgery. During this time, I was slowly getting better, but I felt like no one really knew how bad this journey of mine was. I cried a lot and wondered what I had done with my life. At one point, the neonatologist said, 'Please just try to give the littlest baby your breast milk. We will put the other two babies on formula. If you don't give him your breast milk he could develop necrotizing colitis and die.' This didn't help my stress level. On another occasion, one of the nurses drew up too much breast milk in a syringe to give to one of the babies via NG tube and squirted the excess in the trash in front of me. I absolutely lost it and got hysterical. I tried so hard to pump and make milk, and she just put it in the trash.

"At 6 weeks postpartum I had a grand mal seizure while visiting the babies in the NICU. I was admitted to the hospital for 2 days. I had to quit pumping my breasts because of the medication they put me on. That was when my panic attacks stopped. I was so happy that I didn't have to pump anymore. The NICU we were in was small and it had room for only eight babies. We were all close together and it seemed like you knew everyone's business. All the monitors would go off and my nerves were already on overload, and I was constantly anxious. I guess the biggest thing that helped me most was knowing that the nurses and doctors were taking great care of our kids and loving on them when I couldn't. It was a sense of relief to know someone could love them when emotionally I couldn't.

"One night my littlest boy was dying, and the NICU staff couldn't figure out what was going on with him. The doctors and nurses never left his side for 24 hours. He eventually turned around by prayers and great doctors and nurses figuring out his problem. Two babies came home at 2 months and the third at three and a half months. They did come home, one at a time, which helped me prepare for the next baby and get in a routine. It probably took me 6 months to finally start feeling better. A friend of mine gave me a book that the actress Brooke Shields wrote about her journey with postpartum depression. After finishing that book, I finally felt like someone really knew how I actually felt. My journey finally turned around. Before that, I felt like no one really understood the pain

(*continued*)

(*continued*)

I was going through and that I was all alone. I quit feeling crazy and knew that it was hormonal.

"I have three beautiful children who just turned 12 years old. I am a great mom and am there for them every day. I help other moms who have gone through postpartum depression, when called on. What I learned most of all through this journey is to tell people how you are feeling. You are not crazy, and this too shall pass. Postpartum depression doesn't need to be a taboo subject but something real that with time will get better with the proper treatment and support. I felt like giving up every day, but with my support system, I made it and I'm glad I did."

RECOMMENDATIONS/SUGGESTIONS FOR BEST PRACTICE

1. All NICU care providers should be well educated on the signs and symptoms of perinatal mood disorders.

2. Bedside NICU staff should screen all NICU families within 48 hours for predictors of perinatal mood disorders.

3. Each organization should have a customized screening tool for perinatal mood disorders.

4. Organizations should have a letter they provide families at admission that explain the high rate of perinatal mood disorders among NICU families and the layered levels of support their unit provides families.

5. Units should have layered levels of support available to NICU families:

   a. Trained and adequately supportive staff

   b. Peer-to-peer organization with paid mentor on staff to offer peer-to-peer connection opportunities

   c. Trained mental health providers on staff

   d. Expanded mental health screenings

   e. Mental health professionals providing support to both families and staff

6. Families in the NICU should be continuously monitored and screened for perinatal mood disorders throughout the NICU stay following the American Academy of Pediatrics recommendations (at 1, 2, 4, and 6 months).

7. N.U.R.S.E. or another self-care program should be included as a part of the standard of care in the NICU for families.

8. All families should be encouraged to participate in self-relaxation techniques.

RECOMMENDED RESOURCES

Countless resources are available to staff and families to find support for those struggling with perinatal mood disorders. Our resource list is just a small sample of some of those resources (Figure 12.4).

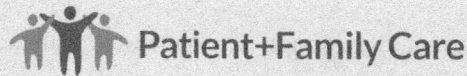

Website Recommendations:

1. http://babybluesconnection.org/finding-help/bbc-groups
2. http://www.mom365.com/baby/moms-health/how-to-beat-the-baby-blues
3. https://www.postpartumdepression.org
4. http://www.postpartum.net
5. http://www.postpartumprogress.com/ppd-support-groups-in-the-u-s-canada
6. http://www.postpartumprogress.com/get-hope
7. https://www.dailystrength.org/group/post-partum-depression
8. http://www.1800ppdmoms.org
9. https://postpartumhealthalliance.org
10. https://www.helpguide.org/articles/depression/postpartum-depression-and-the-baby-blues.htm
11. https://www.acog.org/Womens-Health/Depression-and-Postpartum-Depression
12. https://themighty.com/2016/03/22-ways-to-support-a-mom-with-postpartum -depression-from-moms-whove-been-there
13. http://www.scarymommy.com/support-spouse-postpartum-depression-anxiety
14. http://perinatalsupport.org
15. http://www.themotherhoodcollective.org/pmads
16. http://postpartummen.com
17. http://postpartumdads.org

Book Recommendations:

1. *A Deeper Shade of Blue: A Woman's Guide to Recognizing and Treating Depression in Her Childbearing Years* by Ruta Nonacs
2. *Beyond the Blues: A Guide to Understanding and Treating Prenatal and Postpartum Depressions* by Shoshana Bennett and Pec Indman
3. *Birth of a New Brain: Healing from Postpartum Bipolar Disorder* by Diane Harwood
4. *Depression in Mothers: Causes, Consequences, and Treatment Alternatives* by Kathleen Kendall-Tackett
5. *Identifying Perinatal Depression and Anxiety: Evidence Based Practice in Screening, Psychosocial Assessment and Management* by Alan Gemmill
6. *Perinatal and Postpartum Mood Disorders: Perspectives and Treatment Guide for the Health Care Practitioner* by Susan Stone and Alexis Menken
7. *Postpartum Depression and Anxiety: A Self Help Guide for Mothers* by Pacific Post Partum Support Society
8. *Postpartum Depression for Dummies* by Shoshana Bennett
9. *The Afterglow: A Perinatal Mood and Anxiety Disorder Support Group Curriculum* by Ashley Hanna Morgan
10. *The Hidden Feelings of Motherhood* by Kathleen Kendall-Tackett
11. *This Isn't What I Expected* by Karen Kleiman
12. *The Mother-to-Mother Postpartum Depression Support Book* by Sandra Poulin
13. *Down Came the Rain* by Brooke Shields

Figure 12.4 ■ Recommended resources for helping families separated by neonatal transport.

Case-Based Learning

You have been caring for the family of an infant born at 28 weeks' gestation for a month. Baby is out of the woods respiratory-wise and is progressing well on feedings. In spite of this positive trend, you notice that the mother is becoming less interested in caring for her baby. When she visits, she no longer wants to provide skin-to-skin kangaroo care or participate in caring for baby. She tells you that she is too exhausted to help and that her baby "doesn't like it" when she changes the diaper, anyway.

QUESTIONS

1. What are the warning signs in this scenario?

2. What are your thoughts about why this mother's behavior is changing?

3. What interventions are needed and why?

ANSWERS

This mother may be experiencing postpartum mood disorders such as anxiety and/or depression. The timing is right (baby blues usually resolve around 2 weeks), and her overwhelming fatigue and feeling of worthlessness are consistent with the symptoms seen with depression (Brummelte & Galea, 2016). Screening and referral of this mother for the diagnosis and treatment of postpartum mood disorders is indicated.

The high rates of depression in families enduring the stress of a NICU experience won't be a shock to anyone who has ever worked in a NICU. However, the effects on neonatal neurobehavior and neurodevelopmental outcomes that are associated with gestational depression might come as a surprise. Even more astonishing is that some of these alterations start in utero. In a systematic review, Gentile (2017) describes irregular fetal heart rate, increased levels of cortisol and norepinephrine (stress hormones), decreased dopamine levels, altered EEG patterns, and reduced vagal tone in neonates related to maternal depression. The sequelae can extend into childhood and beyond, manifesting as poor growth, irregular sleep patterns, irritability, and reduced activity. Attachment and psychosocial functioning, as well as the development of cognitive skills, may be altered.

This scenario illustrates the importance of weighing the effects of untreated maternal depression against the concerns associated with in utero exposure to antidepressants.

REFERENCES

Brummelte, S., & Galea, L. A. (2016). Postpartum depression: Etiology, treatment and consequences for maternal care. *Hormones and Behavior, 77,* 153–166. doi:10.1016/j.yhbeh.2015.08.008

Gentile, S. (2017). Untreated depression during pregnancy: Short- and long-term effects in offspring. A systematic review. *Neuroscience, 342,* 154–166. doi:10.1016/j.neuroscience.2015.09.001

REFERENCES

Beck, C. T. (2003). Recognizing and screening for postpartum depression on mothers of NICU infants. *Advances in Neonatal Care, 3*(1), 37–46. doi:10.1053/adnc.2003.50013

Busse, M., Stromgren, K., Thorngate, L., & Thomas, K. A. (2013). Parents' responses to stress in the neonatal intensive care unit. *Critical Care Nurse, 33*(4), 52–59. doi:10.4037/ccn2013715

Cherry, A., Blucker, R., Thornberry, T., Hetherington, C., McCaffree, M., & Gillaspy, S. (2016). Postpartum depression screening in the neonatal intensive care unit: Program development, implementation, and lessons learned. *Journal of Multidisciplinary Healthcare, 9*, 59–67. doi:10.2147/JMDH.S91559

Earls, M. F. (2010). Incorporating recognition and management of perinatal and postpartum depression into pediatric practice. *Pediatrics, 126*(5), 1032–1039. doi:10.1542/peds.2010-2348

Hall, S. L., Cross, J., Selix, N. W., Patterson, C., Segre, L., Chuffo-Siewert, R., . . . Martin, M. L. (2015). Recommendations for enhancing psychosocial support of NICU parents through staff education and support. *Journal of Perinatology, 35*, S29–S36. doi:10.1038/jp.2015.147

Hynan, M. T., Steinberg, Z., Baker, L., Cicco, R., Geller, P. A., Lassen, S., . . . Stuebe, A. (2015). Recommendations for mental health professionals in the NICU. *Journal of Perinatology, 35*, S14–S18. doi:10.1038/jp.2015.144

Mosher, S. (2017). Comprehensive NICU parental education: Beyond baby basics. *Neonatal Network, 36*(1), 18–25. doi:10.1891/0730-0832.36.1.18

Purdy, I. B., Craig, J. W., & Zeanah, P. (2015). NICU discharge planning and beyond: Recommendations for parent psychosocial support. *Journal of Perinatology, 35*, S24–S28. doi:10.1038/jp.2015.146

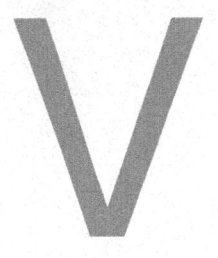

SUPPORTING WITH BEREAVEMENT
AND PALLIATIVE CARE

BEREAVEMENT: SUPPORTING FAMILIES EXPERIENCING A LOSS IN THE PERINATAL PERIOD

13

The death of a child is a devastating life event that no parent ever wants to experience, no matter what time of life the death occurs. Whether a child dies before birth, at birth, shortly after birth, in childhood, or in adulthood, a parent never wants to have to experience saying goodbye to their precious child. However, "the death of a child around the time of birth is one of the most profound, stressful events an adult may experience" (Koopmans, Wilson, Cacciatore, & Flenady, 2013, "Background" section), and at a time when parents anticipate celebrating new life, they find themselves sometimes welcoming their child into and out of this world simultaneously.

Care providers who enter the field of obstetrics, family birthing, and neonatal care typically enter their respective fields because of the joyous outcomes that they get to experience with families. I can honestly say that it is such an incredible honor to be present at the birth of a new life and witness the pleasure and gratification that a new family experiences in that moment. To see a mother hold her baby for the very first time and looking deep into her child's eyes is a moment that not everyone gets to witness, and yet, I have had the honor of seeing it hundreds of times. Watching a father look adoringly down at his wife in admiration as she holds this tiny little life in her arms with pride beaming from his heart is one of the most precious look I have ever seen, and I have seen it more times that I can even count. Watching families crowd around new little babies and try to figure out whose noses they have, whose lips they have, and who they look most like makes me feel nothing but happiness. It's as if when a new baby is brought into their world, no matter what else might be going on, all is right for them in that moment. The only thing they know right then and there is abundant love.

Unfortunately, not every birth ends with a perfect outcome, and not all families get to experience that moment of joy. Some families have to face the devastating reality that not all babies survive birth or infancy. In those situations, not only are families faced with a tremendous moment of grief, but also the staff caring for them are also faced with experiencing a traumatic loss. When I went into neonatal nursing, I knew that not all babies would survive, but I honestly didn't ever really sit and think about what that would mean for me as a nurse. I didn't think about the fact that I would have to witness the same intensity of emotions with families, just on the completely opposite spectrum, and I certainly didn't consider the fact that I would be relied on as the support system to get the family through that grief-stricken time. I realized that I would have to perform postmortem care on the infant, but what I was not at all prepared for was that I would be the one responsible for caring for the entire family during times of infant loss.

Previous practice separated families from their deceased infants in the perinatal period, as the thought was "grief could be prevented if no attachments were formed" (Koopmans et al., 2013, "Background" section). Yet, mothers and fathers build and establish attachment relationships with their child well before birth, throughout the entire pregnancy, so "best practice guidelines recommend that all parents should be offered a choice about whether or not they want to see and hold their [deceased] baby, and that parents should be supported throughout this process" (Koopmans et al., 2013, "Seeing and Holding" section). There is still controversy about whether holding the infant after death helps or hinders the long-term grieving process, yet the reality is that every family is going to grieve differently, and the choice is going to have to be theirs and theirs alone. It is extremely important that staff offer and encourage them to consider seeing and holding their infant after death, since many families that chose not to see or hold their infant share later that they regret that choice.

Throughout the perinatal period, families may experience different types of loss, and each requires intentional support and activities by staff who support the "parents in developing a bond with their baby [and helps] create a sense of identity of the child" (Koopmans et al., 2013, "Memory Creation" section). In the immediate perinatal period, families may experience miscarriage, stillbirth, or neonatal death. Although each type of loss is unique, each is equally devastating to the family, and the loss should never be minimized by staff.

MISCARRIAGE

Miscarriage is a loss that occurs within the first 20 weeks of gestation. Typically, these losses do not occur within the family birthing setting as a woman's pregnancy is considered nonviable and therefore would not necessitate hospital care. Some women, however, are admitted to the hospital prior to 20 weeks, and I would argue that women should be allowed to miscarry in a family birthing center if they desire to. Before you all jump to the part of the book where my contact information is so that you can write to me and tell me what a horrific idea that is, I want to tell you that I have been in the management role and fully understand what a nightmare that would be! Rooms are a hot commodity as it is, and I know what opening the doors to women who were having a miscarriage would do to staffing, room availability, healthcare costs, and so on. So, please understand that I am not starting any national movement here to make this a new practice, but I at least feel it should be a practice that is considered, especially for families who have experienced multiple losses or experience miscarriages further into their pregnancy.

Why? Because families experiencing loss would greatly benefit from the support and the bereavement rituals that are offered within the family birthing center that they won't receive when experiencing the miscarriage at home, isolated and alone. Families who endure miscarriages at home are more likely to suffer in silence and do not receive that sense of identity of their child that the hospital staff are so eloquently able to provide. Families also do not likely receive the same level of social support or a list of available grief resources that they would receive while in the hospital.

Although babies lost before the 20th week of pregnancy are not viable, they still are children potentially wanted, loved, and maybe even desperately tried for. Staff needs to understand that parents grieve both the physical and symbolic loss of that child. In addition, "another common misunderstanding about miscarriage is that a woman will experience less grief if she loses the baby early in her pregnancy. Most researchers have not been able to find an association between the length of gestational loss and intensity of grief, anxiety or depression" (Leis-Newman, 2012, "Early Loss" section), so it is vital that staff understand this and support families who experience a loss at any gestation.

For many families, a fetus becomes a person at a very early gestation "and a miscarriage is as significant as perinatal or neonatal death" (Bryant, 2008, para. 8). If a miscarriage does occur within the hospital setting, staff needs to ensure that families are treated with empathy, respect, and dignity and are given privacy to grieve. Often, women appear in emergency rooms with bleeding and cramping, and because they are carrying a nonviable pregnancy, family birthing units will not admit them for care. Emergency rooms, however, are busy, loud, and rushed, and the staff are not often able to provide the same level of compassionate care. This is another argument for allowing women who show up to hospitals with miscarriage symptoms to be admitted to family birthing units. Patients would then be able to be in the hands of staff who can adequately assess and manage both the physical and emotional symptoms of the family and can provide comprehensive psychosocial support throughout the traumatic process.

STILLBIRTH

A stillbirth is a death that occurs within the womb after the 20th week of gestation, and the infant has to be delivered lifeless. As previously stated, "emotional bonding occurs well in advance of birth, and parents bring with them expectations and dreams about themselves as parents and about the child that they will have. The lost images and projections constitute major secondary losses, which must be mourned no matter what the age of the child; therefore even in death before birth, parents lose much" (van Aerde & Gorodzinsky, 2001, "Special Considerations: Stillbirth" section). Parents enter and then leave family birthing units with not only the physical loss of their child, but also potentially with the feelings of loss of their pregnancy, loss of their dream of parenthood, loss of self-esteem, loss of the anticipated celebration, and for the mother, the feelings that her body failed at being able to protect and save her child. Therefore, parents who experience a stillbirth need support in helping prepare them to experience all of the "pathological responses to bereavement [which] include bereavement-related major depression, post-traumatic stress disorder and complicated grief and it is not uncommon that these conditions co-occur in bereaved individuals" (Koopmans et al., 2013, "Grief Reactions" section).

Staff, immediately after admission, should meet with the family and do everything possible to make the family comfortable. This includes encouraging them to create a comfortable and safe environment if time allows. Just as with any delivery, women should be allowed to have a birth plan that incorporates her cultural, spiritual, emotional, and familiar beliefs and comforts. Families who deliver a stillborn baby should be no exception to this experience and should be asked if they have a birth plan. As long as the safety of the mother is a priority, all birth rituals should be respected and carried out.

Staff also needs to talk to the family about their wishes for after delivery. Many families are unaware of what the after-delivery process can even look like, so explaining what options they have and what to expect is incredibly important so that they can make choices that feel right for them. Points to discuss might include the following:

- After delivery, the infant can be placed immediately up on mom's chest, placed in the arms of a family member, or taken over to the infant warmer.

- There will be no resuscitation efforts made, and a warm blanket will be placed around the infant, who will be cleaned off and dried.

- Describe what the infant might look like and describe the process the body will go through to prepare the family for the changes they will see.

- Inform the family that they can stay with their baby as long as they wish, or the baby can be taken away.

- If the baby is taken out of the room, tell the family exactly where the baby will go.

- Explain to the family that they can have their baby return to their room as many times as they wish, and tell them how they should request that the staff return their baby to them.

- Explain to them they can bathe, dress, and wrap their baby in a blanket.

- Offer and highly encourage bereavement photography (Now I Lay Me Down to Sleep is a national organization that offers free newborn bereavement photography to families). Have them look at the website or fliers ahead of time and read family testimonials if they are unsure of the offer.

- Ask the family if they would like to invite family, friends, or clergy for visits or ceremonial events.

- Connect family with social workers and chaplain services to discuss how burial or cremation plans can be handled.

During all aspects of the conversation, words should be compassionate and guided by what the parent's desire and what they are asking for at the time. All care should be individualized and customized for each family to meet their physical, emotional, cultural, and spiritual needs.

NEONATAL DEATH

Neonatal death, also known as *newborn death*, is when a baby dies within the first 28 days of life. Within the family birthing center setting, neonatal death occurs within the first

72 hours of life, before a mother is discharged from the hospital. Chapter 14 explores what happens when a newborn dies in the neonatal period in the NICU, but here we focus primarily on neonatal death in the family birthing unit closer to the time of birth.

Neonatal death closely following birth may or may not be anticipated. Some deliveries occur for families that come to deliver with a prenatal diagnosis that was known to be incompatible with life. They hopefully have come in with some preparation as to what to expect and have a plan to communicate with the team regarding the postdelivery resuscitative or palliative care treatment. Staff needs to work collaboratively with the family and the obstetrical teams to ensure that all familial wishes are carried out and that respect for their birth plans are maintained. Families who anticipate a neonatal death should be encouraged to have bereavement photographers on site for the delivery; if a child lives for a time after delivery, photos can be captured while the child is alive so that those precious moments will be held in time forever.

Other families come in with a very healthy and normal pregnancy, and at the time of delivery, something very unexpectedly goes wrong and their child suffers a tragic adverse outcome. Despite a team's best effort, not every infant survives resuscitative efforts, and a family is then faced with a very unplanned neonatal death. These families have come to the hospital with a car seat, a packed diaper bag, and a going-home outfit and likely have a nursery set up at home waiting for the baby. Their entire world is turned upside down. They find themselves recovering on a unit among other families who have crying babies and are wheeled out of the hospital with empty arms and an empty car seat, only to go home to an empty crib and empty hearts.

Some families may have a healthy pregnancy, a noncomplicated delivery, and then suddenly find themselves with a child unresponsive hours later because of an undiagnosed congenital heart condition or another disease. These families also experience devastating heartbreak and have to go home with the unanticipated loss and emptiness that comes with a neonatal death.

I have witnessed so many scenarios of neonatal death over my career, and regardless of the reason or the amount of time a family had to prepare before a loss, each and every death was equally devastating to the family and to the staff. Yet, irrespective of the cause or reason for demise, one thing should always be kept as a priority: family support!

FAMILY SUPPORT DURING PERINATAL LOSS

During their birthing experience, every family should be cared for with compassion and individuality, but it is so incredibly important for staff to know that during a time of loss, the actions and environment that healthcare staff provides a family impact their immediate and long-term grieving process. "A patient-centered approach that responds to the sociocultural context and unique needs of each bereaved parent is the foundation of sensitive communication, information provision and supported decision making, all of which are vital elements of perinatal bereavement care" (Flenady et al.,

2014, "Maternity Healthcare Professionals" section). Every unit needs to have a robust bereavement care program in place to care for all families who experience a loss, and all staff needs to be adequately trained and supported to be able to care for families who experience a loss.

Staff who works with families experiencing a perinatal loss should be well educated on how to care for these families in their time of stress and grief and how to have such difficult conversations with them. Thankfully, there are some wonderful training opportunities available to staff on infant and newborn bereavement, and staff must take advantage of the training before caring for families to ensure that optimal care is provided.

Resolve Through Sharing is an organization that not only provides education to frontline staff, but also helps leaders in organizations fully implement a successful bereavement program into their unit through evidence-based, yet compassion-first care. This organization has trained healthcare professionals around the world and has been considered the gold standard in bereavement education for over three decades. The resource section has more information about this organization and the many educational offerings they provide on how to support the families who suffer loss in the perinatal and neonatal periods.

With or without the support of a program such as Resolve Through Sharing, every unit needs to have a complete palliative and bereavement care program that directs staff on how to care for families consistently and comprehensively. These programs must include, but do not need to be limited to, the following:

- A written policy on how to care for bereaved families
  - Family should be allowed to follow birth plans as much as possible.
  - Family should be respected and given privacy to grieve.
  - Family should be allowed to have as many visitors as they wish and at any time of day.
  - Families should be allowed to stay with their babies as long as they want and should never feel rushed.
  - Families should be encouraged to participate in care of their newborn.
  - Ceremonial rituals should be allowed and encouraged within the room/unit.
  - Burial gowns should be provided to families.
  - Infants should be kept in a crib at all times, until it is time for them to be transported to the morgue, and then the body should be transported in an infant Preshand box.
  - Layered levels of support should be provided to the family (bedside staff, family-support specialist, social workers, staff psychologists).
  - A keepsake box should include a card for staff to sign; a small bag to place a lock of hair, a baby ring, or some piece of commemorative jewelry; grief

information; a place for photos; a space to place items used on the baby; and a place for hand/foot molds to give to the parents.

- A similar keepsake box can be prepared by staff for each sibling.

- A way to obtain hand and/or foot molds of the baby should be available.

- Bereavement photography should be available to all families, even if a professional service is not available. This means a high-quality digital camera should be available on the unit at all times so that staff can capture photos for families.

- Grief material, including both local and online resources, should be available and given to all families.

- Some type of identification should be placed on the outside of the door, alerting staff about the demise. Typically, units choose to use a butterfly, which symbolizes a fleeting, yet beautiful life. For some, it is a symbol of eternal life. The symbol on the door is used as a way to sensitize hospital staff and give them time to pause and be mindful of the family's experience of loss beyond the door.

- A written policy on how to care for the infant body (including how to allow families to remain with the body as long as they wish, to have the body taken out of the room when they wish, and then brought back when they wish) should be prepared.

- Social services or clergy on staff should be prepared to walk families through how to make decisions and arrangements with a funeral home.

- Social services should prepare families to anticipate a birth certificate arriving at their house and it showing that the child is deceased, or a death certificate may arrive.

- Families should be educated on the normal grief process and be informed that they should anticipate grief, loss, and mourning.

- Families should be told prior to discharge that the hospital will contact them when the hand and/or foot molds and any other keepsakes are ready.

- Mothers should be set up with lactation support to learn how to deal with either weaning lactation or donating breast milk.

Above all else, and probably the most important aspect of caring for the family during this time of loss, is to allow them the opportunity to create an identity for their child and for themselves as parents. It has been shown that "for many parents, it is the experience of parenting, not mementoes, which is the most valuable in the creation of a bond" (Koopmans et al., 2013, "Memory Creation" section) and can lead to the most beneficial grieving process and healing. Providing families space, time, privacy, respect, and compassion is what staff needs to prioritize during these difficult times.

Author's Personal Story

I was assigned to a role called "baby nurse" one night shift, and my only responsibility was to attend every delivery on our family birthing unit and be just that, the baby's nurse. I would be the one to initially warm, dry, and stimulate the baby on the mom's chest, and if there were any signs of distress, I would take the baby to the warmer and call for my NICU team backup. I would stay with that baby until all postpartum care was completed, which for me included obtaining weight and measurements, administering vitamin K and erythromycin eye ointment, getting baby footprints on the infamous keepsake birth announcement card from the hospital, giving the first bath (I'm dating myself here I know), and completing all initial assessments and documentation.

I was not pleased about being assigned this role, as I had been assigned it the previous night and we were supposed to rotate. Performing the role two nights in a row was not at all common and not something most of us particularly enjoyed doing, since us NICU gals preferred working in the NICU. However, the coworker who was due to rotate to that position that night was far into her pregnancy and was not up to running around the unit for the anticipated nine deliveries. In addition, because of staffing combinations in the NICU that shift, she needed to fill the charge nurse role. Luckily for her, I adored her and considered her such a good friend that I cordially agreed to rotate out of turn for her. I, of course, let her know that she would have to pay me back at some point because the night before I had attended 10 deliveries and never made it to lunch because we were so busy. As a result, I was not super-thrilled about another night of running ragged again.

The anticipated nine deliveries wound up being 13. When you work a 12-hour shift and the baby nurse responsibilities take a minimum of 2 hours per delivery, I will allow you to imagine what my shift looked like. And the first 12 deliveries occurred in the first 10.5 hours of the night. Just as I was handing delivered baby number 12 over to her mother, the neonatal code alarm sounded in the hall and my pager went off. When I looked at the room number on my pager screen, it was a room number that was not a room that had a laboring mother in that I had known about. This told me a new patient had come in that I hadn't been told about and must have been an imminent delivery when she arrived. As I ran over to the room, I was immediately pushed out of the way by a team of staff running in the opposite direction out of the room. The mother was on her bed and they were pushing her toward the operating room, and I noticed a lot of blood on the bed and trailing behind them on the floor. I started to follow them, but the charge nurse met me in the hall and stopped me. She informed me that I wouldn't be needed at this delivery and carefully walked with me into the patient room once everyone had vacated.

I was informed that this mother had suffered an abruption and lost the baby. The baby was delivered stillborn, so the nurse needed me to stay in the room, perform postmortem

(continued)

(*continued*)

care, and, if possible, complete all those cares before the family returned. She gave me these orders with almost a question behind the statement, and I always wonder if she was worried if I would refuse my assignment after the night I had already had. Not to mention the shift was coming to an end and we were short-staffed, so there was no on-time end in sight for either of us. Looking at my pregnant colleague, I wanted nothing more in that moment than to protect her from having to see the trauma of what was happening around us. I imagined her internalizing emotions and questions about her and her own baby, and I hated that we had to witness such tragedy for families in our line of work. I wanted to cry for her and for this poor family who had just experienced such misfortune but also wanted to stay strong and do everything I could do to be a support for all parties involved. I told her I had it all under control and she should go to the operating room and see what she could do.

I stood for a moment in that room alone and looked over at the infant warmer and could see the lifeless body of a baby lying there in a pool of blood. I was afraid to walk over because there was so much blood on the floor that I was afraid I would slip and fall. I used the phone to call housekeeping and asked if someone could quickly come and help STAT clean the room so that when the family did arrive or return, the room would be presentable. I also made a call to the NICU nursing assistant and asked her to bring the baby care supplies, clean linen, a baby outfit, a quilt, and a bereavement kit so that I didn't have to leave that precious baby alone in the room.

Between a hardworking housekeeper and me, we were able to clean the entire room in less than 30 minutes and have a perfectly set up room ready to go for the family to come back. Unfortunately, when I finally had been able to get safely to the baby, I realized the team had the bed-warming mechanism turned on. They must have initially had all of the equipment on and ready to go in the hope that they could resuscitate the baby at birth. Regrettably, that was not that case. The baby was born previable, and in the time she had been on the warmer, her immature skin had warmed to the blankets. In fact, her skin had warmed to the blankets so much so that it was almost stuck to the blankets. As a still fairly novice nurse in bereavement care, I had a moment of panic! I had no idea what to do. I sat there holding this sweet and beautiful baby girl, all alone in this room and was completely frozen with distress. I wanted nothing more than to remain respectful and considerate of this infant's life and body, and to perform some basic care to clean her up for her parents so that she would be all ready to be held and cuddled, and I had absolutely no idea how I was going to get her off the blankets.

I called the family birthing staff for support and they were thankfully extremely helpful in educating me on how to work with such immature skin. We were able to use water to moisten the skin and loosen the material away. I of course insisted on warm water because I told the nurse I would hate cold water to be poured on me, to which she looked at me oddly and said, "It doesn't matter what temperature water you use." Yet to

(*continued*)

(*continued*)

me it did, and it still does. I filled the sink with warm water and gave the little girl a gentle bath to clean her of all the blood that covered her limp little body. Typically, I would ask families if they would like to give the first bath, but in this case, this baby needed to be clean before her mother and father saw her. I figured they could give her another bath if they wished to do so.

After I had her cleaned up and dried, I was able to get some great hand and footprints that were going to be given to the family as special keepsakes. The little girl didn't have any hair, so I wasn't going to be able to get a lock, but I still used the infant brush to brush the little fuzz that was on her head and put the brush in the memory box alongside the footprints. I used a tape measure and marked the little girl's length, abdominal and head circumferences on it, then placed that in the memory box as well. I used the smallest diaper we had and placed it on the infant, carefully wrapped her in an infant blanket, and then made up the infant warmer bed to have a cute quilt on the bottom so that if she needed to be laid back down, she would have a soft place.

I sat in the rocking chair holding the little girl in the room for what seemed like eternity, but in reality, it probably wasn't more than 45 minutes until the staff wheeled the mom back into her room. The father was walking behind the team and I stood up as they all came into the room. I introduced myself to the father and mother and let them know I had been with their daughter the entire time they had been out of the room. I asked if they wanted to hold her and the mother nodded. I gently placed her daughter in her arms and handed care over to the postpartum team.

I wish I could have stayed longer that day to continue providing care to that family. To this day, so many years later, I wonder if anyone offered them photos with Now I Lay Me Down to Sleep, if they allowed the family to give her a bath, if they let them dress her in one of the outfits the NICU secretary had picked out and brought, if they knew that they could keep the quilt we had on the warmer as a keepsake, if a caring nurse wrapped the baby in a warm blanket before taking her down to the cold morgue, and if they knew they were allowed to stay with her as long as they wanted. I also wonder if that family ever went on to have another pregnancy and, if so, if they have had a viable pregnancy.

That night was one of the most memorable nights in my entire nursing career. And it is one that bonded my coworker and me in a way that is unique to just her and me. I would like to say that that was the only night we had that was crazy and memorable, but we continued to have several unforgettable shifts together. Despite the traumatic events and difficulty for all of us, I wouldn't trade it for the world! That night helped mold me into the nurse that I am and has created the journey that I feel so incredibly blessed to be on.

Family Story

Cadie Nagi was pregnant with her second child when she and her husband learned at their 20-week ultrasound that their unborn child was diagnosed with multicystic kidney disease and that the condition would be incompatible with life. Cadie so graciously shares her story about what her experience giving birth to her beautiful baby girl and receiving support from the staff at the time of birth and the hours following.

"My husband and I were expecting our second baby, due May 2011. Our daughter was a year old when we found out we were going to have another one and were so excited. In December, at our 20-week ultrasound, we were informed that our second baby, also a girl, had multicystic kidney disease, meaning that both her kidneys were filled with cysts and not functioning. We were told that she would not survive, and they didn't know if she would even make it full term. I was considered a high-risk pregnancy from then on.

"We began grieving for our child that we could still feel moving in my stomach. We sang, spoke, and prayed fervently for her as the pregnancy progressed. I went into labor at 36.5 weeks, and we were told that they were not sure if she would be born alive. We prepared for the worst. The doctors decided to not monitor her heartbeat during her delivery. I was warned during my pregnancy that this would happen, and although it bothered me thinking about it, I was actually relieved when I finally went into labor with her. I was able to concentrate on my labor instead of being so concerned with her heart rate and if she were still alive.

"The nurses and doctors who were working with me all knew what was going on without me having to inform each one. This was incredibly helpful since it was such a painful time. I was relieved I didn't have to continuously tell each nurse that our baby had a 0% chance of survival. Our main nurse was a godsend, a woman who herself had dealt with the loss of a baby. She warned me of things that I would never have thought of (e.g., expecting the birth certificate to say 'deceased' when it arrived, something that was shocking to her since no one warned her of that). She was empathetic and warm. Becoming more of a friend than just a nurse, she shared stories of her own baby who had passed away and how it affected her and her husband, as well as their other child. She cried with me and made me laugh. She really was an incredible nurse to have during that delivery.

"Our other nurse also meant the world to us. Although she had never lost a baby before, she was compassionate and caring and did everything she could to help us during that time. She also became our friend and was a complete blessing to our family during our delivery, even staying through her shift so that she could help with the delivery. The friendships we made with both nurses were incredibly special to us and they were both able to meet our third and fourth baby, celebrating with us during those times.

"Our daughter was born in the early morning and came out crying, the most beautiful sound in the world. The nurses and doctor were quick to give her to us and wiped her down while I held her. Although there were so many people in the room, they were able to give us privacy and feel like it was just us there holding her. While I had been pregnant, our doctor had mentioned Now I Lay Me Down to Sleep, a company that would come to the

(continued)

(*continued*)

hospital and take photographs for us. My husband and I hadn't really decided whether we would want someone taking photos or not, but that early morning, the nurses informed us that the photographer was there and ready. We were surprised since it was so early in the morning and didn't know how we felt about someone coming in during such an emotional and private time. When the photographer came into the room, we told her we were a little hesitant. She was extremely kind and said that she would stay out of the way and if we felt uncomfortable at any time, she would leave and give us the photos she had already taken. We agreed and she ended up staying the entire time. She was so quiet and respectful of our time with our daughter.

"Our baby lived for a little over 3 hours, and during that time, our photographer captured the most amazing photos, which now mean the world to us. Our family members all were able to hold our baby and get photos of them holding her. We have a beautiful family photo that would not exist if our photographer had not insisted on us giving her a try. During that time, I was so consumed with holding our daughter and telling her everything I wanted to say that I never even thought about taking photos. I am so thankful that we have so many to look at now. Our photographer was so patient and compassionate. She made an incredible video of our photographs set to music that we watch every year on her birthday. Some of the photographs are of memories that I would never remember if she hadn't taken a photo of it. I am so thankful for the time and energy our photographer put into our family and for giving us such a gift that we truly treasure.

"After our daughter was born, our nurse allowed us to stay in the birthing room instead of transferring us to the recovery room. She gently informed us that we would stay so that we wouldn't have to hear all the newborn cries in the recovery rooms. This was a small thing but something that I was so thankful for. It also made it easier to have our family come and visit in large numbers to say hello and goodbye to our baby, considering the room was much larger than a recovery room.

"We were able to keep our baby with us through the night and throughout most of the following day until we decided to let the nurse take her away. Our nurse gently wrapped her in her blanket and gave us time to say goodbye.

"Our time at the hospital has been something I have thought about for years. We could not have asked for better nurses. On our last day, they gave us a memory box filled with everything they had used on our baby: her comb, shampoo, hospital bracelets, gown and hat she had worn, and a special card the nurses had all written on for us. I have opened it often and reread all their messages many times. Our children love to look through it as well and see everything that belonged to their sister. We are so thankful to our nurses and doctor who helped with our delivery and their sacrificial love they poured out on our family, putting themselves in a difficult situation, opening their hearts up to love us through an incredibly painful time, and doing everything within their power to make it as easy of a time as it could possibly be. Our gratitude is beyond measurable."

RECOMMENDATIONS/SUGGESTIONS FOR BEST PRACTICE

1. Have a comprehensive bereavement program embedded within the practice of every family birthing unit.

2. Consider allowing women who are experiencing a miscarriage to receive care within the family birthing center.

3. Allow families who are delivering a stillborn infant to carry out their birth plan as much as possible.

4. Encourage bereavement photography. Have a high-quality digital camera on the unit so photographs can be captured at any time and in the event a professional service cannot be present.

5. Never leave the deceased infant alone.

6. Prepare families for what to expect after the death of an infant.

7. Have layered levels of psychosocial support available for families. This may include bedside nursing, social work, and chaplain support, as well as unit staff psychologists.

8. Have resources, such as social workers, available to assist families with funeral home arrangements.

9. Provide lactation support to mothers to assist with lactation weaning or milk donation.

10. Provide grief and loss resources, both locally and online.

11. Provide keepsake mementos.

12. Find ways to create the identity of the infant and ways for the family to bond with their child.

RECOMMENDED RESOURCES

Remarkable resources are available to both staff and families to help support the process of loss during the perinatal period (Figure 13.1).

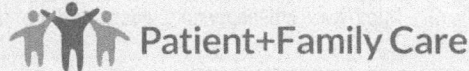 Patient+Family Care

GENERAL SUPPORT SERVICES:

1. https://griefwatch.com/topics/infant-loss.html
2. http://www.springerpub.com/perinatal-and-pediatric-bereavement-in-nursing-and-other-health-professions.html
3. https://glbereavement.dcopy.net/category/memories-unlimited
4. https://glbereavement.dcopy.net/category/perinatal-death-resources
5. https://www.nowilaymedowntosleep.org
6. http://support4nicuparents.org/for-professionals/palliative-and-bereavement-care

Figure 13.1 ■ Recommended resources for supporting families who experience loss in the perinatal period.

7. https://www.nicuhelpinghands.org/programs/angel-gown-program
8. http://nationalshare.org
9. https://www.zoerose.org
10. https://www.mend.org
11. http://babysteps.com
12. http://www.memoryjar.org
13. https://centering.org
14. http://angelnames.org
15. http://skylersgift.org
16. http://www.highriskhope.org/what-we-do/bereavement-support
17. http://babylosscomfort.com/grief-resources
18. http://www.handonline.org

MISCARRIAGES:

1. http://babybluesconnection.org/finding-help/bbc-groups
2. http://www.gundersenhealth.org/app/files/public/5740/RTS-INTE-clinical-guidelines.pdf
3. https://miscarriage/your-feelings
4. https://www.nct.org.uk

STILLBIRTH:

1. https://griefwatch.com/tips-for-caring-for-a-stillborn-infant
2. http://www.gundersenhealth.org/app/files/public/2082/RTS-Position-Paper-Caring-for-
   Families-Experiencing-Stillbirth-English.pdf
3. http://www.perinatalhospice.org
4. http://www.throughtheheart.org
5. https://www.sands.org.uk

NEONATAL DEATH:

1. http://babybluesconnection.org/finding-help/bbc-groups
2. http://www.mom365.com/baby/moms-health/how-to-beat-the-baby-blues
3. http://www.littlefingers.org.uk/support04.html

EDUCATION/TRAINING:

1. http://www.gundersenhealth.org/resolve-through-sharing/bereavement-training
2. http://www.mynicunetwork.com/education_individuals.html
3. https://hearthsidecare.com/services-for-birth-professionals/
   perinatal-bereavement-specialist-certificate-programd

Figure 13.1 ■ Recommended resources for supporting families who experience loss in the perinatal period. (*continued*)

Case-Based Learning

D.L. is a 37-year-old, G5, P4, AB1, L1, who has just delivered at 23 2/7 weeks' gestation (dates are exact since she had assisted reproduction with embryo transfer). This is the farthest she has carried a pregnancy; her previous three very preterm births were losses. Her first pregnancy occurred as a young teen and was electively terminated. The family received prenatal counseling about the outcomes associated with this gestational age. Baby boy L. has severe respiratory distress syndrome requiring high-frequency ventilation. He is 4 days old and has bilateral chest tubes for pneumothoraces, pulmonary interstitial emphysema, and very poor blood gas levels. Seizure activity was evaluated with a cranial ultrasound, which shows bilateral grade III intraventricular hemorrhages. The treatment team has recommended that there be no escalation in care and a do-not-resuscitate status for baby L. D.L. and her partner insist that everything be done.

QUESTIONS

1. What are the contextual elements of D.L.'s emotional state?

2. What may be influencing D.L.'s decision making?

3. How can you best support D.L.?

ANSWERS

The term *trauma-informed care* refers to the practice of trying to understand behaviors in light of previous traumas that the person may have experienced (Coughlin, 2017; Discenza, 2017; Sanders & Hall, 2017). We all bring our pasts with us into each new experience, and the way that we respond can depend on what happened previously and how we coped with it.

D.L. has experienced pregnancy losses that may be influencing her current state of mind and decision making. She may be grieving the losses of her most recent pregnancies and yet feel guilty about the elective termination of long ago. Her age may be playing a role in her decision to continue treatment, as may the difficulty and cost of assisted reproduction.

It is important to support D.L.'s feelings of safety to prevent retraumatizing her (Coughlin, 2017). Her stress response system is on full alert. She is reliving a nightmare that may overwhelm her coping skills. She is staring at yet another loss of a loved one that she worked so hard to conceive.

D.L. may believe that she is protecting her baby from harm, whereas the staff may see the interventions as pain causing and inhumane. This can lead to moral distress in staff caring for the family. An ethics consultation and care conferences can be valuable in these circumstances.

A therapeutic relationship would include open, clear communication about the baby's status, including pain care, and shared decision making. By allowing parental

(*continued*)

(*continued*)

autonomy, the team enhances empowerment and collaboration (Coughlin, 2017; Sanders & Hall, 2017).

Not only do previous traumatic experiences affect coping with a NICU admission, but also the incumbent stress of a NICU stay itself is traumatic and can result in lifelong posttraumatic stress for both families and infants. Coughlin (2017) posits that the undesirable neurodevelopmental outcomes associated with NICU graduates may be considered a hospital-acquired condition (HAC). She contends that evidence-based, trauma-informed, family-integrated care mitigates the lifelong negative effects related to spending one's first days of life in the toxic stress of a NICU environment. Even better is that the entire family can benefit, reducing the likelihood that this hospitalization will be yet another distressing ordeal that leaves a scar on all involved.

REFERENCES

Coughlin, M. E. (2017). *Trauma-informed care in the NICU: Evidenced-based practice guidelines for neonatal clinicians.* New York, NY: Springer Publishing.
Discenza, D. (2017). "Mental health" in the NICU: Time to catch up and provide trauma-informed care for families and pros. *Neonatal Network, 36*(5), 318–320. doi:10.1891/0730-0832.36.5.318
Sanders, M. R., & Hall, S. L. (2017). Trauma-informed care in the newborn intensive care unit: Promoting safety, security and connectedness. *Journal of Perinatology, 38*, 3–10. doi:10.1038/jp.2017.124

REFERENCES

Bryant, H. (2008). Maintaining patient dignity and offering support after miscarriage. *Emergency Nurse, 15*(9), 26–29. doi:10.7748/en2008.02.15.9.26.c8178
Flenady, V., Boyle, F., Koopmans, L., Wilson, T., Stones, W., & Cacciatore, J. (2014). Meeting the needs of parents after a stillbirth or neonatal death. *BJOG: An International Journal of Obstetrics & Gynaecology, 121*, 137–140. doi:10.1111/1471-0528.13009
Koopmans, L., Wilson, T., Cacciatore, J., & Flenady, V. (2013). Support for mothers, fathers and families after perinatal death. *Cochrane Database of Systematic Reviews.* doi:10.1002/14651858 .CD000452.pub3
Leis-Newman, E. (2012, June). Miscarriage and loss. Retrieved from http://www.apa.org/ monitor/2012/06/miscarriage.aspx
van Aerde, J., & Gorodzinsky, F. P. (2001). Guidelines for health care professionals supporting families experiencing a perinatal loss. *Paediatrics & Child Health, 6*(7), 469–177. doi:10.1093/pch/6.7.469

14

PALLIATIVE CARE AND BEREAVEMENT SUPPORT IN THE NEONATAL PERIOD

Perinatal and neonatal palliative care is a practice that has gained acceptance and recognition in recent years, primarily due to an increased need because technology has allowed for more infertility treatments, has led to more accurate diagnosis of nonviable conditions prenatally, and with the ability to care for infants at lower ages of viability. Despite these great technological advances in therapies and treatments, not all pregnancies and babies survive. "Palliative care should be offered to all parents who have been informed of a life-limiting fetal diagnosis, [and] end-of-life care should include individualized bereavement interventions for women with a high-level multiple gestation and their families when the pregnancy may need to be reduced or if there is an intrauterine fetal demise" (Catlin, Brandon, Wool, & Mendes, 2015, "Background and Significance" section). In the NICU, palliative care support should be offered to families whose babies are "diagnosed with life-limiting conditions at birth or who become critically ill during a NICU stay and are not responding to aggressive medical management" (Kenner, Press, & Ryan, 2015, "Abstract" section).

Palliative care, and end-of-life care decisions in the NICU, can be ethically and morally challenging. Yet "palliative care is an approach that improves the quality of life of patients facing life-limiting conditions, and their families, through the prevention and relief of suffering by means of early, impeccable assessment and treatment of pain and other physical, psychosocial and spiritual issues" (Kenner et al., 2015, "Core Concepts and Values" section). Palliative care truly focuses on and "emphasizes quality of life while alleviating the symptoms of medical conditions and their treatments" (Eden & Callister, 2010, para. 8) which can often be a welcoming decision for families and care providers who are looking for an alternative for continuing potentially futile ongoing care. In a unit where babies with complex medical needs are exposed to ongoing aggressive treatments, tracheal intubation, repetitive blood sampling, and invasive catheters are cared for daily and are being treated at younger and younger gestational ages, the uncertainty of immediate and long-term outcomes become a real issue. When infants do not seem to be responding positively to provided treatment, working with families to decide on palliative care can "enhance end-of-life care for newborns through better control of pain and other distressing symptoms and by avoiding futile treatments whose burdens outweigh benefits" (Dighe, Manerkar, Muckaden, & Duraisamy, 2011, p. 104).

PREPARING FOR PALLIATIVE CARE

When a healthcare team feels that palliative care would be warranted as the best care decision for an infant, there are careful considerations on how to approach the family. The provider must continue to have "ongoing assessment of care goals, parents, nurses, and other providers weigh the benefits of shifting the goals of care from focus on cure to provision of comfort for the infant and family" (Catlin et al., 2015, para. 1) and then determine who is the most appropriate person to first talk to the family. It is important to keep in mind that "family is defined as a constellation of people who are related by birth, adoption, marriage or those individuals the parents designate as part of their family unit" (Kenner et al., 2015, "Core Concepts and Values" section). Parents often lean on their extended family as their support network during this stressful time and may want them included in difficult discussions.

When deciding who should speak with the family and how the conversation should be approached, the team should delegate the person who has both the best relationship with the family and is the most comfortable with palliative care discussions. "Even though the neonatology team may have a good rapport with the family, members of the palliative care team may be able to provide additional psychological support to parents and families through these difficult times" (Dighe et al., 2011. p. 104). If a neonatal unit does not have an embedded palliative care team, it is essential that neonatal staff be well trained and comfortable having end-of-life discussions with families, which means that they know how to respectfully, compassionately, and honestly speak with families who are facing such an "immense, heartbreaking responsibility to decide to withdraw life-sustaining treatments for the infant" (Eden & Callister, 2010, "Parent Involvement in Decision Making" section).

Once a staff member is identified, families should be talked to in a private space so that there will be limited interruptions during the conversation. If possible, parents should be warned that the care team needs to have a difficult conversation with them, so if they would like to have anyone else present, they should be encouraged to invite them and schedule the meeting when all individuals can be present, if time allows. When the discussion occurs, parents need to then be given accurate, candid, direct, and thorough information about the condition of their child and the projected outcome of ongoing treatment. Some families decide that ongoing treatment is the best decision for their child, so healthcare teams need to continue caring for the infant and family while navigating the difficult task of either continuing with their wishes until the child can no longer maintain life and the discussion needs to occur again or to escalate the discussion to a hospital ethics committee—a topic for an entirely separate publication.

For families who do wish to proceed with palliative care, the care team in collaboration with the family, must "assist parents in making decisions about treatments their infant may receive" (Eden & Callister, 2010, "Palliative Care and Decision Making" section) as the family is an "integral part of the health-care team, and both work together to plan and implement palliative and/or bereavement care" (Kenner et al., 2015, "Core Concepts and Values" section). Families should be allowed to be involved in every aspect of the palliative care process as possible, including up to the time they choose to remove life support if time allows. This affords family time to invite other family, friends, or clergy members to be present for the passing of their child if they wish. Many units have visitation policies that limit the number of visitors that are allowed to be at a given bedside at a time, but in times of palliative care, families should be allowed to have as many support individuals present that they desire to fully support the family-centered care philosophy.

It often can take families some time to process the news and reality of having to make such a definitive decision for their child, and if time allows, families should never be rushed into their decision and should be led with grace and patience by the care team in making the decisions they need to. Until that point, most parents were envisioning what it would be like to put their baby in their going-home outfit, to put them in a car seat and take them home to their nurseries, and to watch affectionately as they grow up and turn into their own little individuals. Now they are having to say goodbye to all of those dreams and have to picture bathing their baby for the last time, dressing them in a burial or cremation outfit, and knowing that after they leave that hospital, they will never be able to hold or see their precious child again. This is a realization that must be met with compassion, empathy, respect, and understanding.

When time is limited due to a rapidly declining status, care teams must express that time is restricted, that the staff wants the family to have every last minute with their child be as pain free and comfortable as possible, and that the staff wants the family to be as present and involved as they want to be. Yet staff must keep in mind that families may not be able to process everything that quickly and may not be capable of making many decisions in that moment. In these situations, staff need to assist the family in ways that support bonding and honoring the life of the child while being the primary decision makers; they must help walk the family through the process step by step.

Families need to be made aware of what to expect and how to prepare. For example, staff should inform all families of the following prior to removing life support or stopping lifesaving therapies:

- What will happen when respiratory support is removed
- How a baby typically responds during the transition from life to death
  - What respirations may look like
  - What color changes to anticipate
  - What body temperatures to expect
  - What secretions they may see
  - How long the transition may take
- What the team will do for the family during the time of transition
- How the team will be present to support the baby and family, to assess vital signs, and to determine an official time of death
- What will happen after the baby has passed away
  - What care the family can participate in
  - How long they can remain with their baby
  - How the unit will spend time helping collect keepsakes
  - What will happen with the baby's body when families are ready to say goodbye and leave the hospital

- How social workers or other designated staff will help them with the resources they need to make arrangements with a funeral home
- How they will be given wraparound support services for grief and loss, and how they will not be leaving the hospital without the team continuing to support them
- How the option of bereavement photography is available and is highly encouraged

"Parents are often encouraged or expected to be at the bedside of their infant at the time of withdrawal of life-sustaining treatment" (Eden & Callister, 2010, "Palliative Care and Decision Making" section), and many families choose to hold their infant and be with them for the duration of the transition from life to death. However, some families do not feel that they can be witness to the event. Those families should be encouraged to make the decision that feels right for them and should not be shamed for choosing not to be involved. They do, however, need to also receive this information so that they can know what to anticipate for their child, if they wish to know. Parents should be assured that their infant will not be left alone during the transition, and a staff member should be assigned to care for their infant during the time from when the family leaves to when the baby passes. If at all possible, a staff member who has an established rapport and positive relationship with the family should be assigned this role to provide a layer of comfort for the family, who will know that someone they trust will be with their child during the difficult time when they could not be.

TRANSITION FROM LIFE TO DEATH

During the highly stressful and emotional period of transitioning from life to death, "it is important for health-care professionals and families to engage in effective communication and mutual respect" (Eden & Callister, 2010, para. 8) to ensure that families feel that they are being made aware of every new update on their child's condition and current state. This transitional period is one that is foreign and completely devastating for families, and during this time, most parents feel out of control and powerless while they question whether or not they are making the best decision for their child. Staff have the significant responsibility of supporting families in finding ways that they can have control and to acknowledge their parenting abilities and decisions. One highly effective way to provide control is to allow families to be the decision makers and drive the majority of care during this time with the support of staff nearby. Families have "identified nurses as central figures in helping them assume parental roles" (Eden & Callister, 2010, "Parents' Perceptions" section) during the time of transition, so nursing staff should remain present and available to families to help with education about the process, to help with any infant care, and to continuously reinforce the family's positive interactions and actions.

As stated previously, parents should be allowed and encouraged to include other support individuals during this time. Healthcare professionals have become much better at ensuring parents are spending time with their infant, but the importance of including other family members is still less recognized. The grief of parents often is more "validated when their own parents, siblings, children and close friends can be with the baby, however briefly" (van Aerde, Gorodzinsky, Canadian Paediatric Society, & Fetus and Newborn Committee,

2001, "What to Do During the Dying Process" section). These individuals, who will be the ones to support the families after they leave the hospital, will be able to help continue the recognition of the child's life if they are allowed to be a part of the transition process or are allowed to be present prior to the death, which will help them also acknowledge the child and the imprint of the child on the family's life.

During the dying process, staff needs to prioritize respecting any cultural and/or religious rituals. If language barriers exist, all attempts to have an appropriate interpreter on site and in person should occur to truly foster a compassionate and more connected experience for the family. When an interpreter is available, staff may then directly ask families how they can best support any cultural or religious traditions that are important to them during the death and dying process. Not all families associate with a particular religion but may have feelings about how they want to respectfully deal with death and dying based on past experiences or familial traditions. Questions that staff may want to ask families might include the following:

- What are the family's beliefs about what happens after death?
- What does the family consider to be the roles of each family member in handling the death?
- Who should the care team talk to about decisions that need to be made or to provide updates?
- Are baptisms or other religious ceremonies important to arrange prior to death that would be meaningful to the family?
- Are there prayers that can be said over the infant that would be significant?
- Are there treatments or particular cares that should be avoided?
- Are there specific oils or other ointments that they use during the dying process that they should be encouraged to bring in?

The overall importance is to ask questions that will encourage families to open up about what is important to them and how they want to honor the life, death, and dying of the child in relation to their culture, their religion, and their beliefs. In addition, the experience needs to be tailored to meet the needs of each family. When a plan is created, staff should always be flexible and realize that it may need to change as the parents experience various emotions and work through the emotions of the process.

FAMILY SUPPORT AFTER DEATH

Once death occurs, parents should be allowed to remain with their infant for as long as they would like and be given full privacy if they wish. Bereavement photography with the family should be offered during this time, and although many families initially decline because they cringe at the thought of ever wanting to see a photograph of their dead child, staff need to take the time to educate them that "remembrance photography is a very important step in the healing process. Photographs are one of the most precious and tangible mementos that parents can have, showing the love and bond that was given and shared with their baby" (Services for Families, n.d., para. 3). Professional organizations are available in many areas and can be engaged ahead of time to be present if there is time to prepare for the infant's death. In these situations, photography can even be taken during the transition phase when the infant is still alive and spending time with the family. Now I Lay Me Down to Sleep is one of the largest and most reputable organizations that provide newborn bereavement photography. Volunteer photographers are trained at being present in a very discrete and respectful manner so that they do not disrupt the precious time families have with their child, yet can capture amazingly precious moments for them in a photo that will last for generations. When a professional organization or volunteer photographer is not available, staff must step in and fulfill the photographer role. As mentioned numerous times in this text, a high-quality digital camera should be available on the unit at all times so that staff has the ability to capture photographs for families. Now I Lay Me Down to Sleep has a wonderful resource called a "posing guide for hospitals," which shows examples of various photos that are good to take of families, of infants, of close-up features and even of keepsake memorabilia to assist staff who may not have experience or ideas on how to capture bereavement photographs.

NICU staff should continue providing comprehensive psychosocial family support to families as they provide postmortem care to their child. It is also highly encouraged that words such as "postmortem," "expired," and "demise" not be used around families. Families have shared that those terms feel extremely medical and feel harsh when used about their baby. Families want staff to continue "talking to parents about the infant as a person, not the infant's medical condition" (Eden & Callister, 2010, "Parents' Perceptions" section), which in this case, would be *expired* or *demise* in medical terms. Talking to families as if the infant is still alive and treating the infant with as much respect is what families need after the time of death.

Families should be supported by staff to participate in all of the afterlife care that they desire to participate in, including, but not limited to:

- Bathing
- Combing/brushing hair (even if there is just a little amount)
- Dressing the infant
- Participating in photography
- Obtaining a lock of hair
- Obtaining additional footprints/handprints
- Creating hand/foot molds

When families have spent time with their infant and are ready to say goodbye, staff should reassure them that their baby will be cared for after they leave and that there will be close collaboration between the hospital and the funeral home of their choice. Some families may ask details as to what will happen with their baby's body until the funeral home comes to pick them up, and staff should provide an honest answer about the morgue and the process of safely and properly storing bodies. If possible, organizations should use the infant Preshand system as a more respectful way to support the infant's body, rather than using a body bag or just wrapping the body in a blanket with a tag to be taken to the morgue. These beautiful and comfortable boxes provide a peaceful and private place for the infant to lie, wrapped and secure, while being taken off the NICU or family birthing floor and while in the morgue waiting for the funeral home to come. For families who want to see what will happen with their baby, they can help tuck them into the comfortable bed and have a visual of exactly where their child will be after they are separated.

When parents leave the hospital, staff must recognize that they will experience a wide range of emotions. They will be leaving the intensive care unit for the last time, which compounds the intensity of their loss. NICU staff, for some families, has become an extension of their family and has been their support system for days, weeks, or even months. Walking out of the unit after the loss of their child means they are leaving their baby and their entire network of people who knew them as a family (a family they so desperately wanted to be) behind. Families find themselves leaving both an extremely intensive situation and a very intense environment only to enter silence and emptiness. Sending families' home with mementos, photos, and a blanket that was wrapped around their baby can be ways to help them feel a little less empty. Furthermore, staff should tell parents that they will call within a few days to check in with them and see how they are doing. They also help staff anticipate future support, which can be a great comfort.

Having an infant loss in the NICU is a distressing event for both families and staff, so follow-up calls and sympathy cards can be extremely therapeutic for both parties. Often, staff also choose to attend memorial services of patients to help with closure and to also show ongoing support to families. Chapter 15 discusses the impact that loss has on caregivers and the ways that staff can support themselves and one another during tragedy. It is comforting to families to know that their baby's care team truly cared for their child as an individual and not just as another patient on the unit.

Author's Personal Story

I was greeted by Baby L.'s parents in the lobby of our NICU on the afternoon of his 22nd day of life. Each encounter I had with these parents was pleasant. Although baby L. had been through so much in his first 22 days out of the womb, his parents remained optimistic even in the most difficult moments.

L. had a very long journey ahead of him. He had been delivered emergently at 26 weeks' gestation due to his mom's worsening preeclampsia and was fighting the many challenges premature babies must fight to survive. By the radiance in his mother's eyes, the almost giddy tone in her voice, and the ear-to-ear smile on his dad's face, I instantly knew they were going to share a great success story with me that day in the lobby, a story that I was incredibly honored to have been invited to share with them and one that I will never forget.

As a nurse in the NICU, I am given a front row seat alongside families on the roller coaster ride each of them experiences during their NICU journey. I have to buckle up and ride the twists and turns that make me nervous and instill a great deal of fear, but I also get to soar through the easy parts and enjoy the fun and exciting milestones right along with them. L.'s roller coaster ride wasn't much different than any other 26-week-old

(continued)

(*continued*)

neonate's. There were good days and there were difficult days. There were days when he was intubated, then days when he would stabilize on continuous positive airway pressure (CPAP). Yet L. ended up requiring oscillatory ventilation, and it became extremely difficult to wean him from this high level of respiratory support. L. was a very critical patient, no one would argue that. But above the diagnosis and above the many therapies L. was receiving, he was most importantly H.M. and M.M.'s son, their first and only child.

Being in the unique combined role of a neonatal nurse and family-support specialist, I got to share in the most intimate moments with families who were living through very traumatic and emotional birth crises. Whether their child was born at 24 weeks or if their term infant needed a few hours of NICU transition after birth, the stay in the NICU is a parent's worst nightmare.

In the case of H.M. and M.M., I initially met them on the 4th day of their son's life at his bedside. I remember entering the darkened room and seeing his parents visiting him. Both parents were standing at his Isolette staring in what looked like pure disbelief, at this incredibly small life in front of them. There was the traditional introduction of who I was and what I would be able to provide during their stay, and it seemed to be like any other first meeting. Little did I know that that moment was not only the start of an experience that I would never forget, but also was one that would turn into plans for great practice change in our department.

On Day 22 of baby L.'s life, when his parents found me in the NICU lobby, their excitement was contagious. His mother said that baby L. was doing so well that in 2 or 3 days, if he continued to improve, she would be able to hold him for the first time. My heart filled with joy for them. I anxiously watched L.'s progress the next few days right along with them. I frequently checked in with the medical care team and L.'s parents and received updates around the clock on his condition. I couldn't wait to hear when his parents would be able to hold him, and I planned on being present to capture that monumental moment for them with as many photos as our unit's digital camera would hold. Three days passed, and on Day 25 of life, I was there to capture pictures of baby L. in H.M.'s and M.M.'s arms for the first time, but tragically, it was also the last.

On the evening of Day 24, baby L. wasn't acting himself. His beautiful bright eyes didn't look the same; he was having more apnea and bradycardia, and after a septic workup, the providers found that he was very sick. L. was so small and had been so fragile that he didn't have much reserve and sadly continued to get increasingly ill as the hours passed.

As I walked into the unit early in the morning on Day 25, I saw extreme pain on the nurse's faces. As each nurse looked at me, I knew. I found both parents beside baby L. just waiting, praying. The care team frantically worked with baby L. trying to do whatever they could to improve his condition. One nurse had run to the blood bank and returned with blood and fresh frozen plasma, one nurse was administering his current dose of antibiotics, and another nurse was administering a fluid bolus. Baby L. was on 100% oxygen therapy with maximum ventilator support and maximal infusion of nitric oxide. Unfortunately, there was not much more that the care team could do, and L. was quickly slipping away.

(*continued*)

(continued)

The neonatologist asked the family and I to step away into a private room for a few moments and told them that he thought it was time to have a very difficult conversation. I remember him sitting beside the family and so delicately explaining everything that had happened over the past 24 hours and what everything meant in very-easy-to-understand terminology. The parents sat there in disbelief, but the gentle hand that the provider placed on their shoulder and their knee comforted them. I offered tissue, and together the physician and I talked with the family about their two choices. They could either have us continue to provide therapies to see if baby L. would turn around, although all of the efforts up until this point made us believe that he would continue to decline and not respond favorably; he likely would not survive despite our very best efforts, yet this option would prolong how long he would be with them. They also could choose to stop the aggressive therapies and allow their son to be comforted and receive palliative care in his last hours of life; they could spend quality time with him and focus on holding him and loving him without the interruptions of invasive treatments, tubes, and wires. We recognized that the decision was extremely difficult to make, and either choice would be an okay choice to make, but it was up to them to look into their hearts and decide what was most important to them on how to parent and care for their son.

We allowed L.'s parents to have time alone and escorted them back to their son's room where they could talk to one another and call family or friends if they wished. We knew this was an extremely difficult and painful decision and wanted them to have all the support they needed to make the decision that would impact them for their lifetime. Nurses continued to enter the room to provide treatment to baby L. as necessary until his parents had come to a decision; they wanted to end all of the aggressive treatment and allow their son to receive comfort care. The neonatologist acknowledged the parent's difficult decision and their bravery in making such a big decision on behalf of their son, one that he felt was the right decision and one that would end a lot of pain for baby L. He then took the time to explain everything that the parents could anticipate, from how aspects of each care could be discontinued all the way up until the point of them placing baby L. into one of their arms and removing the intubation tube. He shared with them what the dying process in infants was like, so they knew what baby L. would look and feel like and offered to either allow them to be alone in the room or to have him or any one of the nurses stay with them. What was so special is that he said, "Getting to the point of where he passes away is difficult and is a lot to handle right now. Let's just focus on getting from here to there, and then when we get to that point, we can talk about what the next phase of care looks like. Does that sound okay to you?" The parents both nodded yes, and I imagine they were happy with not having to be overloaded with more information at that moment but were relieved to know they would be given the information when they were ready.

The family was present and participated in deciding when the medications were slowly weaned and discontinued and was there when the monitors were removed. Slowly they were able to look down and see more and more of their child, who up until this point they had only seen covered in wires, tubes, and IV lines. As I was capturing some photos of

(continued)

(*continued*)

baby L's last few moments, the physician sat beside the parents and told them it was time. The nurses very compassionately removed the IV lines, assisted the parents in dressing baby L. in his first and only outfit, and then removed him from life support. Baby L. was gently picked up and placed into his mother's arms.

The entire room filled with tears. As I watched H.M. and M.M., my heart ached. I kept reliving the moment 3 days ago when they shared their excitement at the thought of finally getting to hold their son. The pure delight and joy in their eyes were gone and were now replaced with hurt, confusion, sadness, emptiness, and uncertainty. Discretely, I continued to capture photos for the family of what would be their only family photos and hopefully be mementos that they would cherish later on.

Shortly after baby L. was removed from life support, both H.M.'s and M.M.'s parents arrived to not only say goodbye to their grandchild, but also to support and grieve with their children. Over the next several hours, other family members, friends, and church family arrived to also support the family. The social work team worked closely during this time with the father and mother to determine how they would like to proceed with arrangements, and I remember being in awe at the strength and bravery M.M. had in that time. He stepped up and really took on his caretaker role for his wife and his son and made really tough decisions with dignity and confidence.

After many hours and after the parents felt that all of their friends and family who were going to come pay their respects had been by to visit, they were ready to move to the next phase of care. In collaboration with another nurse, I walked H.M. though giving her son a bath, capturing moments of that in photographs as well. She then dried and dressed him, brushed his hair, and even helped clip a small amount to place in her memory box we were putting together for them. After all care was done and when the parents were finally feeling ready to leave, they were given privacy to say goodbye to their son.

Family Story

This first incredibly touching story comes from Megan Walker. Megan graciously shares about her experience with having both compassionate and less than compassionate care team members during their NICU journey when they were faced with the devastating reality of losing their son Simon.

"I remember clearly the moment when I knew Simon was dying. My husband was getting ready to leave the NICU; he was going to go home and try to sleep for a few hours. It was around 8 p.m., and we were standing above our Simon's bed, quietly contemplating how life had brought us to this point in time. His little body was medically paralyzed as a last result to give his failing lungs rest to recover, he was on one hundred percent

(*continued*)

(*continued*)

oxygen support, and there were cords and IVs surrounding him. We hovered there; it was as if our minds could not quite grasp what our eyes were seeing. Suddenly, the monitor beeped loudly beside us; Simon's O_2 saturations were dropping low. Our nurse, and a resident from Simon's first days who was working in a different section of the NICU that night, were there immediately beside us, watching with us and studying the monitors. Our doctors had exhausted every option for his care. We watched silently, helplessly to see what Simon would do. Would he recover? Or would he continue to decline? Simon's saturations wavered, and I begged him to try harder, to keep going, to please not leave me. But then the moment came, one that many of my doctors had prepared me for, when Simon 'told us' he was done fighting. His saturations fell lower than they'd ever fallen, and my heart knew. I turned to the resident, and asked the hardest question I've ever had to ask, 'Is he dying?' Even though we'd only worked with this resident for the first week or so of Simon's life, passed him in the halls on occasion, and spoken briefly with him, in this moment of our journey, he became a crucial person in our lives. His gentle answer, confirming what immediately became my reality, was exactly what I needed in that moment. Perhaps it is not common knowledge for all doctors, nurses, and caregivers, but this very important fact remains: Every working person in an intensive care unit is a key player to suffering families—his or her voice, smile, and the way in which he or she chooses to present himself with language and emotion, even how one handles stress or disappointment will influence lifelong memories for families like ours. Though our interactions with this resident were few considering the scale of our 5-month stay. I remember little details of our association that built the trust and friendship that I needed in that singular, critical moment of my life. I remember his genuine smile and concern with every mundane question I asked, and I remember one instance of passing him in a group in the hallway when he actually stopped to say hello despite his group continuing on. He was never angry, always kind, and he was genuine, confident, and encouraging at appropriate times. He didn't have to be in Simon's room that night. He was assigned in a completely different section of the NICU. But because he could, and because he cared, he was there with us. That, to me, is the epitome of an outstanding caregiver. This man is one of many we cherish in our NICU family. I remember fondly our receptionist too, a stickler to the rules, who kindly and patiently reminded me on countless occasions over 5 months to sign in before going back to Si's room; our RT, who heard my seemingly crazy plea that something was wrong with Simon's tubing and discovered holes twice during our stay; one of our nurses who spent extra time in our room to teach me how to care for a tiny human, who used clips to organize the cords around Simon, always making sure his bed was clean and clear; another nurse who kindly, but firmly, pushed me through my fear to hold Simon when he weighed just over a pound, who wiped down keyboards and tables at the beginning of every shift; yet another nurse, despite her own pain and devastation that last night, who gave me strength to cherish the moments and gave me a voice when I didn't feel like I had one. All of these staff members were exceptional because they treated their jobs like they were truly members of our family.

(*continued*)

(*continued*)

"We were able to hold Simon all night that night, but we knew his lungs were failing him and that our time with him was now measured in moments. I had no idea what would happen next, what death looked like, or how to navigate through this process with Simon. Unbelievably, there were professionals at this point in our journey who failed to guide us. The fellow on call that night, I cannot even remember his name, who always seemed stern, rushed, and panicked, came to talk with us while we were holding Simon. He could barely look at us as he awkwardly explained, 'It's not looking good.' My husband and I looked at each other, and the tender feelings in the room were exchanged with painful awkwardness and kindling anger at this oblivious man. 'He's dying,' I said pointedly, crossly. The fellow seemed to let out a breath at my admission, his face immediately relaxing, and the nurse practitioner beside him loosened up as well. They proceeded to roughly explain that there were no further options to explore for Simon, and that we needed to decide if we wanted to 'wait it out' or pick a time to let him go. I felt dirty and disgusted at the way they treated my son's life; his coming death felt like a business transaction, and I felt like I was negotiating the details with the Devil himself. They said things like, 'I'm sorry this is happening,' and 'this must be hard for you,' as plainly as though they'd read the lines from a book, but without any human feeling. Every kind phrase was followed by 'but we need to know,' or 'let us know when you decide.' The nurse practitioner was impatient, coming in to our room at several points in the evening, asking, 'Have you thought about it? Have you made any decisions yet? We need to know in advance so that we can lift his paralysis. He shouldn't feel anything, but if he does we'll be ready with any medicine he might need. I'll just wait outside; you just let me know.' After three similar occurrences in this form, we felt horribly pressured. I told her that we were not ready, and we'd probably wait for the next shift to be with our doctor. I remember her face, always disappointed, always as if we'd inconvenienced her, like she had a plan already in her mind that was best, and we were doing something wrong. As the morning approached, we eventually made the impossible decision to remove care in the garden at the top floor of the hospital. I wanted my Simon to feel the sunshine that he'd gazed at so fondly through his window for 5 months. The morning was arriving, Simon was fading, and we called in the fellow and nurse practitioner to tell them our plan. They were immediately defensive, arguing that we couldn't use the garden because it would be too complicated and that the time we'd chosen would overlap with shift change and would be too impossible for the staff. I was so angry and hurt; I felt like we'd been set up to fail and that after finally making the most difficult decision of my life and feeling like I had a voice and a plan to do something so completely against my heart and soul, I was rejected and tossed aside. We asked them to leave, without a further word and waited for our team to arrive. Our doctor came directly to us, she hugged us, gave us her deepest sympathies, and granted with ease our desires for Simon's last hours. My broken heart was held together in that moment, my burdens carried a bit, by a capable friend.

"Two things I appreciated that morning in the garden were, first, having faces I loved surrounding us, and second, having a voice and being heard in every step. My team

(*continued*)

(continued)

provided physical help by helping me find my shoes, walking beside me, squeezing my arm, providing tissues, and holding and organizing my things; they also offered emotional support by making eye contact, sharing in my pain, and allowing me moments to cry and express what I was feeling. Everything was made as simple and as straightforward and uncomplicated as it could be, with no judgment, only respect; we were presented with options as they were appropriate to the situation, and we were able to be in control of everything. Our night nurse stayed over and offered to take pictures for us; I am so grateful to have those reminders of how sick Simon was, to help me remember on hard days that I made the best choice for him.

"When the time came, I'm grateful in that experience to have had intelligent and compassionate individuals to explain those hard things to us. One of them looked us in the eyes as he spoke to us, although I know it was terribly painful for him, too. As we gave Simon back to his Father in Heaven, we felt broken in a way no one in this earthly life should have to feel. It is inconceivable. I had no idea; I could not have even remotely fathomed that the pain I felt then and continue to feel now was humanly possible. No description can justify the feeling of once bearing life and then holding that life as it leaves. It was the hardest moment I will ever witness, and if I could take this pain away from any other human being, I would. But on the same token, it was also the most sacred, spiritual experience of my life, and I am equally grateful for the reverence and respect given to us by our team. The staff stayed close to us through it all, and I know we were surrounded by both heavenly and earthly angels that morning.

"The nurse helped me wrap him in a blanket and cover his sweet face, and I carried him back to our room. She guided us to bathe and dress Simon's body. She provided us with every necessity, stayed close, but gave us space. Loving staff members aided her in making gifts with his handprints and footprints. Every single previous doctor of Simon's came to see us. One gave me paperwork to guide me through drying up my breast milk, with information on donating my remaining bottles. After the family had packed up our room, we again said goodbye to our Simon, King of the NICU. The nurse hugged me and cried with me and told me that she would personally make sure Si's body was kept safe.

"Since then, a dozen or so of Simon's nurses and staff came to his funeral nearly 3 hours away. Some sent me gifts soon after and even Christmas cards this past year. They are forever my family. I can never thank them enough for what they've given me—for sharing their intelligence and education to allow my family 5 months with the strongest, most beautiful little spirit I have ever met. It has been 7 months since my last moments with Simon, but I relive that final night, see the faces of every person who surrounded us in those precious last hours, every single day."

This second story is shared by Sherry Graf, who openly shares her experience of having premature triplets in the NICU and having to go through saying goodbye to one of the three, after one became too ill from an infection to survive.

"On February 9, 1997, I gave birth to triplets at 28 weeks. It was an exciting yet scary time for my husband and me. The weights of my three babies were 2 lb 11oz, 2 lb 12 oz,

(*continued*)

and 2 lb 13 oz. I thought that was good since that seemed to be the focus on my doctors at the time When one of the doctors told us this would be an emotional roller coaster ride, they weren't kidding. Naturally, because they were born premature, all of them were on a ventilator. Every hour, it seemed like there was a change in one of the babies' care, whether they were off the ventilator or put back on to something as simple as one needing a blood transfusion. I kept daily logs on all three. Through this experience we dealt with many doctors and nurses. Overall, most were great. When dealing with such high emotions and uncertainty, it is helpful to have people taking care of your, not one baby, but three babies, who have compassion. I understand they deal with so much and see so much; however, in my experience, the ones who showed compassion are the ones that I shall remember and be thankful for. Some of the neonatal doctors talked to my husband and I as if we had gone to medical school. We needed to understand everything that was happening, and yet we felt like some were just reading a textbook to us. I worked in a hospital setting and thankfully understood most, but I needed to feel connected to these people I entrusted to take care of my children.

"The nurses were amazing. For all that they do in taking care of our babies, I was quite amazed. It made it so much more tolerable for when I had to leave the hospital to go home and take care of my 4-year old. I knew they were in good hands. I always called to get updates, and not once did any of them make me feel like I was bothering them.

"After 5 weeks, one of my triplets caught an infection. Despite all the days that we scrubbed our arms and hands, there is never a guarantee that anything can be 100% sterile. Giving antibiotics to a preemie is the only hope we had. In this case, it wasn't enough. The infection attacked my baby viciously and he became septic. His kidneys shut down, and we helplessly watched him deteriorate slowly. The doctor in charge at that time was wonderful. On March 13, 1997, I lost my precious baby. I watched him fight for his life, and in the end, he lost. The hospital we were at during that time had no privacy around each baby. The whole room watched as we suffered our loss. I am a very private person, and that was very difficult to deal with. I tried to be strong, yet I saw everyone around watching and crying with us. When we lost our baby, we knew that he had the best care and that the doctor did everything he could to try and save him. I am thankful for that because I didn't become angry at my loss and want to blame anyone for it. To me, that is huge in the healing process. We all want to blame something or someone when something goes wrong, and we did not. My only challenge was that I did not have time to grieve for my loss because I had two other babies and a 4-year-old who needed me. After the nurses cleaned and dressed my baby, they then did give us a private room where we could hold our baby and spend some time alone with him. I can't tell you how important that time was to us. There were many times I did not hold my baby and I needed to. I took pictures as well and I am so glad I did. I wanted everything I could so that my heart could heal from this loss. It was in fact very difficult giving him back because I knew it would be the last time I would ever see him again, but I did.

(*continued*)

(*continued*)

"The hospital took pictures as well. Those pictures did not turn out good at all and I think I can definitely say they were awful. The mistake the hospital made was, they put my baby in the same position you would see a deceased person in a coffin. Although it is great to have pictures, I think they should have swaddled my baby instead. I offered my opinion to them in hopes that they would change that for the next parent who had to suffer a loss.

"The loss of a baby is traumatic and one a parent will never forget. And like everything, in time it gets easier to cope with but the pain never goes away. My children may never have met their brother, but they know of him. In fact, two of them have tattoos of his name on them in remembrance. The outcomes may not have been what I wanted, but I will always cherish and celebrate his birth."

The final story comes from Sophie Fauveau, who bravely shares her story about losing both of her twin boys—one very shortly after birth and one unexpectedly more than 2 months into his NICU journey and just after they began to anticipate preparations for discharge home.

"I am Sophie, the happiest, saddest mom at the playground. I have been excited to be a mom from as young as I can remember. Daydreaming about my future family, pregnancy, and sometimes even daring to stretch my dreams to a vision of raising twins. After a grueling 7-year battle with infertility and a scorecard boasting six miscarriages, countless infertility procedures, injections, and insemination, my husband Mark and I decided to put the '*US*' back in 'uter*US*' and adopt.

"We naively thought adoption would be an easier road. Instead, what followed was a 3-year trek with many setbacks, false hopes, and crushing disappointments. But, in the midst of our storm, came our rainbow. We were blessed with the privilege to adopt a newborn little girl in Oregon. We named her Zoélie Estrella.

"Shocked, though pleasantly surprised, within a few months we were referred a *second* little girl in Ethiopia who had a rough start in life and needed parents. She was just 5 months younger than Zoélie. The stars were aligning. Several months and mountains of paperwork later, we flew to Ethiopia to adopt our new daughter and named her Azalea Mitike. Life got busy, happy, smelly, and exhausting. With our girls holding hands, strapped in their double stroller, we could see a twin-like bond blossoming. It was perfection. Zoélie and Azalea are 8 years old today and best friends.

"When our 'twins' turned two, life surprised us with a biological son! My belly and my heart grew bigger but unbeknownst to me, Windsor's heart grew weaker. Windsor was born at 35 weeks, with holes in his heart. A large ventricular septal defect and small atrial septal defect. At 3 months old and barely 9 pounds, he underwent open heart surgery and I learned what it really feels like when the heart of a mother is put to the test. It was a traumatic time. Windsor flat-lined when he got extubated postsurgery but was successfully resuscitated, giving me just enough time to know what losing a child would feel like. Complications continued with pneumonia and respiratory syncytial virus, which sent him back in the ICU for weeks, but Windsor is a healthy, thriving 6-year old today.

(*continued*)

(*continued*)

"Two years later I became unexpectedly pregnant with identical twin boys. I was 39. I knew they were twins from the minute I peed on that stick in the bathroom at work. The stick lit up with shiny blue lines in less than a second and the nausea was so severe that I just knew it. I did the math: 5 kids under 5 years old!! And mentally curled in the fetal position. That would scare even the most ambitious of moms! But I felt giddy.

"The first ultrasound was memorable. The OB/GYN only saw one baby and I asked her to look more, it took her 30 seconds but she said 'Oh, yes! Oh, yes!! There is another one!' I cried in disbelief that my intuition was right, I cried out of joy. And out of fear. I was monitored very closely because the boys were identical and because I was well, you know, *geriatric*! The pregnancy was hard with three little kids and a home undergoing a massive remodel, but we were literally 'making rooms' to accommodate a family of 7.

"At my 20-week anatomical scan, everything looked perfect! The boys were so healthy! Because I had a 2-year-old son with coronary heart disease (CHD), I was told that the twins needed an echocardiogram. I was confident that life could only be trending up now. Our suffering bank was full. At 23 weeks, I went in for the echo. Alone—I was confident. The technician was serious, concentrated and not engaging with me despite my attempts. She left the room a few times, came back, and kept taking pictures. I was petrified and freezing cold, but it was not a regular surface cold; it was a 'core cold,' a feeling that everything was about to turn.

"It did."

"The doctor walked in and told me she was sorry. This word 'sorry' never quite fits in the mouth of a doctor. It is way too small and just falls out pathetically. There should be a word solely for doctors and nurses to express how sympathetic and horrified they are to deliver bad news. She told me that Baby A (whom we later named Cyprien) only had half a heart. *Half. A. Heart.* His condition was called *hypoplastic right heart syndrome*. I wrote 'HPRHS' down to Google later. Our family could handle CHDs and open-heart surgeries, we had been there. I immediately tried to be positive. The doctor crushed my hopes with 3 simple words: 'Unfit for life.'

"Armand (Baby B) had a perfectly formed heart, but because I also had the beginning of a placenta abruption and was showing signs of twin-to-twin transfusion syndrome (TTTS), Armand was not getting enough amniotic fluid or blood—and was in utter distress in my uterus. My brain froze. I was getting this news all at once. Alone. In a cold room, dimly lit by neon fluorescents. It was like getting a death sentence. I don't know how else to describe it. I was a deer in headlights that felt shot in the heart.

"I was then walked out and left (once again) *alone* to check myself into the maternity ward for observation. Once in my room, I called my husband, Mark. Words failed me. Everything failed me. The neonatologist came to my room and showed me a statistic chart with what it meant to have a baby at 23 weeks, 24, 25, 26 weeks, and so on. He gave me a cold, dry, and matter-of-fact speech and showed very little compassion or emotion. I was still alone, as Mark was stuck in traffic. The conversation with the neonatologist left me to feel that I too should not have feelings about the decision. I stayed a night in the hospital

(*continued*)

(continued)

attached to two fetal monitors. I was bleeding internally but was offered to go home on modified bed rest. I decided to leave because I desperately needed warmth. I needed my children and my husband to warm my soul and tell me we would be OK.

"My body was covered in red blotches. My belly was visually growing by the day. I was bigger at 23 weeks than I was at delivery with my last pregnancy. I had no room for my lungs or my stomach to function. I was gasping for air and hope; for nutrition and nurturing. I was at the end. I felt I was going to die, but nevertheless I went 'home.' They let me walk out. We were not in our house anymore, as the construction prevented us from living in it. We were in a borrowed place living out of a suitcase.

"With the chart of statistics in hand and the neonatologist still talking in my head, we decided that we would not resuscitate any babies prior to 25 weeks. We decided that we would not try to resuscitate Cyprien because he was 'unfit for life.' Oh, how I felt 'unfit for life' too. And surely 'unfit to decide about life and death' for Armand. It was awful. I felt very lonely and broken. By that point, the hemorrhage inside my uterus had created a clot the size of a third baby. My stomach was enormously distended. Both babies were fighting for their lives inside and I, their vessel, was out of fuel. It felt to me that cabin and cargo were headed for a fatal crash and all I could do was sit in a recliner. 'Sit back, relax and enjoy the crash.' It (I, we) felt like a ticking time bomb.

"At 24 weeks and 3 days, on Labor Day of all days, I went into labor at home. Everything happened extremely fast and in the middle of the night. Our three kids were sleeping, and we had no family around, so my best friend Sue took me to the emergency room. There started a whirlwind of misinformation, rapid contractions, confused diagnoses, magnesium infusion, steroid injections, poor communication, projectile vomiting, debilitating headaches, and utter confusion. In the middle of that walks in our doctor. I liked her, despite the sad little 'sorry' she had to deliver earlier. She greeted me at the head and the tail and said, 'Girl you are 9 cm dilated, we need to make a decision as to how you want to deliver. You have about 5 minutes to decide.'

"She said I could deliver the babies vaginally but that neither baby would survive given their positions. Baby A was breech, and Baby B, transverse. I was informed that a vaginal delivery would be a safer option for me (they were very concerned I might hemorrhage as I had low platelets due to the giant clot). She said a C-section would give us options to save the babies, but the risks for me should not be ignored. She had papers in hand for me to sign.

"Mark and I had already decided not to resuscitate the babies less than 25 weeks, as it was the neonatologist's cold-headed recommendation, so a vaginal delivery would be the proper answer to give them right now. Yet, in that moment, my motherly instincts burst out and took over. I could not follow-through, I had to give Armand a chance. From my bed, which felt like a death bed, I chose a C-section. I didn't weigh the consequences. I was not mentally or physically able too. I chose their life over mine because the promise of hope is far greater than the grip of fear. 'C-section,' I said. I chose the C-section. I was not even done saying the word 'section' when I was handed those papers to sign and got

(continued)

(continued)

wheeled to the OR—numb, scared, and crying for my babies. Crying in fear and disbelief. I wanted to resist, to scream, to go back, yet I was so docile. I felt like a restrained mental patient who is taken away against her will to a mysterious torture chamber. I was lost but had no more fight in me.

"The OR was jammed with people ready to operate. I was praying that the spinal tap would be put in between contractions and not during. I was 10 cm dilated, and contractions were 2 minutes or less apart. I sat on the edge of the operating table and hugged my labor and delivery nurse, Brandy. I hugged her and hung on to her body like a barnacle on a rock holding on as furious waves crash and attempt to make it lose its suction. As the anesthesiologist pierced my skin, Brandy hugged me calmly with a motherly strength. The pain was uncontrollable, and I was wondering if that would be my last memory of being alive.

"I was now lying on my bed, crying, and silently holding my friend's hand. Sue had appeared all suited up in a sterile gown. She looked scared. Sue never looked scared. Tears were streaming down my face, and the warmth of them was the only thing I could feel now; everything else was numb. I was so sad, so lost. An island of stillness and silence among the hustle and bustle. I put 100% of my faith in God that He would work through these strangers' hands. From my vantage point, I looked up at faces to try to connect and be a little present. I could see the kind eyes of the young anesthesiologist and knew she cared. I could see that Nurse Brandy was concealing her worries like a family member would. There was a solemn atmosphere of urgency and sorrow in the operating room.

"I was strapped-in in a cross position and thought of Jesus. No one was going to put nails in my palms and feet, but I was about to be cut open and witness my child dying. Maybe I would die too and meet Jesus or I would go crazy. My babies, my precious babies, what would happen to them? Would we all enter Heaven together? Those were the thoughts going through my head. Sue's firm grip on my hand brought me back to earth. The babies' heart rates were going down; everyone panicked. I was calm while shoved, cut open, tugged, and pulled. Sue's gown and shoes were splattered with blood. I could hear the squishy sound of rubber soles walking in my blood on the floor. Babies were out, I heard 'he is beautiful,' then I heard nothing. There were no baby sounds, there were no cries, no signs of any infant, no noise anywhere. I saw that Mark had appeared, Sue had disappeared. I cried for my babies. For Mark. For me.

"Once sewn back up and wheeled to my room, it all got blurry. Within some time, we got an internal call from the NICU to tell us that 'Baby A' was not doing well. Our sweet Cyprien's heart was failing. We were asked what we wanted to do, and we both said we didn't want him to suffer and that we wanted to let him to go. We didn't confer, but we both talked in unison. Minutes later, we were in the NICU to meet our son who was alive. *Living*! It was the first time I saw him.

"Numb from the chest down, in my giant bed on wheels, I entered the NICU. I have no recollection until I saw Cyprien as he was being unhooked, unplugged, and carried to my chest. We lay there in my bed, just him and me, then Mark leaned over and stayed

(continued)

(continued)

with us very close. Brandy had brought her big camera and took a picture that I cherish today. I am so thankful that they wheeled me in before unplugging. I am so thankful our nurse was prepared. So thankful she took that photo of Cyprien alive.

"Cyprien died on my chest, peacefully. I was kissing his head, telling him how I loved him. I felt at peace. Finally, the dreaded moment had come and gone; it was over. I was alive, he was in Heaven, yet I felt that we were still together and would always be.

"For the next 8 hours he stayed with us in the room. After a while, Brandy took him, washed him, got him little clothes, and dressed him. He looked so beautiful. So peaceful. She took his hand and footprint, busied herself with him like a nurse would with any 'live' newborn. She had a gentle touch and a caring voice. From my bed, I watched her caring for our son, and it looked like any scene in any postpartum room. I am grateful she gave me that moment. Despite the fact that there were no cooing and cries, seeing her with him was healing.

"A couple of close friends came and loved on Cyprien. I felt at peace. I could not think of anything besides being here in the moment. I did not think about Armand, our other kids, or anyone else. Just us now, in that room. This day is all we would ever get, and we had to make it count by being present. Mark held him and cried, quietly. I could not cry anymore. I went into a zone, a place where all of this was not sad, and a place of peace. I enjoyed my 8 hours with Cyprien. I didn't want to be a sad, sobbing mom. I do not know what superpower allowed me to have a good day with my son. All my preconceived ideas of 'acceptable,' 'normal' behavior for a mom holding her dead child was challenged. I will never judge how someone acts when they are shocked out of their body by trauma, grief, and pain.

"I cuddled Cyprien in bed for 6 hours. All sadness was repressed and thoughts of death kept at bay. My brain was doing a great job protecting my heart, but I could not ignore what my hands were now starting to feel. Cold. His body was getting cold. Time was up. From that point on, I could no longer look at his face. I had to hold him wrapped up a little more, with the blanket covering almost all of his face. He was starting to change physically and I was starting to change emotionally. For the first time, I saw myself as a mom holding a dead baby. I didn't want to remember him not looking alive and I didn't want to remember me feeling that way.

"Mark felt like he was ready to say goodbye. I held Cyprien in his blue blanket and, after Mark had said his goodbyes and left to go back home to care for the kids, I stayed a couple more hours with him but didn't look at him straight on. When it was time for me to say my final goodbyes, I told the nurse (a new one) that I was ready. She called the morgue and someone came up with a body bag. I heard the ruffle of plastic and the sound of a zipper. I froze, felt anger, and said I did not want this in our room. The person and their horrid piece of plastic of death swiftly disappeared.

"Even if my son had been dead for hours he was not 'that dead' to me. Body bags are for other people, for movies, not for precious babies whose souls were still way too close to their bodies. That moment made me have visions of suffocation in a bag. It is something

(continued)

(continued)

I still have nightmares over. Cyprien went to the morgue and I never saw him again. The only comforting thought was that my 2 babies and I were all still in the same building. I asked my brain to not think of the morgue or of anything related to what happens after death. My brain listened. Our nurse printed the photos she had taken during the day and put them in a beautiful keepsake box with other memorabilia.

"The next day I had a friend help me build a 'shrine' in my room. I was never a 'shrine person,' but in this moment, I had the urge to express my pain, and a shrine in my room was helpful. As someone who had zero experience with grief, I had always thought that shrines were 'creepy' and that they kept people 'stuck.' Now, I understand the power they have. They provide a place to pray, to meditate and to focus our grief so it doesn't suck all the oxygen out of life. I put pictures up, flowers, an old Bible, a precious rosary, and a statue of the Virgin Mary that various friends had brought over. I do not consider myself religious, but my Catholic upbringing and convent-school education provided an anchor in the storm.

"With Cyprien now 'safe,' I needed to see Armand. I wanted to go to the NICU but could not sit in a wheelchair yet. I was severely anemic due to the blood loss and needed a transfusion. Mark went to see Armand, but words failed him, and he could not report back on what he saw or felt. He kept saying, 'You will see; he is small, but he is strong.' The 6-hour transfusion literally pumped life back into my veins and put me in an unexpected state of euphoria. I am not sure whose blood I got, but that was some amazing blood! I am thankful to all the blood donors, especially those who share their 'happy blood.' I had oodles of energy and the giggles, which was hurting so bad in my stitched and stapled lower abdomen. Finally, like a reinflated balloon, I felt good enough to move and was told I could be transferred to a wheelchair and go to the NICU.

"As I was 'refueling' at the blood station, Mark was asked to sign lots of paper, pick a funeral home, and make impossible final arrangements for Cyprien's transport and cremation. I could not help emotionally, as I had to focus solely on *life*. I wish that there had been a person dedicated to handle such things. 'Paperwork of death' is a horrible thing to ask a parent to do right after they said goodbye to their child. Mark handled it all through many tears, but he did it without asking me to be much involved. It was hard to see him cry, but I was so relieved not to have to look at those papers. Cyprien's soul felt present, very present to me. I am immensely thankful that Mark took care of the sad and 'down-to-earth' realities of dealing with bodies after death.

"Now, in my wheelchair, ready to head to the NICU, I felt terrified. I feared I would find Armand in a state that my heart would not be able to handle. I was afraid that seeing him would send me into a panic attack with uncontrollable anxiety and spasms. With the wound on my abdomen and the one in my heart, I was not sure I could take either. But nevertheless, I went in.

"Entering the NICU felt like entering a high-security sci-fi research lab. Special badges, special access. The light, the smells, the noises. Nothing felt familiar. It is a world within a world, with its own staff, its own hours, its own culture and language. Time doesn't exist.

(continued)

(*continued*)

There are no windows, no reference to anything that the outside world is busying itself with. The earth keeps turning, the world keeps churning, but the NICU stands as its own ecosystem. I felt like I was sucked into a vortex every time I entered. I learned to love that vortex. Over time, it became a cocoon. A warm and safe cocoon where everyone knew what we were going through. A cocoon full of superheroes cut away from daylight, time, and distraction.

"I was wheeled to Armand's area. I approached carefully, feeling so sorry that I did this to him. Everything looked foreign. The plastic incubators felt like no match for a womb. I felt so sorry that I subjected him to this. I felt broken and responsible for my broken womb that had forced him out and into *this*. I remember thinking that it would be better if the incubators were filled with warm water. At least it would make me feel better.

"Then I met him. My little man. Smaller than a baby cat, with all his tubes and lines, all wired. I saw him, and as hard as I tried not to fall in love, I did. Wholeheartedly. Desperately. Right there and then, the minute I laid my worried eyes on his 575 g of strength and perfection. Armand's size scared me because he had a lot to accomplish in this body to remain alive. Cyprien was the same size, but nothing was required of him. He was not asked to live in that size of a body. I felt immeasurably helpless but unconditionally in love.

"I wish someone had prepared me for what I was going to see though. I wish there had been a movie in my room like the one in the plane. 'Buckle up, you are about to enter a new universe, you will see things that will change you forever, you will be pushed to your limits but always remember that you are not alone, meet the friendly crew with decades of experience, meet the passengers, many are feeling just like you, review the safety procedures, map of the facility, blah blah.'

"What I mean is that I wish someone had gone over the unique language of the NICU, explaining the pumps and PICC lines and blood gases and what each number on each monitor was indicating. I really wish someone had walked me through the setups and what a typical day would look like. I would have wanted a tutorial about all the alarms and learn what they really meant. To this day I have an inner fear every time I hear the 'ping' of an elevator because it sounds so much like one of the alarms. In the first few days, I craved stats and success stories. Even just realistic stories. I wanted context, a roadmap for my brain to not feel so lost and for my body to not feel so inadequate. I wish there had been a nurse, a therapist, or social worker with me to check on my emotional health and detected signs in me indicating I needed help when I could not recognize or express it. I had millions of questions that I didn't dare to ask. I felt like all the babies in the other incubators were *huge,* but when I asked if they had started as small as mine, I was given vague answers.

"Mothers on recliners were holding babies or pumping; grandmas were smiling and cooing. It seemed that all the fully grown humans I could see were acclimatized and comfortable. No one was in the same state of stress, despair, and shock that I was in. I felt like an unassimilated alien, and surrounded by all the Isolettes, I was the one feeling utterly isolated. By Day 4, it was apparent that Armand was a special kind of preemie. He

(*continued*)

(*continued*)

hit many milestones early. He was strong. Our strong, tiny, baby miracle. I was so proud of him and would allow myself to catch glimpse of hope that he would make it and come home. We named him 'Armand Cyprien Williams.' This way, he would know his guardian angel by name.

"I poured all my positive energy into my little warrior. I loved him so ferociously. Cyprien's ashes were in a heart-shaped urn inside Armand's incubator. It made me feel good to see my boys together, and I believed it gave Armand strength. I needed to believe a lot of things to survive. I didn't care if it was real or not. I taped a picture of our family in Armand's area. I wanted him to feel that he was part of our strong tribe, but most of all, I wanted the nurses and doctors to see him as a member of a family. That was so important for me to know that those who cared for him saw him as a full-fledged human being with parents and siblings rather than just as a patient on a shift. I felt that seeing us all would make them remember him more easily, relate to our family—trauma and dreams—and with that, maybe they would grow to love him.

"I was on unpaid extended maternity leave and spent 8 hours a day in the NICU. I was dropping our three kids off at day care and spending the day with Armand. Life was entirely scheduled and all consuming. I lived hour by hour in the NICU as a caretaker and in a construction site back in our home with no gas or water. I didn't care. I lived for kangaroo care.

"Milk did not come easy; I pumped for hours on end. My lactation consultant Kathy was a godsend. I really struggled with my pumping schedule on top of everything else. She had seen me with breasts bigger than my head when I was engorged, brought me cabbage leaves, and helped me through mastitis day after day. I could share everything with her. She was my lactation confidante.

"There was absolutely zero time for self-care for me, and if I did take 30 minutes to eat in the cafeteria, I felt guilty. All my time was spent caring for my children. I desperately needed to feel that everyone *loved* my son and would care for him like I would if I could. I wanted him to be surrounded by love, and until I felt that, I couldn't leave his side and feel at peace. My nurses Ruby, Audrey, Rachel, Jenni, and Joy took turns caring for and loving on him.

"Each time a new nurse was a bit rough (or perceived rough), I felt like they were hitting me. I felt every discomfort as if it was done to my body. I tried not to comment or ask for anything as I didn't want to be the annoying mom and aggravate them. I cried every night but in the NICU, I was strong. I was Armand's advocate, and advocates don't cry. Soldiers don't cry.

"Here I was, day in and day out, with all the ups and downs other parents have described in the other stories, the roller coaster of bad blood gases, surgeries, coding, resuscitations, and so on. There were the good days where I felt almost high on hope—and bad days when I was in despair, gasping for air. Hyperventilating happened a few times. We had some big scares.

"By Day 74, we finally started talking about 'when Armand goes home.' The delicious word *home*. I had never heard that word in one sentence with 'Armand' before and that was

(*continued*)

(continued)

music to my ears. It gave me so much hope. Two days after that, at 76 days old, Armand took an unexpected turn for the worse. All his levels were out of whack. Everything that needed to rise, dropped, and everything that needed to drop, rose. All attempts to stabilize him failed. He was given blood, platelets, blood pressure medication, insulin, morphine, and 100% oxygen. We could not support him enough. Armand's spirit was still strong but his body was failing. Mark and I held his hand on both sides of the bed. He was showing us he wanted us right there by refusing to close his eyes and doing slightly better when we were around, so we stood by his side every minute. We sang, hummed, and talked to him out loud while praying in our heads. He was incredibly alert for being on so many drugs. I started to sing religious hymns through my tears. The nuns of my youth would be proud.

"Both Mark and I were dropping big tears all over his bed. He didn't want to go to sleep. The doctors and nurses were puzzled as to how he could still have his eyes open and connect. His stare was very intense. We didn't know what to do for him. The priest and chaplain came, and I prayed with them. I was begging God to intervene. The harpist who had been part of our 77-day stay also came to play for him. Armand loved it when she played, but this time, over the loud noises of his oscillator, he could not hear her. We conferred with all the professionals around us, trying to figure out how best to care for him, how best to help him. We talked to the doctors and surgeon, the nurses, and therapist. We reached out to anyone for input/advice/guidance—anything, from anyone. It was utter desperation.

"We were seeing more pain on his face, and he was maxed out on morphine as it was, lowering his blood pressure too much. We understood that there was really nothing medically that could be done, so we decided to ask Armand to help us help him. He had given us such strong responses and eye contact for the entire day. He had even reached for Mark's face with pleading eyes. We knew he could talk to us. We knew he had a say in this. So we asked him.

"We told him we were so proud of him and that we loved him beyond this body, beyond life. I asked him to open his eyes really big if he needed us to take him off all the support and let him rest. He opened his eyes really big. Maybe a burst of pain, maybe a response, but he did, and we felt we knew what to do.

"The doctors and nurses were still trying to do things to help him and support him. It was so busy around his bed. More drugs were being ordered, blood was ready to be drawn, and someone was preparing to add more things to the IV in his head. I felt like we had instructed them to stop, but I guess it was not official enough, so I gathered the last bit of strength I had in me and said: 'We want to discontinue support.' It took everything out of me to say those words. My last heroic act as his mother. And with these words, my world collapsed.

"The privacy screen showed up and surrounded us immediately, leaving a 2-foot radius around his bed. The world was shrinking, the walls were literally closing in. I was suffocating and started to have a panic attack. By the grace of God (and cell phones), Nurse Ruby and Kathy magically appeared and joined Audrey who was our nurse on this

(continued)

(continued)

final shift. Audrey and Ruby really had been part of 'Armand's Army' and supported him for 77 days. Now they were the ones disconnecting him from life support. I felt that even though the machine stopped, the love and respect was continuing to flow from them to him. That was so important for me to feel.

"First the monitor went dark, then the humming of the ventilator stopped, and all went silent. Until I heard this primal and cavernous sound. I didn't understand immediately what it was and that it was coming out of me. I was wailing in a way I had never heard myself or anyone before. It came from the pit of my stomach. It was controlled by instinct. It was the sound of despair. I collapsed and was lifted to a chair. It was like the floor opened up to swallow me whole. All the adrenaline that had held me up for 77 days vanished, and I became a shell. I was empty. I had no strength and temporarily no purpose. I picked myself up because I wanted to be present for Armand while he was still alive and give him the mom he deserved. Once again, I feel like I was spiritually lifted to be able to be present.

"Armand was free; they wrapped him and handed him to Mark. We were ushered in hush-hush ways to a little private room out of the way. I felt so bad for any families in the NICU who witnessed us that day and accidentally got a vision of the dreaded nightmare scenario.

"Once in the room, I rested Armand's head on my bare skin. He felt so good and finally closed his eyes. I swear he smiled a bit. After a few minutes, Audrey listened to his heart. It was still beating. I asked to listen for it with the stethoscope and heard a sad slow, peaceful beautiful and barely audible beat. 'Pom … pom … pom … pom.' I sensed an irrational hope building up and imagined that it would turn into a 'pom-pom' … 'pom-pom' … 'pom-pom' … 'pom-pom' … 'pom-pom.'

"I had fantasies that the heartbeat would be back, strong, that Armand would suddenly move and start crying. He was so perfect. How could he be dying?

"After 10 minutes, Audrey listened again and declared time of death. I continued to bargain with God for several minutes, asking for the ultimate miracle. I felt guilty for bargaining, seeing the disapproving faces of nuns. I couldn't stop squeezing his body and kissing him. I was making up for lost time. I rocked him, talked to him. I kissed his head over and over again. Mark and I cried over him, told him everything we wanted to tell him. It was sad but peaceful. We felt we had followed through and honored him. I even felt proud that we did that.

"Audrey took pictures of us. We brought a heater so his body would not get cold so fast because I now knew I could not handle that. I bathed him. It was excruciatingly painful. Mark wanted him to have a bath but didn't feel strong enough to do it himself. I did it for him but made it short because it was beyond my capabilities too. I then dressed my clean baby in the same rocket ship striped outfit he was in when he was healthy. He looked so gorgeous and perfect. He looked like Mark, a lot. He was perfect. He is perfect.

"Our NICU team of nurses came in the room. Audrey, Ruby, and Kathy were surrounding us. Others had come in with tears in their eyes and wide-open arms. Everyone was very

(continued)

(*continued*)

supportive. I ran my fingers on Armand's skin, his perfect face. So soft, so peaceful, and his eyes so firmly shut. With our team in the room, Mark and I decided it was time to let him go. We handed him over and thought he would be taken straight out of the NICU and to this place I didn't want to think about.

"We went by his bedside to collect our belonging and stopped. Armand was still there, laying in his bed with the privacy screen around it, all dark, all quiet … all *dead*. So much more dead than 5 minutes before. I wish I had not seen him again like that. When a parent has said goodbye in their own term, they cannot have a surprise sighting.

"All of our stuff was there by his bedside. All the pictures and cool scrapbook pages that the nurse made that had accumulated for two and a half months. All taken down and piled up with everything else … all there, with our dead baby, it was the saddest sight. I cry every time I think of it. I wrapped Armand in his quilt, gave him a last kiss, and walked away. I never saw him again but in my dreams.

"I felt evicted. Nicely evicted by a landlord who deeply cares but still needs to kick you out, because you no longer belong or qualify.

"We left the unit walking by busy, crying nurses and others oblivious to the tragedy. We hugged, we kissed. It was horribly sad yet comforting to see so much sadness. At least it matched how we felt. Our cocoon was feeling with us. Our tribe was vibing with us. My legs were shaking. Mark held me in his strong arms. I could not believe how sad it was that this was our last walk out of there.

"No balloons or ceremony for those who leave without a baby. All I had was a baby in the morgue and Cyprien's ashes in my pocket. That is as close to 'walking out with a baby' as it got. How sad can this be? *Why?* Why us? Why me? I wish a nurse had walked out with us all the way to the car. Going through these doors for the last time was simply the hardest walk out of anything and anywhere ever.

"Two days later I asked if I could come back to the NICU with a big basket of treats for the nurses. I got invited back in. Now it was by invitation only. I wanted to thank everyone but mostly I *needed* to go back so I could walk out again. I didn't want that last walk out to be my last memory of this 'temple.' The NICU had shifted from feeling like a cocoon to being a temple. A temple erected in the place where my baby lived his entire life. I have gone back many times since with treats and hugs. I beat the sadness with gratitude and kindness.

"Within days, I also picked up my frozen milk and donated it to a friend who had just adopted a baby boy. It felt good to donate it, yet quite painful, as I was very attached to it. It represented my love and my hopes. Hours and hours and hours of hard work had been 'poured' into those tiny bottles. Literally. Donating my milk was in a desire to make good come out of pain. Within a few weeks, I had partnered with an NGO [nongovernmental organization]and was fundraising to build a NICU in a children's hospital in Ethiopia. I devoted my energy to the cause of helping other babies. I felt that if my sons could not have a legacy, then I needed to be that legacy for them.

(*continued*)

(*continued*)

"Eleven months after Armand died, a little NICU opened in rural Ethiopia with a sign that says, 'In Loving memory of Armand and Cyprien Williams.' I was able to share this with some nurses in the NICU when I went back for the remembrance ceremony. A ceremony held yearly in the basement of the hospital for all the babies who had died that year. It was healing to tell them, and when I registered for my badge at the ceremony, I was handed a card from Nurse Brandy. This was 11 months after that fateful day when I delivered my sons, and she had been my labor and delivery nurse. Rock star Brandy, pillar of strength. I do not know how she knew I would be there that day as we had not kept in touch, but her card meant the world to me.

"I am now 4 years into this grief journey, and my days are mostly joyous. I feel our sons all around us. I cherish memories of my time in the NICU because I choose to focus on remembering the love and the good times more than the pain and trauma. Post-traumatic stress is rearing its ugly face from time to time, but it is manageable.

"There is one more twist to our family story that I want to close with. In January 2016, we found out that our daughter Azalea is a twin!! She was separated from her brother at birth, and he remained in Ethiopia with his grandparents. In January 2018, we headed to Ethiopia to meet him in his village. We hope to have an ongoing relationship and help him thrive and go to school.

"So in the end, miracles do happen. They happened with our adoptions, with Windsor's resuscitation, with the inspiration brought to us by Armand and Cyprien and with this newfound twin brother for Azalea. Miracles are not always what we pray for, but I do get to be a mom of twins in so many ways today. A piece of my heart is in Heaven, but I have learned to live in the present. A sign hangs near our bed, under a shrine I made for Armand and Cyprien, and it says: 'Cherish yesterday, dream tomorrow, live today.' I do all 3.

"Losing a child who never got to meet the outside world and never got to be met by the outside world is a unique loss experience. It is a hidden and invisible kind of loss. There are few pictures parents can share and almost no shared memories to remember fondly with friends and family. It is a very complicated kind of grief and so isolating.

"Because I felt that none of the bereavement support groups locally or online were a good fit for this unique loss, I got inspired to create my own group. First it was for myself, and then it became a healing way to offer a helping hand to other bereaved parents. The group is called Bereaved Mothers of NICU Angels, but we do have a few dads, a few grandmothers, and even a few NICU nurses in it! We are now hundreds from many parts of the United States and abroad. I personally talk to each mom. Every one of them is where I used to be at some point, and some are where I am now (or beyond) and help out. I email, phone, message, or meet with mothers to offer a listening ear and a shoulder to cry on, on a daily basis. At times it feels more like a suicide-prevention helpline, and at other times, we are just proud mothers sharing stories and pictures. The biggest reward is to hear that I eased their isolation and loneliness.

"I have immense gratitude for compassionate medical personnel around the world.

"For all that you are to so many people, Thank you."

RECOMMENDATIONS/SUGGESTIONS FOR BEST PRACTICE

1. Include families as equal members of the care team and allow them to be highly involved in the palliative care decision-making process.

2. Allow families to have as many support people present at the same time during the last hours/minutes of life and at the time that life support is withdrawn.

3. Use in-person and on-site interpreters at all times possible when language barriers exist.

4. Respected and honored religious and cultural rituals.

5. Have a private space for families in the NICU to be with their child as their child passes, or offer to allow them to take their infant to a place where they feel comfortable.

6. Empower families to be the primary care providers during the time of transition from life to death and during the bereavement care process.

7. Staff needs to provide encouraging words to families highlighting their positive parenting skills and decisions.

8. Highly encourage bereavement photography, which should be available to all families.

9. Have a high-quality digital camera on the unit so that photographs can be captured at any time and in the event a professional service cannot be present.

10. Have a comprehensive bereavement program that all neonatal staff are competent and comfortable following.

11. Use the Preshand boxes to transport and store infant bodies.

12. Never leave the deceased infant alone.

13. Prepare families for what to expect after the death of an infant.

14. Have layered levels of psychosocial support available for families. This may include bedside nursing, social work, and chaplain support, as well as unit staff psychologists.

15. Have resources, such as social workers, available to assist families with funeral home arrangements.

16. Provide grief and loss resources, both locally and online, for families.

17. Provide keepsake items and mementos for families.

18. Provide lactation support to mothers who are breastfeeding and/or pumping to assist with lactation weaning or breast milk donation.

19. Send a condolence card, signed by all the care team members who cared for the family during their child's life, to the family 1 to 2 weeks after the patient's death.

RECOMMENDED RESOURCES

Remarkable resources are available to both staff and families to help support the process of loss during the neonatal period (Figure 14.1).

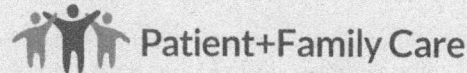
Patient+Family Care

Websites:
1. https://www.nowilaymedowntosleep.org
2. http://www.perinatalhospice.org
3. https://www.projectsweetpeas.com/bereavement-support.html
4. http://www.zoerose.org
5. http://connected4ever.org
6. http://www.october15th.com
7. https://www.mend.org
8. https://www.compassionatefriends.org
9. http://www.heavenlyangelsinneed.com
10. http://www.twinlesstwins.org
11. http://www.handonline.org
12. http://www.journeyofhearts.org
13. http://www.hopeafterloss.org
14. http://www.labelledame.com/infantlossjewelry
15. http://nationalshare.org
16. http://www.3hopefulhearts.com
17. http://www.copefoundation.org

Books:
1. *Grieving the Child I Never Knew: A Devotional for Comfort in the Loss of Your Unborn or Newly Born Child* by Kathey Wiennenberg
2. *Waiting with Gabriel: A Story of Cherishing a Baby's Brief Life* by Amy Kuebelbeck
3. *Angel Baby: A Journal of Healing After the Loss of an Unborn, Born Still, or Newborn Child* by Carey Knifong
4. *Given in Love But Not Mine to Keep: Finding Strength in the Loss of a Newborn Child* by Jan Wolfe Rosales
5. *Shattered: Surviving the Loss of a Child* by Gary Rose
6. *Little One Lost: Living with Early Infant Loss* by Glenda Mathes
7. *Love and Loss: A Guide to Family Healing After the Loss of Your Baby* by Karen Shipp
8. *Seasons of Change: Life Lessons in Grief and Loss* by Kenneth Fallin

Figure 14.1 ■ Recommended resources for supporting families that experience loss in the neonatal period.

Case-Based Learning

S.P. is a 32-year-old primigravida whose fetus has been diagnosed with trisomy 13. In preparation for the birth of her child with a limited life span, she and her partner have met with the genetic counselor, perinatal clinical specialist, and palliative care team to prepare a care plan for their son, whom they have chosen to name Carter.

(continued)

(continued)

QUESTION

1. What are some of the components that you might expect in this family's care plan?

ANSWER

The goal of palliative care is to prevent, treat (as much as possible), and provide support for (as early as possible) the pain, symptoms, and incumbent emotional distress related to life-limiting conditions. Palliative care is about putting quality into the time one has left. A palliative care team provides an extra layer of support to the family and the bedside care team by drawing on the evidence for best practices in this arena. Unfortunately, death sometimes arrives in close proximity to birth. Fortunately, there is a rapidly developing body of knowledge on this topic.

The care plan for a baby with trisomy 13 can be difficult because the immediate outcome is unknown. Perinatal demise is not uncommon, and there is unpredictability about the length of the expected lifetime.

Often, palliative care is involved to help bridge the unknown in preparation for the potential outcomes. One of the most important things that a palliative care consult can provide is a plan for the care of the baby and family. It is important for all team members to be on the same page to provide a consistent approach to care. A documented care plan goes a long way toward this end. Integration with bereavement and grief support is also a benefit of palliative care (Kenner et al., 2015; Parravicini, 2017).

This family will need ongoing information, privacy, unobtrusive emotional support, and possibly, home hospice care. The planning should encompass siblings, grandparents, and other people the parents designate.

Since this family will experience an expected loss, anticipatory guidance regarding the care and grieving process can be provided. Planning will likely include the following:

1. Labor and delivery planning such as whether there will be fetal monitoring of the fetus or C-section for fetal distress

2. The baby's expected appearance and experience

3. Comfort measures and the family's desires for participation in care

4. Identified psychosocial support systems (including peer-to peer)

5. Bereavement rituals—their own, as well as the NICU's

6. Home follow-up: hospice as needed, NICU staff contact

7. Clinical follow-up such as autopsy results

REFERENCES

Palliative care team members have an amazing skill set. It is likely that we could all benefit from a rotation with the palliative care team, as suggested by Henner and Boss (2017).

(continued)

(continued)

Henner, N., & Boss, R. D. (2017). Neonatologist training in communication and palliative care. *Seminars in Perinatology, 41*(2), 106–110. doi: 10.1053/j.semperi.2016.11.003

Kenner, C., Press, J., & Ryan, D. (2015). Recommendations for palliative and bereavement care in the NICU: A family-centered integrative approach. *Journal of Perinatology, 35*(Suppl. 1), S19–S23. doi:10.1038/jp.2015.145

Parravicini, E. (2017). Neonatal palliative care. *Current Opinion in Pediatrics, 29*(2), 135–140. doi: 10.1097/MOP.0000000000000464

REFERENCES

Catlin, A., Brandon, D., Wool, C., & Mendes, J. (2015). Palliative and end-of-life care for newborns and infants. *Advances in Neonatal Care, 15*(4), 239–240. doi:10.1097/anc.0000000000000215

Dighe, M., Manerkar, S., Muckaden, M., & Duraisamy, B. (2011). Is there a role of palliative care in the neonatal intensive care unit in India? *Indian Journal of Palliative Care, 17*(2), 104. doi:10.4103/0973-1075.84530

Eden, L. M., & Callister, L. C. (2010). Parent involvement in end-of-life care and decision making in the newborn intensive care unit: An integrative review. *Journal of Perinatal Education, 19*(1), 29–39. doi:10.1624/105812410x481546

Kenner, C., Press, J., & Ryan, D. (2015). Recommendations for palliative and bereavement care in the NICU: A family-centered integrative approach. *Journal of Perinatology, 35*(Suppl. 1), S19–S23. doi:10.1038/jp.2015.145

Services for Families. (n.d.). Retrieved from https://www.nowilaymedowntosleep.org/families/services-for-families

van Aerde, J., Gorodzinsky, F. P., Canadian Paediatric Society, & Fetus and Newborn Committee. (2001). Guidelines for health care professionals supporting families experiencing a perinatal loss. *Paediatrics and Child Health, 6*(7), 469–477. doi:10.1093/pch/6.7.469

15

SUPPORTING STAFF AND SELF-CARE AFTER A PATIENT LOSS

Neonatal care providers face the daily challenge of caring for and working with intensively ill patients and their families. Each day, staff reports for a shift, during which they are responsible for achieving optimal outcomes for their patients by providing state-of-the-art medical care requiring meticulous attention to detail and very thorough assessments. Staff manages this critical role on top of having to provide physical, spiritual, and emotional care to families at highly emotional and stressful times in their lives. The dual role of providing both exceptional medical care and psychosocial support at such a high standard is a difficult task, and staff often have to accomplish this in spite of overwhelming workloads, heavy assignments, long shifts, growing lists of regulatory requirements they must meet, electronic medical record check boxes that need to be completed, and ongoing best practice guidelines they need to remain up-to-date with and adapt practices to. Nursing in the NICU is a difficult and demanding job and one that requires resilience if one is to sustain in the field without experiencing compassion fatigue or burnout.

With an already stressful job, adding the responsibility of caring for a family that experiences the loss of their child adds to the level of stress that nurses endure. Not only does the added intensity of the situation add weight to the nurses' shoulders, but it also can cause the care provider to experience personal grief, which often goes undersupported. Neonatal providers should be well educated on how to support families who face a neonatal loss and on how to care for themselves when they, or a colleague, experience the loss of a patient. "Literature indicates that nurses experience stress and moral discomfort in the provision of end-of-life and bereavement care [and] ethical issues related to withdrawal of treatment and futile treatments are major contributors to nursing stress" (Zhang & Lane, 2013, p. 2). "Caring for the dying takes a physical and emotional toll on caregivers" (Kobler, 2014, "Article Content" section), and ongoing stress, if not properly managed, can impact the care that a nurse provides to families.

Prior to caring for families who experience the loss of a child, it is important that nurses learn how to support those who have to face the challenges of losing a child, know how to identify and recognize their own grief, practice regular self-care practices, and adequately support their colleagues during times of tragedy and grief in the unit.

Together, these components help reduce the incidence of compassion fatigue and burnout among caregivers and ensure that staff has the infrastructure to have longevity in their career specialty.

PREPARING STAFF TO CARE FOR FAMILIES WHO EXPERIENCE LOSS

"Nurses need to be knowledgeable about bereavement and end-of-life issues and need to be comfortable in their interactions in order to provide quality bereavement and end of life care" (Zhang & Lane, 2013, "Introduction" section). Often, in general nursing school curriculums, limited education is provided on supporting bereaved family members, if it is provided at all. If nurses are lucky, when they are hired into a job, they have mentors who are comfortable and effective in their interactions with families during palliative and bereavement care. However, there is rarely intentional education and mentoring surrounding supporting the bereaved family because the education usually is focused more on how to perform postmortem care of an infant and how to prepare keepsake mementos for families. If nurses witness palliative and bereavement care being provided to a family by a nurse who may not be as effective or supportive, then younger and newer NICU nurses have no other example to learn from and may never get the opportunity to witness great psychosocial support in the end-of-life period.

"Several studies have shown that both nurses and physicians feel ill-prepared to have conversations with families regarding end-of-life issues" (Kenner, Press, & Ryan, 2015, "Staff Education" section). Therefore, units should provide purposeful education for staff on how to communicate and support families and then extend that education on how to provide care for the self in times of loss and grief. There are numerous, and very effective, educational opportunities for NICU professionals, that have been shown to be effective and beneficial to increase a staff member's confidence in caring for families in times of loss.

One nationally recognized educational program is Resolve Through Sharing. This program provides a relationship-based approach to neonatal bereavement care that helps develop a staff member's knowledge, skill level, and personal awareness for providing end-of-life care to patients and their families. Their course provides an opportunity for class participants to learn techniques to help reduce fear and uncertainty about what to say in times of death and loss, reduce compassion fatigue, and reduce feelings of being overwhelmed. Their program is comprehensive in its ability to educate the student on how to care for the patient and for self.

A second educational opportunity is through My NICU Network, which offers a credit course (1.0 continuing education units [CEUs]) on bereavement and palliative care and a credit course (1.0 CEU) on caring for staff as they care for families. These courses were uniquely developed in a collaboration with NICU professionals and NICU graduate families. The aim of this collaborative was to ensure that the NICU family voice was at the forefront of the creation, development, and ongoing assessment of the courses to ensure that class participants hear and understand how their care truly impacts the patients they serve. The course is cofacilitated by a NICU nurse and a NICU graduate parent to foster engaging discussion and thought-provoking dialogue.

A third educational program is Education in Palliative and End of Life Care (EPEC), offered by Feinberg School of Medicine. The vision of their educational program is to prepare healthcare professionals of all varieties to be able to provide all patients with the primary palliative care they need by receiving the essential clinical competencies of palliative and end-of-life care. EPEC's core curriculum was developed in 1997 and has developed over the years to now include population-based adaptations to expand their scope into other areas of illness and specialty.

A fourth recommended educational program, is the End-of-Life Nursing Education Consortium (ELNEC), which is a project supported by the American Association of Colleges of Nursing in partnership with the Hospice and Palliative Nurses Association. ELNEC's education initiative is to provide professionals who care for palliative care patients with the essential information they need to be prepared to improve palliative care both within the United States and internationally. The pediatric module was created by 20 pediatric palliative care experts and launched in 2003. Every year, a minimum of three national training courses are offered within the United States and cover both perinatal and neonatal content.

SELF-CARE PRACTICES

Caring for patients and families is only one component of the equation for successfully providing optimal palliative and bereavement care. The other component is knowing how to care for oneself after a loss in the neonatal unit. Grief and its impact on staff is part of daily healthcare practice. As far as NICU professionals are concerned, they may grieve either of the following:

- A sudden loss of a baby and not understand the reasons why the team was unable to maintain life
- A loss of a long-term patient who they grew attached to and formed a meaningful relationship with
- A loss of having to discharge a family home, knowing they are leaving empty-handed and they won't be returning to the unit the next day

Staff members react to grief in their own unique ways and need to work through and deal with their grief in a way that suits their own personalities and belief systems. Every staff member should be respected, supported, and acknowledged by both NICU administration and by one another when they are suffering from a loss.

Administrators can, and always should, support staff who experience a loss of a patient. This safeguards staff emotional and physical health. Leadership can support staff in many ways and need to individualize the support based on how individuals need to be supported based on personal and spiritual needs. One way that department leaders can support staff is by being present in the unit during times of patient demises. The leaders do not need to participate in care of the patient and family but can be present to support the staff with anything it is they may need. It may help to order food for the staff if the team looks as though it may not be able to leave the family's side for quite some time. It can be helpful to fill water bottles to remind staff to stay hydrated. Running to get supplies so that staff can remain with the family can be incredibly helpful. Just being a support for the staff has been shown to be incredibly appreciated and valued. In addition, leadership can provide time off in between shifts, which will encourage staff to participate in self-care rituals and get plenty of rest before needing to return to work to care for other families. They also can provide flexibility in staff schedules to be able to attend funerals or memorial services, which will allow formal opportunities for staff members to remember babies who have passed away. Last, administrators can schedule and coordinate unit debriefing sessions for staff, which are "specifically aimed at providing emotional support and increasing one's ability to manage grief [in a structured format]" (Keene, Hutton, Hall, & Rushton, 2010, para. 2). A unit's embedded psychologist or the attending neonatologist can facilitate debriefing sessions (Figure 15.1), and the goal of these "facilitated gatherings [is] to process shared experiences of a sudden patient death [to provide] a unique avenue for caregiver validation, support and restoration" (Kobler, 2014, "Team Processing" section).

www.support4NICUparents.org

A GUIDE TO DEBRIEFING SESSIONS IN THE NICU

FOR THE PURPOSES OF STAFF SUPPORT

Sometimes when we have a particularly difficult case, providing care to baby and family can be distressing and/or discouraging, leaving us drained or upset because of our unresolved questions and emotions. It may be hard for us as staff to go forward after such a case, whether or not it resulted in the baby's death. The purpose of this type of debriefing is for everyone involved to have a chance to process their emotions, ask and answer questions related to the situation, give each other feedback, acknowledge the challenges we faced as a community, and provide support to each other. We may also find out things we could have done better.

Who should be a facilitator? (There are many choices.)
• Preferably a mental health professional (psychologist, social worker)
• A NICU medical director
• A neonatologist on service at the time of the baby's death or problematic issue
• Someone from the palliative care team

Who should attend?
• Any staff mental health professionals
• All staff involved in baby's care, from all disciplines, especially those involved in the event being discussed such as a death
• Someone from chaplain service and someone from palliative care, if appropriate

When should it be held?
• This type of debriefing should be held within a week or two after the patient's death (or other issue being discussed). This gives staff a chance to give the family and their patient care

Figure 15.1 ■ A guide to debriefing sessions in the NICU.

responsibilities their full attention at the time of the incident, and then collect their thoughts afterward while not under the immediate stress of the situation.
- It should be held when the maximum amount of involved staff can participate.

Welcome and introduction
- Review purpose of debriefing session.
- Invite participants to give names and answer the question, "How were you involved in care for this patient and family?"

Factual information
- Review time of death circumstances.
- How long was the patient ill before death?
- Was death expected or unexpected?

Case review
- What was it like taking care of this patient?
- What was the most distressing aspect of the case?
- What was the most satisfying aspect of the case?

Grief responses
- What have you experienced since the death? (Elicit physical, emotional, behavioral, cognitive, or spiritual responses.)

Emotional responses
- What will you remember most about this patient/family?

Strategies for coping
- How are you taking care of yourself so that you can continue to provide care for other patients and families?
- Provide grief coping strategies.
- Provide available resources.

Lessons learned
- What lessons did we learn from caring for this patient/family?

Conclusion
- Acknowledge care provided.
- Provide bereavement support available for families and staff.

It's important to remember that team leaders and debriefing facilitators will also experience the emotions of grief, guilt, pain, and sadness no matter how many times we have had a patient die. We need to look out for each other and help each other cope with these emotions.

Source: Adapted from Keene, E. A., Hutton, N., Hall, B., & Rushton, C. (2010). Bereavement debriefing sessions: An intervention to support health care professionals in managing their grief after the death of a patient. *Pediatric Nursing, 36*(4), 185–189.

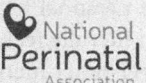

Figure 15.1 ■ A guide to debriefing sessions in the NICU. (*continued*)

When it comes to staff caring for themselves, they need to take time when they are grieving to participate in self-care practices that feel most beneficial to them. They need to provide themselves with self-nurturing thoughts, attitudes, and habits. Some examples of self-care practices that may be constructive include, but are certainly not limited to, the following:

- *Relaxation therapies*: Yoga, meditation, hot baths, and guided imagery are all examples of relaxation therapies that can help reduce stress symptoms when staff need to find respite from grief and loss. These techniques "will not only [help] reduce physical suffering, but will give [one's] mind a place to rest" (Stang, 2017, para. 2).

- *Humor*: Laughing and finding ways to find humor in things can reduce stress and anxiety. In fact, "the good feeling that you get when you laugh remains with you even after the laughter subsides. Humor helps you keep a positive, optimistic outlook through difficult situations, disappointments, and loss" (Robinson, Melinda, & Segal, 2018).

- *Journaling*: "Journaling is a tried and true coping tool for exploring grief, as well as other complicated emotions" ("Grief Journals," 2017, para. 1). Sitting down and writing about the emotions and feelings about the loss experienced can provide the opportunity to reflect and attempt to understand actions, moods, and behaviors toward the experience. Sometimes, writing a letter to the one lost can be beneficial.

- *Exercise*: Grief and sadness can cause many physical ailments and symptoms, and exercise is a way to help reduce those symptoms. In addition, exercise "is one of the most effective prevention and treatment strategies for depression" (Mercola, 2014, para. 8). Walking, biking, hiking, swimming, yoga, dance, or any other form of healthy movement that gets the heart rate moving will be beneficial for self-care.

- *Praying or drawing strength from spiritual beliefs*: Everyone has a personal spiritual and/or cultural background and beliefs that impact how death, dying, and the afterlife are viewed and how honoring the deceased should be done. Many are able to find comfort and strength from their spiritual beliefs and spiritual communities, and "[t]he path to spiritual wellness may involve meditation, prayer, affirmations, or specific spiritual practices that support [one's] connection to a higher power or belief system" (University of California, Riverside, n.d., para. 5).

- *Talking with coworkers*: Even though it may feel uncomfortable to share thoughts and feelings with others, just saying emotions out loud can have many benefits. Not only does it help someone start to make more sense of personal feelings, but it also allows one's "muscles [to] relax a bit, and [one] can literally feel like a weight has been lifted. Feeling good physically makes [one] feel better mentally" ("Benefits of Talking," n.d., para. 9).

HONORING MEMORIES OF PATIENTS AND THEIR FAMILIES

Many NICU staff members want to find ways to honor the memories of patients who were lost either in the care of the NICU, sent home on hospice, or passed away from complications of prematurity sometime after leaving the neonatal unit. Staff tends to become bonded with patients and families, and especially with longer-term patients, staff can become deeply affected by the loss of these young patients.

There are numerous ways to honor the memories of patients and families, both individually and as units. Individually, nurses can attend funeral or memorial services or write cards of condolences to the family. As a unit, there are even more ways to honor the lives of past patients. Some ideas include, but are not limited to, the following:

- *Moments of silence*: Staff can hold a moment of silence for the patient and family at a staff meeting, or another gathering.

- *Remembrance celebrations*: Staff can host an annual remembrance celebration in which families who have lost a child are invited back to the unit to be with staff; together, they celebrate the lives and memories of the precious little lives they all cared for together. Candles can be lit during this celebration, small pieces of memorial jewelry can be gifted to parents, or memorial plaques can be given with names engraved as a memento for families.

- *Memorial walls/plaques*: A wall, plaque, or even stones that line a walkway can have names of deceased patients engraved on them as a way to memorialize them. Some units call these "Angel Walls" or "Always Remember Plaques." When staff walks by them, it affords them the opportunity to stop and remember the precious little ones that had to leave this earth too soon.

- *Remembrance walks*: Organizing a walk annually where families walk in memory of their child is a great way to bring families together and can often be in conjunction with a local grief support group. Some grief groups decide to combine a remembrance walk with their local March for Babies event and dedicate a section of the walk to Angel Babies to honor all of the babies the March of Dimes is working so tirelessly at trying to save through their fundraising efforts.

- *Ornaments*: A way to memorialize and honor patients annually is to write down the names of each patient who passes away every year on their own individual ornament, and decorate a special Angel Babies tree in the NICU with these ornaments. Families can then be invited to come and pick up their ornament before Christmas to place the ornament on their own tree as a gift from the unit, letting them know that the staff will be thinking of them on their first Christmas without their child, or the staff can mail them the ornament if the family does not feel comfortable coming back to the unit.

Author's Personal Story

I was caring for three patients in our level II nursery one night shift and the night was going well. I had completed two rounds of cares and was just getting ready to head out to lunch when the charge nurse informed me she was going to have me change assignments. She shared with me that she wanted me to take over the care of Baby M., who was rapidly declining and was likely going to pass away quickly. My heart dropped.

Baby M. was born to a family I knew well. They had suffered infertility for years and, after the support of in vitro fertilization (IVF), they finally became pregnant with twins and delivered them prematurely a few years prior. Because of their prematurity, they spent time in our unit. C.M. and E.M. delivered a boy and a girl. The little boy didn't survive, but I had the honor of being a primary nurse for their little girl. She spent months in our unit before going home happy and healthy, and the C.M. and E.M. were already looking forward to trying for more children with the assistance of another round of IVF.

C.M. had a successful round of IVF just over 5 months before, and she and her husband were thrilled that they were expecting another set of twins, this time boys. Unfortunately, C.M. went into premature labor at 24 weeks into the pregnancy, and her providers were unable to stop the progression despite their best efforts. That is why she was here this particular day. When I arrived for my shift that day, I saw their name on the master assignment sheet. I knew they were expecting twins, so I knew something wasn't right when I saw only one name on the paper. I learned immediately that several hours after birth, their first son passed away. He was too small and too sick to survive despite respiratory support and medication administration. The second twin however, Baby M., was still alive and stable for the time being. He was ventilated and on many medications to keep him that way, but the fact that he was still alive was a good sign from what we could all tell.

I started the shift with the assignment I had been with the previous two nights for consistency, otherwise I would like to think I would have started out being assigned to Baby M. Halfway through the shift, Baby M. took a turn for the worse. His little body was shutting down despite all of the support the team was providing for him. The neonatologist went to C.M.'s room to let her know what was happening, and she was quickly wheeled into the room in a wheelchair. After having a cesarean section, she wasn't able to move very well, so she needed some assistance from her postpartum nurse to get out of bed and situated in the unit. She called her husband, but he was home with their daughter, and they did not feel that it would be good to wake her in the middle of the night to bring her into the hospital to witness the passing of her baby brother. So C.M. was going to be facing withdrawing life support of her second son that night all on her own.

Because I knew C.M. so well, and had such an established relationship with her, the charge nurse felt it would be best for C.M. if I were the one caring for her and Baby M. for the remainder of the shift. She also shared with me much later that another reason she reassigned me that night was that she felt I had a gift for caring for babies and families

(continued)

(*continued*)

who were facing end-of-life care. I chuckled a little because some nurses had actually mocked me for some of my practices in the past. For example, before I took infants down to the morgue, I would make sure they would have hats on, and be wrapped in blankets. Nurses would laugh and say, "You know it doesn't matter, right?" But to me, it did. I also would talk to the infants when I would perform care and explain everything I was doing. Again, some of the nurses would tell me that I didn't need to do that because it wasn't as if they could hear me or understand what I was saying, so it didn't matter. But to me, it did. I appreciated the charge nurse's sentiment, and more than anything, I was honored to have been with C.M. so that she didn't have to face that grave decision and the devastating ordeal without someone who knew her so well.

I quickly gave report to another nurse and then went up to meet with C.M. As soon as our eyes met, she burst into tears. I walked closer over to her and she reached her arms out to give me a hug. It seemed like eternity before she let go. She just needed to have someone's shoulder to cry on and let out her devastation. It was so intense that I could feel it pouring from every inch of her being and it was pouring into me. I was not a mother yet myself, but, at that moment, I felt her emotions, and think I could feel the level of pain she felt for losing her child. I remember being so overwhelmed by sadness, grief, and ruin. I felt as though I could crumble to the floor beside her and be swallowed by the anguish right along with her. Yet, I wanted to be strong for her and be the support she desperately needed. I held my emotions within and with only small tears in my eyes, I talked with C.M. and explained to her everything that she could choose to do and when. Unfortunately, Baby M. was slipping away quickly, so we didn't have much time. She was able to voice that she just wanted to hold him, so the team and I worked quickly to make that happen.

As we untangled wires, lines, and tubing, I remember looking at this beautiful baby boy and thinking it just wasn't fair. He was so wanted and so loved by such an incredible family. Why did this have to happen? And why did it have to happen to the same family that already had suffered such insurmountable loss? I then looked over at C.M., who looked pale, weak, and exhausted. I handed her the precious little boy and she just held him close to her chest. As I turned off all of the machines and turned back around, a sad reality hit me at that point. I wanted to start to explain to her what she could expect as Baby M.'s body would transition from life to death; but I didn't have to. She had been through that exact process mere hours before. Instead, I wrapped a warm blanket around the two of them, pulled up a chair, and just sat quietly next to C.M. with my hand on her shoulder.

From time to time C.M. would reach over and grab my hand, as if she wanted to make sure she was still not there alone, and I would reassure her I was right there. It took Baby M. 45 minutes to pass away after he was removed from life support, and it honestly felt like hours. The minutes ticked by slowly as we wondered if each heart beat would be his last. Yet, Baby M., was so peaceful and comfortable on his mother's chest, and as each minute passed, C.M. also became calmer. It was as if her heartbeat slowed with his. It was one

(*continued*)

(*continued*)

of the most heartbreaking moments I had witnessed up to that point in my career, yet it was also one of the most beautiful. C.M. comforted her son with such beauty and such grace when her entire world was falling apart. The strength I saw that night, strength that only a mother could muster when her child needed her the most, was so awe inspiring. I remember looking at her, and the pale, weak, and exhausted woman who entered the unit now looked rested, had color to her skin, and even had a slight glow to her. The change wasn't from joy by any means, but I believe it was from the love she shared with her son in those last moments.

After Baby M. passed, and C.M. was ready to put him back to bed, she made the decision to wait and bathe him, dress him, and perform other cares until her husband could return later on. I assured her I would stay with Baby M. until my shift was over and he would be there in the same bed waiting for her and her husband when they were ready to come back. We exchanged another long hug, and she was wheeled back to her room. I sat with Baby M. the rest of the shift, as promised, but I was numb and emotionless the rest of the night.

I don't remember my drive home that day and I don't remember how long it was until I finally fell asleep. I just remember that I went home and crawled into bed and lay there with an image of that sweet baby cradled in his mom's arms stuck in my head for hours. I was angry and confused and sad that Baby M. and his brother had died. It wasn't fair. How could that have happened? Why couldn't they have stopped her labor with all of the technology and medications they have today? Why couldn't we save the babies in the NICU with all of the technologies and medications we have? Did we miss something? It just wasn't right. I did eventually fall asleep and slept for a very long time.

I woke up groggy and still distressed. I recognized that I was experiencing my own grief and was going to need to take care of myself on my few days off before returning to work for a 4-day stretch. I made myself a cup of warm tea and then got into a nice hot bubble bath. Baths always help me wind down and relax. I even put on some relaxing music to help distract me from the images still haunting my mind. After my bath, I got myself outdoors and went for a walk. Getting outside and exercising was something I was told would be a healthy and beneficial way to deal with grief. It helped, and when I returned home I took a friend up on an offer to get together for dinner and shopping. While out together, we laughed and had such a nice time, and it turns out it was the distraction I needed to get through the rest of my day. By the time I got home that night, I was able to crawl into bed feeling a little better. I was still sad, hurt, and down about the events that had occurred the night before. Yet I was able to put into perspective that I was given a gift.

I was given the opportunity to know Baby M. for the short amount of time he was with his family here on earth and provide care to him when he needed it the most. I was also given the extreme honor to be beside C.M. as a crutch and a safety net when she was desperate for support and comfort. I was the one that got to witness the abundance

(*continued*)

(continued)

of a mother's love and what a bond between a mother and child can do for someone, even someone facing the worst nightmare of all. I was able to appreciate through my faith that although Baby M. and his brother were no longer here on earth, they were rejoicing above with their older brother and God and would surely watch over their family. I knew that I had done my job as a nurse that shift and provided not only the best medical care I could, but also the psychosocial support the family needed in the most critical time of all.

STAFF STORY

These stories are shared by Erika Bracken Probst, RNC, MSN. Erika is an author and nurse educator. From 2000 to 2016, she worked in a high-risk maternity unit, in a large metropolitan city, where over 5,000 deliveries occurred every year. She is currently a nurse educator and nurse consultant. To learn more about Erika, you can visit http://www .brackenprobstconsulting.com, and you can learn more about her very popular children's book on her active Facebook page at https://www.facebook.com/FriendsonmyStreet.

"I remember their names. Of the thousands of babies who have passed through my arms over the course of my career, the ones who didn't survive are the ones I carry in my heart. I think of them often. I think of their families. I think of the lost hopes and dreams. I attended only one funeral. After that, I knew my heart couldn't handle any more.

"Baby C. was born at term after a normal pregnancy. He was stable and doing well, and all aspects of his assessment were within defined normal limits. At just over 24 hours old, the emergency call light for his room went off, and I and another nurse rushed in. Baby C. was limp and in his grandmother's arms. He appeared to have a bluish color and did not appear to be breathing. We quickly placed him in his crib, opened the cabinet with emergency supplies, and established that there was no respiratory effort or heartbeat. We immediately began neonatal resuscitation. This was the only full neonatal resuscitation I actively participated in the 16 years I worked acute care. I provided respirations with a bag and mask while my teammate provided compressions. One, and two, and three, and breath . . . one, and two, and three, and breath. We got a heartbeat back, but we did not know how long he was without oxygen. The NICU code team arrived quickly, and Baby C. was rushed to NICU. He was intubated and placed on life support. Despite our ability to revive a heartbeat, the EEG showed no brain activity. Two days later, the decision was made to take him off life support. However, his parents were able to give an amazing gift by donating his organs.

"I remember watching Baby C.'s dad walking through the halls of the maternity unit during those 2 days prior to Baby C. being taken off life support. The maternity unit was a 'happy' unit, yet he was in a daze. Shell shocked. We would ask if he needed anything, and his only response was, 'Can you bring my baby back?' I would see him walking and feel

(continued)

(*continued*)

like we had failed him. It felt like a punch to the gut watching him. His son's funeral was the one funeral I attended. It was beautiful, and devastating. I still have the card from the funeral. What was meant to be a birth announcement was turned into an announcement of both the birth and the death of a very loved little boy. Several staff nurses attended the funeral, as having a newborn code at just over a day old was unusual, unexpected and affected us greatly. A seemingly healthy infant having sudden cardiac arrest on a maternity unit is very rare. The ruling was SIDS and that there was nothing that could have been done. We were told that our actions in resuscitation gave the family time to say goodbye, but that didn't help us. We had several debriefs, and those of us first responders had a bond. Sometimes we would just share a look and a nod and know that we were thinking about Baby C.

"Another experience that significantly impacted me was caring for a baby who had passed just prior to delivery. I was asked to perform 'baby support' for Baby Z. Baby support is generally a role in which the baby is assessed, resuscitation need is evaluated, and if the baby is stable, it is weighed, measured, and bathed after delivery. In this case, because the baby was already a known demise, the situation was different. The tasks of weighing, measuring, and bathing would all still need to be done, but there would be no other assessment. Baby Z.'s mother was, understandably, very distraught. Upon delivery, she requested that Baby Z. be taken to a different room so that she did not have to see her bathed. I took Baby Z.'s father and maternal grandfather to another room to measure, weigh, and bathe her. I remember holding her and being as gentle as I could. I talked to her; I let her dad hear me talking. I told her that her mom and dad loved her. I did extra footprints and cut a lock of hair for the family to keep in a remembrance box. And, I cried. I cried in front of Baby Z.'s dad and grandfather. I had asked Baby Z.'s dad if he was really OK being there. His response, through tears, was, 'I said in the birth plan that I wanted to give the first bath. I just can't give her bath, but I want to be here for her.' I told him that we cry too and to know that she would carry on in our memory, not just her family's memory. Over 13 years ago, and I still remember her as clear as day. In this situation, the obstetrician was also very affected by the delivery. We spoke often about Baby Z. Talking helps. It helps make it real, and it helps process the grief. However, those who are not in healthcare and who have not experienced the loss of a patient cannot fully comprehend the grief that is felt by the nurses.

"One of my other losses was a preterm baby in the NICU. Baby H.'s family was Spanish speaking and I had spent time caring for his mother after delivery. We had done a lot of work with the birth certificate and other paperwork, knowing that the likelihood of Baby H. surviving was low. I was off work for a couple of days, and, the day I returned, I was asked to care for the family again, since I had a good relationship with them. However, at this point, the mom had been discharged and she was with Baby H. in the NICU's bereavement room, as life support had just been removed. He was still alive, but his respirations and heart rate were slowing. Throughout the shift, as I cared for my other patients, I would

(*continued*)

(*continued*)

spend as much time as I could with my family in the bereavement room. I checked Baby H.'s heart rate as often as his mother requested, but at least every hour. At about 3:30 a.m., there was no longer a heartbeat. Although we all knew it would happen and expected it to happen, there were still tears with the finality of it. He was gone.

"Neonatal losses became harder emotionally when I became a mother myself. It was never easy, but once I had carried my own babies, the grief of watching a family lose their baby was so much harder. I got it. I understood the love you could feel for your child even before you knew them. And it made it that much more impactful to realize how strong the families experiencing loss were.

"When I reflect back on the many babies (and families of babies) I cared for who did not make it, I often think of how old the children would be now. What would they be like? For me, knowing that I think of them, that they made a difference in my life and made me want to do better and be better, helps me realize that they were impactful. Their families may never know how much they and their babies impacted me. They taught me how to be more compassionate. They showed me such strength in their darkest hours. They were brave. I am a better person because of them. My way of grieving is by honoring and remembering these amazing babies and families. I recognize them for making me a better nurse and person."

RECOMMENDATIONS/SUGGESTIONS FOR BEST PRACTICE

1. Staff need to be provided intentional education on end-of-life, palliative, and bereavement care prior to caring for a family facing losing a child.

2. Staff should be assigned mentors to witness positive examples of psychosocial support during palliative and bereavement care with NICU families.

3. Staff should be encouraged to practice self-care therapies after the loss of a patient and the resultant grief.

4. Department leadership needs to support staff when they are experiencing grief after the loss of a patient.

5. Units should routinely hold debriefings after every patient death that occurs in the unit.

6. Units should determine ways to honor the memory of deceased patients and their families.

RECOMMENDED RESOURCES

Some good resources are available for staff to help support themselves and families after experiencing a loss during the neonatal period (Figure 15.2).

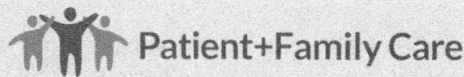
Patient+Family Care

Websites:
1. http://www.gundersenhealth.org/resolve-through-sharing
2. http://www.mynicunetwork.com
3. http://bioethics.northwestern.edu/programs/epec
4. http://www.aacnnursing.org/ELNEC/About/ELNEC-Curricula
5. https://whatsyourgrief.com/course/grief-101-a-primer-for-helping-professionals
6. https://whatsyourgrief.com
7. http://support4nicuparents.org/for-professionals/palliative-and-bereavement-care
8. https://vimeo.com/18714302
9. https://onlinedegrees.bradley.edu/resources/articles/
helping-nurses-come-to-terms-with-patient-deaths-strategies-for-nurse-managers
10. http://www.workingnurse.com/articles/how-nurses-can-grieve-the-loss-of-a
-loved-one-or-special-patient
11. https://griefwatch.com/self-care
12. http://www.hellogrief.org/taking-care-of-yourself-helps-you-grieve
13. https://www.centerforloss.com/2016/12/nurturing-youre-grieving
14. https://tinybuddha.com/blog/
dealing-with-loss-and-grief-be-good-to-yourself-while-you-heal
15. https://psychbc.com/clinical-blog/caring-for-yourself-after-the-death-of-a-patient
16. http://www.usurnsonline.com/grief-loss/grief-self-care-44-tips-for-healing-comfort-peace
17. http://mindfulnessandgrief.com/9-self-care-tips-for-grief
18. https://www.mindbodygreen.com/0-28350/selfcare-strategies-for-healing-from-
heartbreakgrief.html
19. https://www.hrrv.org/patients-caregivers/grief-support/importance-self-care-grief
20. http://drsmoliak.com/self-care-tips.html

Figure 15.2 ■ Recommended resources for staff who experience the loss of a patient.

Case-Based Learning

Refer to the family story in Chapter 14 about baby Simon and his family's experiences while he was dying. His mother is very frank about encounters she had with a couple of the NICU staff that she perceived as extremely negative. She describes these healthcare professionals as cold, lacking empathy, and being insensitive. Their questions were rapid fire, and their responses were emotionless—as if read from a script. They were overly business-like and left her feeling that they were too busy to provide the emotional support she needed.

(continued)

(continued)

QUESTIONS

1. Do you think that the NICU staff was aware of the effect of their words and questions on Simon's mother?
2. What could be affecting the care providers' ability to be empathetic?
3. What kinds of coping mechanisms may be at play in these NICU caregivers?
4. What might be some next steps for this NICU?

ANSWERS

The stress surrounding a baby's death takes an enormous toll, not only on the family, but also on the staff caring for the family. This is called *secondary traumatic stress*, which can lead to compassion fatigue, a condition in which caregivers lose their nurturing ability for their patients, as well as themselves (Beck, Cusson, & Gable, 2017; Coughlin, 2017; Discenza, 2017; Greiner & Poskey, 2017).

NICU staff may be unaware of the risk factors and symptoms and may not even know that they are experiencing compassion fatigue. Taking care of families who are going through the saddest experience of their life can impart feelings of failure and sorrow in care providers. They indirectly suffer trauma by witnessing what their patient's family is going through. They feel loss and internalize the family's grief. Over time, they may begin to lack the ability to support the family and unintentionally come across as callous and impersonal. In spite of this, they may be in denial that they are susceptible to their compassion and empathy being compromised. They may think that they are coping well with the suffering they encounter on a regular basis in the NICU and that they are not vulnerable to the chronic strain that comes with caring for patients with life-threatening illnesses (Beck et al., 2017; Greiner & Poskey, 2017).

Regenerative self-care is invaluable to the caregiver, as well as the patient. Both benefit from the NICU staff's psychological health associated with recognizing and preventing compassion fatigue. Self-care includes rest, nutrition, relaxation, and work–life balance (Discenza, 2017).

Environmental considerations that support healing for patients and positive behaviors in NICU staff include aesthetics, lighting, noise, and space. Noise attenuation and light cycling are part of the design standard for neurodevelopmental care for ill newborns. These conditions also reduce stress in the family and healthcare providers. Exercise rooms, Internet access carrels, and communal gathering areas with kitchens can also help families cope with the trauma of ICU life. Secluded rooms, peaceful gardens, and meditation suites are some further options. In addition, organizational culture is important to employee mental health resilience. Commitment to open communication structures, a culture of safety, proper staffing ratios, team building, and recognition of employee contributions

(continued)

(continued)

are just a few of the ways leadership can support frontline staff (Beck et al., 2017; Coughlin, 2017).

It is incumbent on us all to take care of ourselves to promote authentic, caring relationships with those we care for.

REFERENCES

Beck, C. T., Cusson, R. M., & Gable, R. K. (2017). Secondary traumatic stress in NICU nurses: A mixed-methods study. *Advances in Neonatal Care, 17*(6), 478–488. doi:10.1097/ANC.0000000000000428

Coughlin, M. E. (2017). *Trauma informed care in the NICU: Evidenced-based practice guidelines for neonatal clinicians.* New York, NY: Springer Publishing.

Discenza, D. (2017). "Mental Health" in the NICU: Time to catch up and provide trauma-informed care for families and pros. *Neonatal Network, 36*(5), 318–320. doi:10.1891/0730-0832.36.5.318

Greiner, B. S., & Poskey, G. A. (2017). Fatigue: Has it affected your compassion? *Neonatal Network, 36*(5), 289–293. doi:10.1891/0730-0832.36.5.289

REFERENCES

Benefits of talking to someone: Getting help. (n.d.). *ReachOut.com.* Retrieved from https://ie.reachout.com/getting-help-2/face-to-face-help/things-you-need-to-know/benefits-of-talking-to-someone

Grief Journals: Should picking a grief journal really be this complicated? (2017, March 28). Retrieved from https://whatsyourgrief.com/grief-journal-can-picking-a-grief-journal-really-be-this-hard

Keene, E. A., Hutton, N., Hall, B., & Rushton, C. (2010). Bereavement debriefing sessions: An intervention to support health care professionals in managing their grief after the death of a patient. *Pediatric Nursing, 36*(4), 185–189. Retrieved from https://www.scha.org/files/101615_bereavement_debrief_sessions.pdf

Kenner, C., Press, J., & Ryan, D. (2015). Recommendations for palliative and bereavement care in the NICU: A family-centered integrative approach. *Journal of Perinatology, 35,* S19–S23. doi:10.1038/jp.2015.145

Kobler, K. (2014). Leaning in and holding on. *MCN, The American Journal of Maternal/Child Nursing, 39*(3), 148–154. doi:10.1097/nmc.0000000000000028

Mercola. (2014, June). Sweating out sadness: How exercise can help the grieving process. Retrieved from https://fitness.mercola.com/sites/fitness/archive/2014/06/27/exercise-grief.aspx

Robinson, L., Melinda, S., & Segal, J. (2018, March). Laughter is the best medicine. Retrieved from https://www.helpguide.org/articles/mental-health/laughter-is-the-best-medicine.htm

Stang, P. B. (2017, July 17). Coping with grief in your body: A relaxation exercise. Retrieved from http://mindfulnessandgrief.com/coping-with-grief-relaxation

University of California, Riverside. (n.d.). Spiritual wellness. Retrieved from https://wellness.ucr.edu/spiritual_wellness.html

Zhang, W., & Lane, B. S. (2013). Promoting neonatal staff nurses' comfort and involvement in end of life and bereavement care. *Nursing Research and Practice, 2013,* 1–5. doi:10.1155/2013/365329

VI

THERAPEUTIC STRATEGIES FOR CAREGIVERS AND PATIENTS

16

CARING FOR THE CAREGIVER: HOW TO AVOID BURNOUT

The definition of *burnout* is a "condition of fatigue, detachment and cynicism resulting from prolonged high levels of stress. In the critical care setting, burnout rates may be driven by high workload, frequent changes in technology and guidelines, endeavors for high-quality care and emotional challenge of dealing with critically ill patients and their families" (Tawfik et al., 2016, "Introduction" section). When one thinks of this definition, it is no surprise to hear that burnout rates may affect up to 54% of staff in a NICU (Profit et al., 2014) because the neonatal unit typically is staffed with 12-hour shifts, high-acuity assignments, frequent changes in policies and procedures, changes in electronic medical records, and systems changes with upgrades occurring frequently. The NICU is one of the most stressful units where staff are caring not only for incredibly critically ill patients, but also providing very in-depth psychosocial support for families in crisis on a continual basis.

To prevent burnout, nurses need to place a high priority on caring for themselves. "Nurses are knowledgeable regarding the importance of health-promoting activities such as healthy eating, physical activity, stress management, sleep hygiene, and maintaining healthy relationships" (Ross, Bevans, Brooks, Gibbons, & Wallen, 2017, "Abstract" section), yet too often do not put themselves and their health as a priority. I know, personally speaking, that I am the last one who can say I am a good role model for placing myself as a priority. In fact, I can't count how many times I would stay late on shift to remain with a patient to see a traumatic event through or would pick up extra hours when the unit was short-staffed. I stay up way too late and compromise my own sleep to help get extracurricular work accomplished or finally find the time I need to get housework done because I jam-pack my days with so many other things that I have to wait until I get my kids into bed to do anything around the house. I don't know why I ever question the reasons why I am tired, exhausted, overweight, overwhelmed, and flustered the majority of the time. I don't eat right, I don't make time for exercise, I don't drink enough water, and I certainly don't get enough sleep.

Sadly, I am not alone in my self-destructive habits, and I hear over and over again that nurses are the worst at practicing what they preach. Nurses convey to patients on a daily basis how important self-care practices are, yet do not always do a good job at showing patients how serious they are about it when they don't follow those practices themselves. When it comes to practicing nursing in the neonatal specialty, burnout is found to be highest among "daytime workers and experienced workers" (Tawfik et al., 2016, "Conclusion" section). which is typically the nurses who have been practicing the longest and are likely most knowledgeable and skilled at caring not only for the most critically ill babies but also for families. The nursing profession, NICU patients, and NICU families rely on these nurses not only to provide exceptional care, but also to be an example for the more novice nurses. Organizations need to recognize the real issue of burnout, and all of the stages that lead up to burnout, to help prevent nurses from reaching such a stage in their career and either practicing at a subpar level or leaving all together.

Cheryl Milford, who has been a practicing educational psychologist for over 36 years, has spent the past 34 years providing psychological, neurodevelopmental, and infant mental health services in NICUs and developmental follow-up clinics. Milford has taken a great interest in the topic of caring for the caregiver and has worked closely with physicians, nurses, early intervention professionals, and mental health professionals and has seen firsthand how important caring for the self is in the helping profession. As the Director of Development and Outreach for the National Perinatal Association, Cheryl has been instrumental in helping bring to life the best practice recommendations for psychosocial support of NICU parents come, and she is graciously willing to share her expertise on the topic of caring for the caregiver.

MESSAGE FROM CHERYL MILFORD

It is clear that providing care to neonates, their families, and our coworkers can be stressful and challenging (Cricco-Lizza, 2014; Milford, 2016b). NICU caregivers are exposed to ongoing trauma, pain, and suffering as they engage in their daily practice. This exposure impacts each provider and can have a cumulative effect over time (Coughlin, 2017). Therefore, it is crucial that NICU caregivers understand how work impacts not only their work life, but also their personal life and their attitudes, behaviors, and relationships in both aspects of their lives (Milford, 2016a). We often tell parents that they cannot care for their baby if they do not take care of themselves. This is true for caregivers as well. If they do not have a good work–life balance and practice good self-care, they will not be able to provide the best care to neonates and their families and be a strong team member for their coworkers (Milford, 2016a).

Dedication to their profession and their practice requires caring for themselves and their coworkers to provide optimal care to neonates and families they serve. It really is all about individuals and their mental and physical health (Milford, 2016a).

PATIENT RELATIONSHIPS AND BOUNDARIES

Because of the extended lengths of stay in the NICU, caregivers and family members often develop close relationships. Caregivers learn the family's story and become part of the journey while the baby is hospitalized (Milford, 2016a). Families come to trust their caregivers and depend on their advice and support (Coughlin, 2017). This relationship is the foundation of caring in healthcare professions. Caring is both reducing suffering and pain while moving toward wellness. Because of the intense emotions that occur with suffering and pain, the family perceives the caregiver as an important person in their life, providing healing and comfort (Coughlin, 2017). It is imperative that the caregiver provide an environment that is professional and provides boundaries to support a healthy caregiver–parent relationship (Coughlin, 2017; Milford, 2016a). In a healthy caregiver–parent relationship, caregivers respect the values, emotions, and concerns of the parent in a positive, supportive manner. Sharing of thoughts on the neonate's medical and developmental needs, parent education on care, and supporting parents in their journey are all appropriate topics (Milford, 2016a). Chatting about the weather, local events, and parent support opportunities is also appropriate. Boundaries are crossed when caregivers discuss their personal life in terms of concerns, issues, or difficulties. A relationship between nurses and families is a professional relationship, not a personal one. The boundary can be challenging for parents to understand; however, it is necessary to reduce the risk of emotional harm and role expectations for families and caregivers (Coughlin, 2017; Milford, 2016a). Starting each interaction with a parent by asking how they are (a typical way we greet people) and proceeding from there can facilitate the relationship as one of support and caring while maintaining professionalism. Greeting families with a smile, positive interactions, and conversations; respecting the neonate as a unique individual; and treating the parent as the most important person in the baby's life are keys to happy families and good outcomes (Cozolino, 2014; Sanders & Hall, 2017).

UNDERSTANDING HOW WE RESPOND TO STRESS

We have developed into the people we are based on the relationships we have had and currently have in our lives (Siegel, 2012). The science of interpersonal neurobiology offers us a theoretical structure for how we relate to others and how we handle challenges and stress in our life. It is important to understand that our brain interacts with the brains of everyone we connect with, which directly impacts our attitudes, behaviors, and resilience (Siegel, 2012). It is beneficial to comprehend how our brains work so that we can improve how we care for ourselves and others (Milford, 2016a).

Daniel Siegel has explained how the brain works using one's hand as a model.

- **The Wrist and the Palm:** The wrist and the palm of the hand represent the brain stem. The brain stem is the autonomic control center of the brain, regulating heart rate, breathing, and other survival responses such as fight, flight, or freeze in the face of dangerous situations.
- **The Thumb:** This is the midbrain, where emotions are generated and where storage and integration of all types of memory occur.
- **The Fingers Over the Thumb:** This is the cortex, where all the information from the brain stem and thumb are processed into perception, motor action, speech, and thinking.
- **The Fingernails:** The orbitofrontal cortex/prefrontal cortex, which lies approximately behind the eyes in the head. This is the primary integration center for all

the information from the other parts of the brain. The prefrontal cortex has many functions, including:

- Regulation of the body through the autonomic nervous system
- Emotional regulation
- Regulation of interpersonal relationships
- Response flexibility
- Intuition
- Mind sight
- Self-awareness
- Morality (Siegel, 2012, pp. 20–21).

"Flipping your lid" is how Siegel describes the brain's response to stress: feeling overwhelmed or dealing with traumatic and painful events. In response, the prefrontal cortex shuts down. The fingers go up and now all of the regulation processes we just discussed are unavailable to the individual. It is a temporary situation, but it takes a toll on both the body and the brain, requiring the individual to calm down and bring the fingers back over the thumb and palm to maintain self-regulation and executive function. This occurs often in the NICU for both families and caregivers and requires self-care and behavioral changes to engage in more productive responses (Siegel, 2012). Research has demonstrated that the NICU nurse encounters many demands and stressors during their daily practice. Long hours, lengthy standing, moving of equipment, critically ill neonates, overwhelmed and terrified parents, and exposure to pain, suffering, and intense emotions can result in physical and mental health complications (Cricco-Lizza, 2014). Caring for caregivers involves acknowledging these issues and providing assistance to reduce their negative impacts on the provider.

Each individual is unique in what triggers stress response and what supports self-regulation. Caregivers deserve the opportunity to develop self-awareness skills to know themselves, their triggers, and their happy places (Milford, 2016a). Self-awareness can develop through telling one's story, discussing why one is a caregiver, and seeking professional satisfaction. Understanding the physiological, behavioral, and emotional response to situations that one perceives as stressful can support the integration of different and more effective approaches (Coughlin, 2017; Milford, 2016a). Caregivers must be able to recognize the stressors in their work and their personal lives and be able to reduce the negative effects from them to be effective care team members.

VICARIOUS TRAUMATIZATION, COMPASSION FATIGUE, AND BURNOUT

The work of NICU caregivers in dealing with the trauma and stress of neonates, their families, and their coworkers can cumulatively result in significant mental health issues. Many research studies have demonstrated that working in ICUs can be traumatic as well as stressful for caregivers (Cricco-Lizza, 2014). Exposure to trauma among healthcare providers impacts how their world looks to them and how their work impacts their perception. When exposure to trauma results in changes to how one sees the world as a less safe place and they begin to have feelings of powerlessness to make changes, caregivers become controlling, emotionally unavailable, and intolerant (Sansbury, Graves, & Scott, 2015). Over time, researchers and clinicians have defined these behaviors and attitudes. Treatment modalities include psychotherapy, nurturance, self-care, and appreciation by NICU and hospital administration (Milford, 2016b; Sansbury et al., 2015).

As discussed earlier, working in the NICU is both physically and emotionally stressful. Vicarious traumatization occurs because of the daily exposure to suffering, pain, and emotional crises. Compassion fatigue arises when nurturance, self-care, and administrative support are not available (Sansbury et al., 2015). Compassion fatigue is manifested in sleep disturbances, irritability, numbing to one's own and other's emotions, feelings of powerlessness, and avoidance of many interpersonal interactions (Milford, 2016b; Sansbury et al., 2015). Caregivers who are experiencing compassion fatigue need support from their coworkers and administrator, psychotherapy, and a positive self-care plan (Milford, 2016a). If intervention is not provided at this point, many caregivers can proceed into burnout, which can result in eating disorders, substance abuse, gastrointestinal complications, anxiety, and depression.

Burnout is a gradual, progressive process that results in emotional and physical exhaustion. Caregivers experiencing burnout are disengaged from not only the neonates and families, but also their coworkers. Their negativity, behaviors, and attitudes can result in decreased family satisfaction, coworker bullying, and a hostile work environment (Milford, 2016a). A caregiver in this situation needs psychotherapy and medical treatment, often psychotherapeutic medications. They may even require a mental health disability leave for treatment and healing. Return to work should be based on the recommendations of their healthcare providers, especially therapists and physicians (Porges, 2011; Sansbury et al., 2015). Compassion fatigue and burnout can be prevented by work–life balance, good self-care habits, strong coworker support and engagement, and NICU and hospital administration prioritization of caregivers' value and needs (Milford, 2016a).

SELF-CARE: IT IS ALL ABOUT YOU

Good self-care habits are the foundation for not only the body, but also the brain (Arden, 2014; Cozolino, 2014). Without this foundation, a caregiver does not have energy for positive behaviors and attitudes that are protective factors against stress (Siegel, 2012). Positive self-care habits need to be encouraged as part of the educational and organizational values of the NICU. Caregivers ought to be acknowledged as unique, important people in the lives of their families, their NICU, and their community. They are needed and loved, and reminding caregivers of this regularly inspires them to feel validated and valued not only for work, but also as individuals (Milford, 2016a). This value aids in the development and maintenance of healthy self-care habits for everyone.

Sleep

Sleep is the foundation for the body and brain to renew, reenergize, and reregulate (O'Brien, 2011). A healthy sleep life supports all other aspects of life, making it the first priority for healthy self-care. It is important to make sleep a priority in life, and understanding how to develop good sleep habits is vital to being able to care for others, as well as oneself. There are many aspects of sleep hygiene that one can control, and these include the environment, nutrition, behavior, and attitudes.

The environment in which one sleeps is important to facilitating both REM and NREM stages of sleep (Milford, 2016a; O'Brien, 2011). The room should be dark and cool. One way to create an even darker room is to turn the alarm clock around so that the light is not shining on your face. Some researchers suggest that keeping the feet warm and the head cool provides the right temperature control for restorative sleep (Arden, 2014). A quiet environment can enable one to go to sleep and stay asleep (Arden, 2014; O'Brien, 2011), yet many people prefer to have white noise while they sleep. The use of white noise machines or music specifically developed to promote sleep can be very helpful in noisy environments such as cities (O'Brien, 2011) to quiet the mind and can be a sleep promoter, rather than a hinder. The bedroom should be for sleep and sexual activity. It should not be a place to watch TV or work. It is very important to create an environment that triggers your body to become prepared to sleep.

What we eat and drink within 3 to 4 hours before bedtime is also of great consequence (O'Brien, 2011). One should restrict caffeine use after 1 p.m. because stimulants such as caffeine can impact sleep stages and patterns. Alcohol can also inhibit sleep and should not be used after dinner. Do not drink liquids 1 to 2 hours before bedtime to eliminate the possibility of having to wake during the night to eliminate the bladder, and if one is hungry at bedtime, a light snack of healthy complex carbohydrates and protein (i.e., wheat crackers and yogurt) helps one sleep. A heavy or spicy meal within an hour of bedtime often leads to indigestion and other gastrointestinal issues (O'Brien, 2011), so those choices should be avoided.

Not only is preparing for sleep with a routine important for children, it is also vital for adults, especially as we age (Milford, 2016a). Going to bed when one is sleepy helps one keep a routine for sleep times 7 days a week (O'Brien, 2011). Sleeping in on weekends can be lovely, but it interferes with sleep patterns. Exercising in the late afternoon, such as a brisk walk, has been found to support sleep initiation (Arden, 2014; O'Brien, 2011). The most difficult habit to develop is no screen time, including TV and cell phone use, for at least an hour before bedtime. This is the time to be engaging in relaxing routines, such as taking a warm bath, reading a book (not an e-reader), performing oral hygiene, and completing your "to do" list for the next day (Arden, 2014; O'Brien, 2011).

Finally, a positive attitude toward sleep is just as crucial as the other areas that have been addressed. If one is anxious about sleep, one will have sleep difficulties. Going to bed when sleepy is helpful. If someone is not sleepy, engaging in a relaxing activity and avoiding screen time should help bring on the tiredness. One night of poor sleep is not a major issue and it happens to everyone. Yet one should let daily worries go by writing them down with solutions and acknowledging the need to address them the following day (Milford, 2016a; O'Brien, 2011). An attitude of sleep as a positive and restorative aspect of life will go far in helping to create a good sleep environment and healthy sleep habits (Arden, 2014; O'Brien, 2011).

Nutrition

The food we put in our bodies is the fuel for our energy and levels of arousal. There are foods that support high levels of energy, arousal, and attention, and there are foods that interfere with high levels of energy, arousal, and attention. It is crucial to eat healthy foods and have nonhealthy foods only occasionally. Eating regular meals, especially breakfast, helps maintain energy and arousal levels throughout the day (Arden, 2014; Milford, 2016a).

Breakfast really is the most important meal of the day. Your body and brain have slept and now need nutrition for fueling the energy, attention, and arousal that it needs throughout the entire day. A breakfast of complex carbohydrates, good fats, protein, and fruit provides you with both short- and long-term energy and arousal requirements. At lunch, which should be the largest meal, eating lean protein, good fats, vegetables, fruit, and complex carbohydrates with plenty of water sustains high levels of energy and arousal throughout the afternoon and into the evening (Arden, 2014). A dinner of vegetables and complex carbohydrates encourages the body to prepare for restorative sleep.

We all like occasional treats of chocolate, dessert, chips, and other unhealthy snack options. These should be viewed as treats and we should eat them only occasionally. Processed sugar and fried foods interfere with high energy and arousal and are bad for health in more ways than one. A diet that includes these items frequently can interfere with optimal sleep patterns, energy, arousal, and attention and can lead to numerous health complications (Arden, 2014). Developing good nutrition habits can take time if you prefer these types of foods. Speaking with a dietician and engaging in behavior change with a support group are all ways to assist one in developing and maintaining healthy nutrition habits (Arden, 2014).

Exercise

Exercise is crucial to one's self-care. It is just as vital as good sleep and nutrition habits. Exercise is a necessity and needs to be part of the daily routine (Arden, 2014; Milford, 2016a). Walking for just 30 minutes enhances physical and mental health, energy, attention, and arousal (Arden, 2014; Siegel, 2012). To integrate daily exercise into a routine, find an enjoyed activity and develop a schedule for it. Exercise can be broken into time periods as small as 10 minutes. The key is to increase the heart rate and respirations for at least 10 minutes. Perspiring is a good indicator of raising the heart rate and respirations. At a minimum, 30 minutes of exercise every day is essential for both the body and the brain (Arden, 2014).

Walking is an excellent form of exercise and does not require special equipment or fitness memberships. A brisk walk gives energy and helps focus attention (Arden, 2014; Milford, 2016a). Researchers continue to report that exercise can be neuroprotective and reduce the probability of developing dementia and other degenerative brain diseases (Arden, 2014).

Hobbies

Participating in pleasurable activities supports optimal mental health. Hobbies can be individual or group activities, and there are so many things one can do, both in terms of social interaction and in terms of creativity. Playing and attending sporting events, attending music and art performances, participating in philanthropy, painting, drawing, knitting, and cooking are all wonderful ways to engage with others and to express oneself (Arden, 2014; Milford, 2016a). Everyone should find something they love to do and incorporate that into their lives on a regular basis. Giving of one's time and creations can be very fulfilling and rewarding (Coughlin, 2017; Milford, 2016a).

Attitude

Attitudes are how one approaches the world. A positive attitude is a foundation for a healthy and rich life (Arden, 2014). Positive attitudes start with the belief that problems are temporary and solvable. Making one's automatic thoughts (thoughts that occur when being challenged) positive rather than negative is a key aspect. The most crucial positive thought is optimism. Optimism reduces worry and aids one in visualizing being the best person one can be by thinking about the future and the way that everything has gone as well as it possibly could (Arden, 2014). Positive attitude comes from positive thinking. Positive thinking is based on problem-solving, shifting of attention from the negative, and acceptance of self and others. It is acknowledging oneself as a valuable and unique individual with much to contribute to family, coworkers, community, and world (Milford, 2016a).

Positive thinking and attitudes require new habits. One is called the *positive face*, or the old saying "fake it until you make it." Smiling has been found to lower negative activity in the prefrontal cortex and increase positive activity in the prefrontal cortex, resulting in positive thoughts and moods (Arden, 2014; Siegel, 2012). Smile even when not feeling like it to feel more positive and approachable (Siegel, 2012). Individuals should be open and flexible to new experiences and opportunities; see problems as solvable and new experiences as adventures; and think of themselves as important and valuable individuals (Milford, 2016a).

Finally, meditation is a wonderful activity that enhances positive attitudes. Meditation is simple and difficult at the same time (Milford, 2016a). Meditation is as simple as concentrating on one's breathing in a quiet and calm environment. It is difficult, however, to keep concentrating and not let thoughts intrude. When those thoughts do intrude, going back to concentrating on breathing helps refocus the session. It takes a great deal of practice, so starting with 10 minutes and increasing session times until a session reaches 30 minutes is good practice.

Meditating before bedtime and on awakening engages successful integration of meditation into one's daily routines (Siegel, 2012). Meditation has been found to optimize brain functioning by reducing activity in the amygdala and orbitofrontal cortex (Siegel, 2012). Research has demonstrated that it can increase feelings of acceptance and control over stress while also providing chances to be calm and positive in mood and attitude (Arden, 2014).

RESILIENCE: PROTECTION FROM CAREGIVER MENTAL HEALTH COMPLICATIONS

Resilience is how an individual positively adapts to adversity, trauma, tragedy, family or relationship problems, health complications, and professional or financial stressors

(Milford, 2016a). It means being able to recover from difficult experiences and situations. Resilience is a valuable skill in negotiating life and its challenges. Being resilient doesn't mean one doesn't feel negative feelings or feel pain or suffering. Resilience simply is how one responds to feelings, pain, and suffering. The most resilient people have often suffered significant adversity (Arden, 2014). A combination of factors contributes to developing resilience, including, but not limited to, the following:

- Having caring and supportive relationships with family, friends, and coworkers
- Having a positive attitude
- Being confident in personal strengths and abilities

Problem-solving, in which one can make realistic plans and can take the appropriate actions to implement them, supports an understanding that adversity and stress can be overcome (Arden, 2014).

Self-regulation, the ability to control strong feelings and impulses, is the foundation for problem-solving and development of action plans (Milford, 2016a). Becoming more resilient is a personal journey, and strategies successful for one person may not be as effective for another. Methods for improving resilience focus on having a positive attitude and self-esteem, finding a sense of purpose in life (such as spirituality, community activities, professional development), and cultivating strong, positive social networks. Being flexible and accepting change is a key component of resilience. By learning how to adapt to all experiences and situations, one can improve the ability to respond to a life crisis. Resilient people often find opportunities for new directions in their lives after a life crisis (Arden, 2014; Coughlin, 2017). It is beneficial to establish goals because life crises can be overwhelming. Resilient people, however, view such crises as manageable when broken down into smaller activities and tasks (Coughlin, 2017). Everyone should try to monitor their accomplishments of goals and realize that the resolution of an issue can take time (Arden, 2014).

CONFLICT RESOLUTION WITH COWORKERS

Professionals often disagree, and this can become a source of stress in the workplace. Learning positive conflict-resolution skills is important for a healthy, positive work environment and is advantageous in all areas of life. Conflicts occur as a result of different values, ideas, or perceptions. It is important to recognize these differences and the emotions that they can generate. Conflict resolution begins with understanding and respecting the other party's issues and concerns (Milford, 2016a). The ability to remain calm and focused on the situation can help relieve the stress, and relaxing and providing an emotionally safe space for everyone with both words and body language are key.

Controlling emotions and not becoming defensive help reduce negative emotions, especially anger. Being conscious of both the words that are spoken and the body language that is used can assist one in understanding the issues and respecting the needs of others. The relationship, the current situation, and the ability to forgive and forget are all indispensable to positive conflict-resolution skills (Coughlin, 2017). There is a place for humor as well. Humor can support the ability to make statements that could be difficult to express without creating conflict. It is important that the humor be shared with other individuals and not made at their expense. When humor and playful communication are used to reduce stress, reframe the problem, or put the event in perspective, conflict resolution can become a foundation for positive relationships and emotions (King, 2015).

SUPPORT FROM ADMINISTRATION AND COWORKERS

Caring for caregivers includes care from the healthcare administration and coworker. The administration is responsible for caring for the caregiver with healthy work schedules, appropriate meal breaks, open communication opportunities, and mentoring (Hall et al., 2015). NICU administration can support staff with no tolerance for staff or family verbal or physical threats or abuse. When a caregiver is struggling, it is imperative that the administration supports them with counseling, employee assistance programs, or mental health therapy. NICU administration has to be cognizant of the caregiver's needs for frequent communication on unit operations, scheduling, policies, and appreciation for the work of each caregiver (Hall et al., 2015; Milford, 2016b). Communication in the form of reports from clinical data collected as part of unit quality assurance and benchmarks supports caregivers in understanding the impact their work has on family and infant outcomes (Coughlin, 2017).

Opportunities to debrief from adverse medical events and infant deaths should be available with all team members and with mental health professionals as needed (Hall et al., 2015; Hynan et al., 2015). Bereavement events and remembrances should be offered to caregivers, as well as families (Hall et al., 2015), to support the emotional health of caregivers.

Coworker support enhances positive and healthy workplaces. They are the support system in the professional lives of nurses and providers. Nurturing each other is just as important as nurturing families and babies. Being available to listen and support each other through the challenges and successes of our work can be inspiring and energizing (Coughlin, 2017). Mentoring or requesting mentoring, no matter what one's level of experience and expertise is, nurtures each caregiver in the process and should be encouraged. Building strong, positive relationships with coworkers is a necessary value in the culture of the NICU. Regular staff meetings and social activities such as picnics, holiday celebrations, and meals acknowledging both professional and personal accomplishments create a feeling of belonging and acceptance (Milford, 2016a).

Supporting one another in healthy self-care activities and implementing group self-care activities encourage all caregivers to take care of themselves. Each person needs to be responsive to their coworkers' communications and behaviors. Changes in either, which may be a negative or concerning new behavior, requires them to be supported and encouraged to discuss their feelings; work–life balance may need some additional support. Being mindful of coworkers' attitudes, emotions, and behaviors can reduce the incidence of compassion fatigue and burnout (Milford, 2016b). Sometimes, a smile, an understanding nod, or a pat on the shoulder or back provides a coworker with the knowledge of being valued and important to each professional.

CHERYL MILFORD'S SUMMARY

The NICU is a challenging workplace, so decreasing stress, increasing energy, and improving arousal is the foundation for caring for the caregiver. Caring for the caregiver is the responsibility of the individual professional, coworkers, and the NICU administration. For professionals, self-care is critical to being able to care for others, as well as themselves. Healthy habits regarding sleep, nutrition, exercise, attitude, and work–life balance are part of the commitment to providing the best possible care to babies, families, and coworkers. The old saying, if you don't take care of yourself, you can't take care of anyone else is true. It is why it is an old saying. Self-care starts with the acknowledgment that one is valuable, unique, and loved. A positive self-esteem and attitude are essential for a fulfilling and rich professional and personal life.

Part of self-care is becoming resilient. Being able to work through adversity, trauma, and stress protects one from mental health complications and medical illness that are associated with them. Being flexible and adaptable with a sense of humor and the ability to laugh are excellent traits in all aspects of life, not only work. Coworkers nurture and care for each other by respecting and validating themselves as people, professionals, and valued members in the work of the NICU. Providing opportunities to listen, assist, and advocate for coworkers is an important role. Caregivers do not need to be best friends with every member of the NICU team, but they need respect and appreciate one another. Coworkers are the first people to observe when a fellow caregiver is struggling and at risk for mental health complications. Assisting their fellow caregiver in obtaining the assistance they need for work–life balance is the responsibility of not only administration, but also coworkers. Ultimately, it is the responsibility of the healthcare institution and NICU administration to set the tone for the culture providing care to babies, families, and staff. Scheduling, staffing, and provision of equipment and supplies to enable best practice and care are their responsibilities.

The NICU administration is also responsible for providing training and professional development opportunities that are both mandatory and voluntary. Their role in validating and respecting the work of the NICU caregiver should be an essential and imperative part of their work. Initiation of a structured debriefing and bereavement program for caregivers validates the psychological and emotional needs of those who witness and experience trauma, pain, and suffering with families and their babies. It is incumbent on administration at all levels to comprehend all the factors that impact how neonatal care is provided and its effect on the staff, as well as babies and their families. Administrators also require validation and respect in their work. NICU caregivers are in a unique position to acknowledge and appreciate the work of the NICU administration and advocate for them not only in the NICU, but also in the healthcare institution as a whole. A reciprocal, respectful relationship between caregivers and administrators advances the goals and objectives of providing the highest quality care to babies and families. The reality is we are all on the same team, even when that may be difficult to articulate.

The families and babies NICU caregivers work with will always remember the efforts and the support staff provide them. Many believe that without their staff, their child would not be with them today. Professionals who engage with these families after discharge are told this every day. The influence one has on their family will continue to be communicated across generations. That influence is very powerful and is a clear reason for NICU caregivers, coworkers, and administration to prioritize caring for caregivers as a tenet of the culture and operation of the NICU (Figure 16.1). The work is very significant to the families, the community, and society. The babies usually grow up to be amazing, contributing members of the community. What a wonderful result for all the hard work.

RECOMMENDATIONS/SUGGESTIONS FOR BEST PRACTICE

1. Administration and NICU leadership need to support staff in being able to practice good self-care practices while at work.

    a. Leadership needs to provide space on the unit where staff can take quiet and restful breaks.

    b. Leadership needs to support adequate staffing and provide appropriate coverage.

    c. Leadership needs to support staff after stressful and emotional events that occur in the unit and in one's personal life.

2. Staff need to adhere to professional boundaries with patients and families.

3. Staff need to recognize their own responses to stress.

4. Caregivers need to have good self-care practice routines.

5. Everyone should develop good sleep hygiene practices and habits.

6. Healthy meals and good nutrition should be priorities.

7. Staying hydrated during shifts and at home is important.

8. Getting plenty of exercise and staying active should be foci for all staff.

9. Participating in hobbies that bring joy should be encouraged.

10. Positive attitudes in the workplace are key to creating a positive environment.

11. Developing ways to have positive conflict resolution between coworkers need to be defined, implemented, and supported by staff at all levels across the organization.

RECOMMENDED RESOURCES

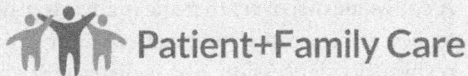 Patient+Family Care

Online Education:
1. www.mynicunetwork.com
2. https://www.nurse.com/ce/from-distress-to-destress-with-stress-management
3. http://www.dandlelion-webinars.com
4. http://aihcp.net/stress-management-ce-courses-program

Website Recommendations:
1. http://www.ahna.org/Resources/Stress-Management
2. http://www.stress-relief-choices.com/stress-management-for-nurses.html
3. http://www.healthleadersmedia.com/nurse-leaders/stress-management-nurses
4. http://www.onlinemsnprograms.com/stress-management-tips-for-nurses
5. https://www.mayoclinic.org/healthy-lifestyle/stress-management/in-depth/caregiver-stress/art-20044784
6. https://elizabethscala.com/stress-management-for-nurses
7. https://celebrateyoga.org/stress-management-techniques-nurses
8. https://www.jacksonvilleu.com/blog/nursing/how-to-reduce-stress-nursing
9. https://www.ausmed.com/articles/stress-in-nursing
10. http://dailynurse.com/stress-management-rescue-strategies-self-care-nursing
11. http://www.linkcapital.com/blog/stress-management-for-nurses
12. http://www.nursingdegrees.com/nursing-articles/tips-for-first-year-nurses/stress-management-and-nursing-burnout
13. http://www.nursingdegrees.com/nursing-community/humor
14. https://sleepfoundation.org/sleep-tools-tips/healthy-sleep-tips
15. http://bettersleep.org/better-sleep/top-15-better-sleep-tips
16. https://www.mayoclinic.org/healthy-lifestyle/adult-health/in-depth/sleep/art-20048379?pg=1
17. https://www.sleepassociation.org/patients-general-public/insomnia/sleep-hygiene-tips
18. https://www.americannursetoday.com/nutrition-tips-for-nurses-who-work-shifts
19. https://www.firsthealth.org/lifestyle/news-events/2015/05/nutrition-tips-for-nurses

Books:
1. *The Joy of Burnout: How the End of the World Can Be a New Beginning* by Dina Glouberman
2. *Spiritual Housecleaning: Healing the Space Within by Beautifying the Space Around You* by Kathryn L. Robyn
3. *Overcoming Job Burnout: How to Renew Enthusiasm for Work* by Beverly A. Pottery
4. *Practice Safe Stress: Healing & Laughing in the Face of Stress, Burnout & Depression* by Mark Gorkin
5. *Restore Yourself: The Antidote for Professional Exhaustion* by Edy Greenblatt

Figure 16.1 ■ Recommended resources for caring for the caregiver.

Case-Based Learning

A colleague discovers that she inadvertently administered the wrong dose of narcotic to her 26-week-gestation patient after a patent ductus arteriosus ligation, causing respiratory depression. She is distraught and crying in the lounge. She tells you that she can't take the constant pressure anymore and wants to quit working in the NICU and change to a clinic job with less stress.

QUESTIONS

1. What are the contextual elements of your colleague's emotional state?
2. What are some approaches that may help?

ANSWERS

Errors and/or adverse events take a toll on providers, causing emotional distress and impacting the professional quality of life. Winning et al. (2018) describe how coworker support can reduce the harmful anxiety and depression associated with these occurrences.

The inherently stressful nature of the intensive care environment impacts families and staff. So that they can nurture families in the face of daily workplace exposure to pain, illness, and death, the multidisciplinary team needs to be nourished too. One of the tenets of the Newborn Intensive Parenting Unit (NIPU) concept addresses this dilemma and suggests solutions. Staff well-being, physical and emotional, is an essential feature of the NIPU. Hall et al. (2017) describe the importance of work culture, the way everything from education to environment to relationships and respect is indispensable to providing support and preventing burnout. As described in Chapter 15, including a psychologist on staff to assist both parents and staff is ideal. Debriefing of traumatic events should be readily available and can be very beneficial. Enhancements to the physical environment with calming space to promote relaxation and adequate meeting space to promote interaction are also recommended. Last, but certainly not least, following best practices in staffing can reduce stress and overwork.

REFERENCES

Hall, S. L., Hynan, M. T., Phillips, R., Lassen, S., Craig, J. W., Goyer, E., ... Cohen, H. (2017). The neonatal intensive parenting unit: An introduction. *Journal of Perinatology, 37*(12), 1259–1264. doi:10.1038/jp.2017.108

Winning, A. M., Merandi, J. M., Lewe, D., Stepney, L., Liao, N. N., Fortney, C. A., & Gerhardt, C. A. (2018). The emotional impact of errors or adverse events on healthcare providers in the NICU: The protective role of coworker support. *Journal of Advanced Nursing, 74*(1), 172–180. doi:10.1111/jan.13403

REFERENCES

Arden, J. (2014). *The brain Bible: A plan to stay vital, productive and happy for a lifetime.* New York, NY: McGraw-Hill.

Coughlin, M. E. (2017). Meeting the needs of the neonatal clinician. In M. E. Coughlin (Ed.), *Trauma- informed care in the NICU.* New York, NY: Springer Publishing and the National Association of Neonatal Nurses.

Cozolino, L. (2014). *The neuroscience of human relationships: Attachment and the developing social brain* (2nd ed.). New York, NY: W. W. Norton.

Cricco-Lizza, R. (2014). The need to nurse the nurse: Emotional labor in neonatal intensive care. *Qualitative Health Research, 24*(5), 615–628. doi:10.1177/1049732314528810

Hall, S. L., Cross, J., Selix, N. W., Patterson, C., Segre, L., Chuffo-Seiwert, R., . . . Martin, M. L. (2015). Recommendations for enhancing psychosocial support of NICU parent through staff education and support. *Journal of Perinatology, 35*(Suppl. 1), S29–S36. doi:10.1038/jp.2015.147

Hynan, M. T., Steinberg, Z., Baker, L., Geller, P. A., Lassen, S., Milford, C., . . . Stuebe, A. (2015). Recommendations for mental health professionals in the NICU. *Journal of Perinatology, 35*(Suppl. 1), S14–S18. doi:10.1038/jp.2015.144

King, B. (2015). *Healthy habits of happy people.* Concord, CA: Institute for Natural Resources.

Milford, C. A. (2016a). *Caring for families and ourselves in the NICU* (Educational Program). Huntington Beach, CA: Cheryl Milford Consulting.

Milford, C. A. (2016b). Supporting NICU staff mental health. *Neonatology Today, 11*(5), 5–6.

O'Brien, M. (2011). *The healing power of sleep* (2nd ed.). Concord, CA: Biomed Books.

Porges, S. W. (2011). *The polyvagal theory: Neurophysiological foundations of emotions, attachment, communication, and self-regulation.* New York, NY: W. W. Norton.

Profit, J., Sharek, P. J., Amspoker, A. B., Kowalkowski, M. A., Nisbet, C. C., Thomas, E. J., . . . Sexton, J. B. (2014). Burnout in the NICU setting and its relation to safety culture. *BMJ Quality & Safety, 23*(10), 806–813. doi:10.1136/bmjqs-2014-002831

Ross, A., Bevans, M., Brooks, A. T., Gibbons, S., & Wallen, G. R. (2017). Nurses and health-promoting behaviors: Knowledge may not translate into self-care. *AORN Journal, 105*(3), 267–275. doi:10.1016/j.aorn.2016.12.018

Sanders, M. L., & Hall, S. L. (2017). Trauma-informed care in the newborn intensive care unit: Promoting safety, security and connectedness. *Journal of Perinatology, 38,* 3–10. doi:10.1038/jp.2017.124

Sansbury, B. S., Graves, K., & Scott, W. (2015). Managing traumatic stress responses among clinicians: Individual and organizational tools for self-care. *Trauma, 17*(2), 114–122. doi:10.1177/1460408614551978

Siegel, D. (2012). *The developing mind: How relationships and the brain interact to shape who we are* (2nd ed.). New York, NY: Guilford Press.

Tawfik, D. S., Sexton, J. B., Kan, P., Sharek, P. J., Nisbet, C. C., Rigdon, J., . . . Profit, J. (2016). Burnout in the neonatal intensive care unit and its relation to healthcare-associated infections. *Journal of Perinatology, 37*(3), 315–320. doi:10.1038/jp.2016.211

INDEX